Instant Notes *in*

IMMUNOLOGY

The INSTANT NOTES series

Series editor
B.D. Hames
School of Biochemistry and Molecular Biology, University of Leeds, Leeds, UK

Biochemistry
Animal Biology
Molecular Biology
Ecology
Genetics
Microbiology
Chemistry for Biologists
Immunology

Forthcoming titles
Neuroscience
Psychology
Developmental Biology

Instant *Notes in*

IMMUNOLOGY

P.M. Lydyard

Department of Immunology,
Royal Free and University College Medical School,
University College London, London, UK

A. Whelan

Department of Immunology, Trinity College and
St James' Hospital, Dublin, Ireland

and

M.W. Fanger

Department of Microbiology,
Dartmouth Medical School,
Lebanon, New Hampshire,
USA

BIOS

© BIOS Scientific Publishers Limited, 2000

First published 2000

A CIP catalogue record for this book is available from the British Library.

ISBN 1 85996 077 4

BIOS Scientific Publishers Ltd
9 Newtec Place, Magdalen Road, Oxford OX4 1RE, UK.
Tel. +44 (0) 1865 726286. Fax +44 (0) 1865 246823
World Wide Web home page: http://www.bios.co.uk/

Published in the United States of America, its dependent territories and Canada by Springer-Verlag New York Inc., 175 Fifth Avenue, New York, NY 10010-7858, in association with BIOS Scientific Publishers Ltd

Published in Hong Kong, Taiwan, Singapore, Thailand, Cambodia, Korea, The Philippines, Indonesia, The People's Republic of China, Brunei, Laos, Malaysia, Macau and Vietnam by Springer-Verlag Singapore Pte. Ltd, 1 Tannery Road, Singapore 347719, in association with BIOS Scientific Publishers Ltd.

Production Editor: Andrea Bosher
Typeset by and illustrated by J&L Composition Ltd, Filey, UK
Printed by Biddles Ltd, Guildford, UK

CONTENTS

ABBREVIATIONS

5HT	5'hydroxytryptamine		GM-CSF	granulocyte-monocyte CSF
αMSH	α-melanocyte stimulating hormone		HAMA	human anti-mouse antibody
Ab	antibody		HEV	high endothelial venules
Ach	acetylcholine		HHV8	human herpes virus 8
ADCC	antibody dependent cellular cytotoxicity		HIV	human immunodeficiency virus
AFP	alpha-fetoprotein		HLA	human leukocyte antigens
Ag	antigen		HPA	hypothalamus/pituitary/adrenal
AICD	activation induced cell death		HPV	human papilloma virus
AIDS	acquired immune deficiency syndrome		HSC	hemopoietic stem cell
			HSPs	heat shock proteins
AIHA	autoimmune hemolytic anemia		HTLV	human T cell leukemia virus
ANA	antinuclear antibodies		IFNs	interferons
ANCA	antibodies to neutrophil cyto-plasmic antigen		Ig	immunoglobulin
			IL	interleukin
APC	antigen presenting cell(s)		ITP	immune thrombocytopenia purpura
BALT	bronchus-associated lymphoid tissue		Its	immunotoxins
BAS	basophil		KARs	killer activation receptors
BCR	B cell receptor		KIRs	killer inhibitory receptors
BsAbs	bispecific antibodies		Kr	keratinocytes
CEA	carcinoembryonic antigen		LAK	lymphokine activated killer
CGD	chronic granulomatous disease		LCMV	lymphocytic choriomeningitis virus
CMI	cell-mediated immunity		LGLs	large granular lymphocytes
Co	chondrocytes		LPS	lipopolysaccharide
CRDs	carbohydrate recognition domains		LRR	leucine rich repeat
CRH	corticotrophin-releasing hormone		LT	leukotriene
CRP	C-reactive protein		mAbs	monoclonal antibodies
CSFs	colony stimulating factors		MAK	macrophage activated killer
CTL	cytotoxic T lymphocyte		MALT	mucosa-associated lymphoid tissue
CVID	common variable immuno-deficiency		MBP	mannose binding protein
			MCP	membrane cofactor protein
DAF	decay accelerating factor		MCP-1	monocyte chemotactic protein-1
DNA	deoxyribonucleic acid		M-CSF	monocyte colony-stimulating factor
DPT	diphtheria, pertussis and tetanus		MDP	muramyl dipeptide
EAE	experimental allergic encephalomyelitis		MHC	major histocompatibility complex
			MØ	macrophages
ECF-A	eosinophil chemotactic factors of anaphylaxis		Mo	monocytes
			MS	multiple sclerosis
EGF-R	epidermal growth factor receptor		MTb	*Mycobacterium tuberculosis*
ELISA	enzyme-linked immunosorbent assay		MZ	marginal zone
			NALT	nasal-associated lymphoid tissue
En	endothelial (cells)		NBT	nitroblue tetrazolium
FasL	Fas ligand		NGF	nerve growth factor
Fb	fibroblasts		NK	natural killer (cells)
FDC	follicle dendritic cells		NO	nitric oxide
GALT	gut-associated lymphoid tissue		NSAID	nonsteroidal anti-inflammatory drug
G-CSF	granulocyte colony-stimulating factor		PAF	platelet activating factor

PAGE   polyacrylamide gel electrophoresis
PALS   peri-arteriolar lymphoid sheath
PCR   polymerase chain reaction
PMNs   polymorphonuclear cells, neutro-
           phils
PPD   purified protein derivative
PRR   pattern recognition receptors
RA   rheumatoid arthritis
RAST   radioallergosorbent test
RBCs   red blood cells
RFLP   restriction fragment length poly-
           morphism
RhD   Rhesus D
RIA   radioimmunoassay
RP   red pulp
SAA   serum amyloid protein A
SCF   stem cell factor
SCID   severe combined
           immunodeficiency
SDS   sodium dodecyl sulphate
SLE   systemic lupus erythematosus

SRS-A   slow reacting substance of
           anaphylaxis
SV   splenic vein
TAA   tumor associated antigen
TB   tuberculosis
TBII   thyrotropin binding-inhibitory
           immunoglobulin
Tc   T cytotoxic
TCR   T cell receptor
TGFβ   tumor growth factor β
TGSI   thyroid growth-stimulating
           immunoglobulin
Th   T helper
TIL   tumor infiltrating lymphocytes
TLRs   toll-like receptors
TNFα   tumor necrosis factor α
TNFβ   tumor necrosis factor β
TSA   tumor specific antigen
TSH   thyroid stimulating hormone
tTG   tissue transglutaminase

PREFACE

Immunology as a science probably began with the observations by Metchnikoff in 1882 that starfish when pierced by a foreign object (a rose thorn) responded by coating it with cells (later identified as phagocytes). Immunology – the study of the way in which the body defends itself against invading organisms or internal invaders (tumors) – has developed rapidly over the last 40 years, and particularly during the last 10 years with the advent of molecular techniques. It is now a rapidly moving field that is contributing critical tools for research and diagnosis, and therapeutics for treatment of a wide range of human diseases. Thus, it is an integral part of college life science courses and medical studies.

For ease of understanding, we have divided the subject matter in this book into five main areas: Components of the immune system (Sections A–G); Mechanisms involved in the development of immunity (Sections H–N); The immune system in action (Sections O–R); When the immune system goes wrong (Sections S–U); and Immunotechnology (Section V).

The first area begins with an overview of the immune system. This is followed by the details of the origins and properties of the important cells and molecules of the innate and adaptive immune systems, including the structure and function of antibodies. The cellular components, their interactions and modulation, as well as the mechanisms by which effective immune responses develop are presented in the second area: this includes the way in which the immune system distinguishes self from non-self in order to mount an immune response. In the third area, the role of immune responses in infection, cancer and transplantation are considered along with a description of our current understanding of vaccination. We describe in the fourth area what can and does go wrong with the immune system. This is divided into immunodeficiency, particularly important now with regard to the world wide epidemic of AIDS, hypersensitivity (the commonest form being allergy) and autoimmune diseases. In the last section we describe how antibodies, because of their fine specificity and properties, are used as tools in diagnosis of diseases and identification and purification of antigens.

In order to test your understanding of the subject, we have included 120 multiple choice questions with answers at the back of the book. These questions are in the format used in the US National Boards (USMLE) Step 1, and in degree courses in the UK.

We would like to acknowledge the help of Dr. Michael Cole and Dr Peter Delves for looking at sections of the manuscript, and in particular, Professor Paul Guyre who helped enormously with advice and support on the whole manuscript. We also thank Professor Randy Noelle who allowed us to use diagrams and tables he currently uses in teaching and Professor Eamon Sweeney for his helpful suggestions. Finally, we would like to thank our wives, Meriel, Annette and Sharon for support and understanding during the preparation of these Notes in Immunology which have been 'Far from Instant' in terms of time of preparation!

A1 THE NEED

Key Note

The ubiquitous enemy	Infectious microbes and larger organisms such as worms are present in our environment. They range from being helpful (e.g. *E. coli*) to being major pathogens which can be fatal (e.g. HIV).
Related topics	Immunity to different organisms (O2) Pathogen defense strategies (O3)

The ubiquitous enemy

Microbes are able to survive on animal and plant products by releasing digestive enzymes directly and absorbing the food, and/or by growth on living tissues (extracellular), in which case they are simply bathed in nutrients. Other microbes infect (invade) animal/human cells (intracellular), where they not only survive, but also replicate, in this case utilizing host-cell energy sources. Both extracellular and intracellular microbes can grow, reproduce and infect other individuals. There are many different species of microbes and larger organisms (such as worms) which invade humans, some of which are relatively harmless and some even helpful (e.g. *E. coli* in our intestines). Many others cause disease (human pathogens), and there is a constant battle between invading microbes and the immune system (Topic O1). Some microbes can even cause the death of their hosts, although this should not be the property of the most successful microbes. *Table 1* shows the range of organisms that can infect humans.

Table 1. Range of infectious organisms

Worms (helminths)	e.g. tapeworms, filaria
Protozoans	e.g. trypanosomes, leishmania, malaria
Fungi	e.g. Candida, aspergillus
Bacteria	e.g. *E. coli, Staphylococcus, Streptococcus*, mycobacteria
Viruses	e.g. polio, pox viruses, influenza, hepatitis B, HIV

A2 EXTERNAL DEFENSES

Key Notes

Physical barriers to entry of microbes	Microbes gain entrance into the body actively (penetration of the skin), or passively (ingestion of food and inhalation). They have to pass across physical barriers such as the skin or epithelial cells which line the mucosal surfaces of the respiratory, gastrointestinal and genitourinary tracts.
Secretions	Secretions from epithelial surfaces at external sites of the body are important for protection against entry of microbes. They include sweat, tears, saliva and gastric juices; all contain antimicrobial substances such as enzymes, small peptides (defensins), fatty acids and secreted antibodies.
Microbial products and competition	Nonpathogenic bacteria (commensals) colonize epithelial surfaces and by releasing toxic substances, utilizing essential nutrients, and occupying the microenvironment, they prevent invasion by pathogenic bacteria.
Related topics	Mucosa-associated lymphoid tissues (D3) The microbial cosmos (O1)

Physical barriers to entry of microbes

Before a microbe or parasite can invade the host and cause infection, it must first attach to and penetrate the surface epithelial layers of the body. Organisms gain entrance into the body by an active or passive means. For example, they might burrow through the skin, or be ingested in food, inhaled into the respiratory tract or penetrate through an open wound. In practice, most microbes take advantage of the fact that we have to breathe and eat to live and therefore enter the body through the respiratory and gastrointestinal tracts. Whatever their point of entry, they have to pass across physical barriers such as the dead layers of the skin or living epithelial cell layers which line the cavities in contact with the exterior such as the respiratory, genitourinary or gastrointestinal tracts. In fact, the main entry of microbes into the body is via these tracts.

Many of the epithelial cells at the interface with the outside world are mucosal epithelial cells which secrete mucus. In addition to the physical barrier, in the case of the respiratory system, epithelial cells of the nasal passages and bronchi have **cilia** (small hair-like structures) which beat in an upward direction to help remove microorganisms as they enter during breathing. This is the **mucociliary escalator** (*Fig. 1*).

Secretions

A variety of secretions at epithelial surfaces are important in defense (*Table 1*). The overall aim is to provide a hostile environment for microbial habitation. Some substances are known to directly kill microbes e.g. lysozyme by digesting proteoglycans in bacterial cell walls; others compete for nutrients (e.g. transferrin, Fe), and others interfere with ion transport (e.g. NaCl). Mucus (containing mucin) secreted by the mucosal epithelial cells coat their surfaces

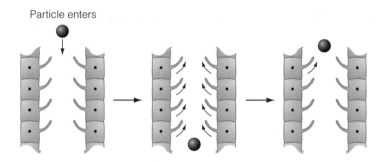

Particle enters

Fig 1. The mucociliary escalator. When a particle is inhaled, it comes into contact with cilia of the bronchial or nasal epithelia which beat in an upwards direction to a position where the particle can be coughed up or sneezed out.

and make it difficult for microbes to contact and bind to them – a prerequisite for entry into the body.

The washing action of tears, saliva and urine also helps to prevent attachment of microbes to the epithelial surfaces. In addition, tears and saliva contain IgA **antibodies** which are secreted across epithelial cells and prevent the attachment of microbes. These antibodies are also secreted across epithelial cells in the respiratory, gastrointestinal and genitourinary tracts. Gastrointestinal, respiratory epithelia and phagocytes throughout the body are also known to produce a number of small peptides which have potent anti-bacterial properties (**peptide antibiotics**). These include cecropins, magainins and defensins and are part of the body's innate defense mechanisms against microbial infection. These peptides (molecular weights 3–5 kD) are effective against both Gram positive and Gram negative bacteria, although their mechanisms of action are different. Whereas **cecropins** and **magainins** cause lysis, others interfere with ion transport. Secretion of these peptides is upregulated as a result of bacterial infection. These peptides are highly conserved throughout species and probably represent one of the most primitive defense mechanisms against microbes.

Microbial products and competition

Normal commensals (**nonpathogenic bacteria**) also help to protect from infection. These nonpathogenic microorganisms are found on the skin, in the mouth and in the reproductive and gastrointestinal tract. The gastrointestinal tract contains many billions of bacteria that have a symbiotic relationship with the host. These bacteria help to prevent pathogens from colonizing the site, by preventing attachment, competing for essential nutrients and releasing antibacterial substances such as **colicins** (antibacterial proteins) and short-chain fatty acids.

Table 1. Secretions at epithelial surfaces

Site	Source	Specific substances secreted
Eyes	Lacrimal glands (tears)	Lysozyme, IgA and IgG
Ears	Sebaceous glands	Waxy secretion – cerumen
Mouth	Salivary glands (saliva)	Digestive enzymes, lysozyme, IgA, IgG, lactoferrin
Skin	Sweat glands (sweat) Sebaceous glands (sebum)	Lysozyme, high NaCl, short chain fatty acids
Stomach	Gastric juices	Digestive enzymes (pepsin, rennin), acid (low pH, 1–2)

Escherichia coli and bactericidal intestinal anaerobes secrete these, respectively. Gut flora also perform such house keeping duties as further degrading waste matter and helping gut motility. Normal microbial flora occupying the site of entry (e.g. throat and nasal passages) of other microbes probably function in a similar manner. Some bacteria such as lactobacilli, which inhabit the vagina, cause their environment to become acidic (pH 4.0–4.5) which probably discourages the growth of many microorganisms.

A3 IMMUNE DEFENSE

Key Notes

The immune system

The immune system protects us from attack by microbes and worms. It uses specialized organs designed to filter out and respond to microbes entering the body's tissues and a mobile force of molecules and cells in the bloodstream to respond rapidly to attack. The system can fail, giving rise to immunodeficiency, or 'over-react' against foreign microbes giving rise to tissue damage (immunopathology). It has complex and sophisticated mechanisms to regulate it.

Innate versus adaptive immunity

The innate immune system is the first line of defense against infections. It works rapidly, gives rise to the acute inflammatory response, and has some specificity for microbes. In contrast, the adaptive immune system takes longer to develop, is highly specific for antigens, including those associated with microbes, and remembers that it has encountered a microbe previously (i.e. shows memory).

Interaction between innate and adaptive immunity

The innate and adaptive immune systems work together through direct cell contact and through interactions involving chemical mediators, cytokines and chemokines. Moreover, many of the cells of the innate immune system are the same cells used by the adaptive immune system.

Clonal selection

All immunocompetent individuals have many distinct lymphocytes, each of which is specific for a different foreign substance (antigen). When an antigen is introduced into an individual, lymphocytes with receptors for this antigen seek out and bind it and are triggered to proliferate and differentiate, giving rise to clones of cells specific for the antigen. These cells or their products specifically react with the antigen to neutralize or eliminate it. The much larger number of antigen-specific cells late in the immune response is responsible for the 'memory' involved in immunity.

T and B cells and cell co-operation

There are of two major types of lymphocytes, B cells and T cells. T cells mature under the influence of the thymus and, on stimulation by antigen, give rise to cellular immunity. B cells mature under the influence of bone marrow and/or gut associated tissues and give rise to humoral immunity, immunity that involves production of soluble molecules – immunoglobulin. Interactions between T and B cells, as well as antigen presenting cells, are critical to the development of specific immunity.

Related topics

Adaptive immune system:
  lymphocytes, lymphoid organs
  and tissues (D)
Antibodies (F)
Cytokines (G)

Antigen recognition (H)
The acute inflammatory response (I)
The antibody response (J)
Lymphocyte activation (L)
Self and non self discrimination (M)

**The immune
system**

The immune system is much like the other body systems, e.g. respiratory and reproductive systems, in that it is composed of a number of different cell types, tissues and organs. Many of these cells are organized into separate lymphoid organs or glands (Topic D2). Since attack from microbes can come at many different sites of the body, the immune system has a mobile force of cells in the blood stream which are ready to attack the invading microbe wherever it enters the body. Although many of the cells of the immune system are separate from each other they maintain communication through cell contact and molecules secreted by them. For this reason the immune system has been likened to the nervous system. Again like the other body systems, the immune system is only apparent when it goes wrong. This can lead to severe, sometimes overwhelming infections and even death. One form of dysfunction is **immunodeficiency** which can result from infection with the human immunodeficiency virus (HIV) causing AIDS. On the other hand, the immune system can be 'hypersensitive' to a microbe (or even to a substance such as pollen) and this itself can cause severe tissue damage sometimes leading to death. Thus, the immune system must strike a balance between producing a life-saving response and tissue-damaging reactions. This regulation (as in other systems) is maintained both within the immune system and from without through nonimmune cells, tissues and their products (Section N).

**Innate versus
adaptive systems**

Having penetrated the external defenses, microbes come into contact with cells and products of the immune system and the battle commences. A number of cell types and defense molecules are usually present at the site of invasion or migrate (**home**) to the site. These constitute the 'first line of defense'. This is called the '**innate immune system**' since it is present at birth and changes little throughout the life of the individual. The cells and molecules of this innate system are mainly responsible for the first stages of expulsion of the microbe and may give rise to inflammation (Section I). Phagocytes are important cells in the innate immune system since they ingest and kill microbes.

The second line of defense is the '**adaptive immune system**' and this is brought into action while the innate immune system is dealing with the microbe and especially if it is unable to remove the invading microbe. The key difference between the two systems is that the adaptive system shows far more specificity and remembers that a particular microbe has previously invaded the body. This leads to a more rapid expulsion of the microbe on its second and third time of entry. The cells, molecules and characteristics of innate and adaptive immune systems are shown in *Table 1*.

Table 1.   The innate and adaptive immune systems

Characteristics	Cells	Molecules
Natural immunity		
Responds rapidly	Phagocytes (PMNs and	Cytokines
Has some specificity	macrophages)	Complement
No memory	Natural killer cells	Acute phase proteins
	Mast cells	
	Dendritic cells	
Adaptive immunity		
Slow to start		
Highly specific	T and B cells	Antibodies
Memory		Cytokines

Interaction between innate and adaptive immunity

Although, innate and adaptive immunity are often considered separately for convenience and to facilitate their understanding, it is important to recognize that they frequently work together. For example, macrophages are phagocytic but produce important **cytokines** (Section G) that help to induce the adaptive immune response (Sections J and K). Complement components of the innate immune system are activated by antibodies, molecules of the adaptive system. The various cells of both systems work together through direct contact with each other and through interactions with chemical mediators, the cytokines and chemokines (Section G). These chemical mediators can either be cell bound or released as localized **hormones**, acting over short distances. Cells of both systems have a large number of surface receptors: some are involved in adhesion of the cells to blood endothelial walls (e.g. leukocyte function antigens – LFA-1), some recognize chemicals released by cells (e.g. complement, cytokine and chemokine receptors) and others trigger the function of the cell such as activation of the phagocytic process (Section I).

Clonal selection

All immunocompetent individuals have many distinct lymphocytes. Each of these cells is specific for a different foreign substance (**antigen**). This specificity results from the fact that each lymphocyte possesses cell surface receptors all of which are specific for a particular antigen. When this antigen is introduced into an individual, lymphocytes with appropriate receptors seek out and bind the antigen and are triggered to proliferate and differentiate into the effector cells of immunity (i.e., they give rise through division to large numbers of cells). All members of this **clone** of cells are specific for the antigen initially triggering the response and they, or their products, are capable of specifically reacting with the antigen or the cells that produce it and to mediate its elimination. In addition, there are a much larger number of cells specific for the immunizing antigen late in the immune response. These cells are able to respond faster to antigen challenge giving rise to the '**memory**' involved in immunity. That is, individuals do not usually get infected by the same organism twice, as their immune system remembers the first encounter and protects against a second infection by the same organism. Furthermore, in an immunocompetent individual, there must exist enough different specific lymphocytes to react with virtually every antigen with which an individual may potentially come in contact. How this diversity is developed is considered in Topic F3.

Clonal selection as it applies to the B cell system (see below) is shown in *Fig. 1* and is presented in more detail in Section J. In particular, when antigen is introduced into an individual, B cells with receptors for that antigen bind and internalize it and receive help from T cells (below and Topic J1). These B cells are triggered to proliferate, giving rise to clones of daughter cells. Some of these cells serve as memory cells, others differentiate and become **plasma cells** (Topic D1) which make and secrete large quantities of specific antibody (*Fig. 1*).

T and B cells and cell co-operation

The lymphocytes selected for clonal expansion are of two major types, B cells and T cells, each giving rise to a different form of immunity. T lymphocytes mature under the influence of the thymus and, on stimulation by antigen, give rise to cellular immunity. The B lymphocyte population matures under the influence of bone marrow and/or gut-associated tissues and gives rise to lymphoid populations which, on contact with antigen, proliferate and differentiate into **plasma cells**. These plasma cells make a humoral factor (**antibody = immunoglobulin**) which is specific for the antigen and able to neutralize and/or eliminate it.

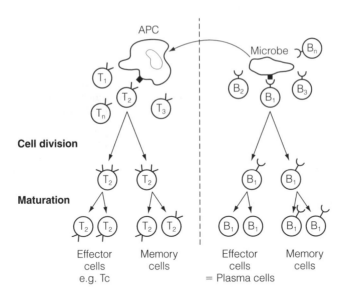

Fig. 1.   Clonal selection. From a large pool of B and T cells, antigen selects those which have receptors for it (e.g. T2 and B1) and stimulates their expansion and differentiation into memory and effector cells. Although B cells can recognize and bind native antigen, T cells only see antigen associated with MHC molecules on antigen presenting cells (APC).

The development of the immune response to an antigen also requires cell co-operation. T and B cell populations, as well as macrophages, interact in the development of specific immunity. In particular, subpopulations of T cells regulate (e.g. help) humoral and cellular immune responses. Although immune responses to most antigens (especially proteins) require cell co-operation, some antigens (**T-independent**) are able to initiate an immune response in the absence of T lymphocytes.

A4 ANTIGENS

Key Notes

The range of antigens

Invading organisms have antigens which are recognized by the immune system. Antigens are defined as substances which induce an immune response. They include proteins, carbohydrates and lipids.

The structure of antigens

An antigen molecule may contain a number of the same or different antigenic determinants to which individual antibodies or cell responses are made. The smallest unit (antigenic determinant) to which an antibody can be made is about three to six amino acids and about five to six sugar residues. All large molecules are multideterminant. Antibodies bind to conformational antigenic determinants (dependent on folding of the molecule) whilst T cells recognize linear amino acid sequences by their T cell receptor. Molecules which can stimulate an immune response ('immunogens') should be distinguished from those which react with antibodies but cannot initiate an immune response (haptens or individual antigenic determinants).

Related topics   Antigen recognition (H)   B cell activation (L3)

The range of antigens

The first stage of removing an invading organism is to recognize it as being foreign i.e. not 'self' (Topic M1). The immune system sees the invader as having a number of antigens. An antigen is any substance which induces an immune response in the form of proliferation of lymphocytes and production of antibodies specific for the antigen introduced. This usually includes proteins, carbohydrates, lipids and nucleic acids. Responses can be made to virtually anything when introduced in an appropriate form. Even self molecules or cells can act as antigens under appropriate conditions although this is quite well regulated in normal healthy individuals (Topics M1 and N1).

The structure of antigens

On the structural level, an antigen must be sufficiently unique for the immune system to warrant making an immune response to it. It is usual that an antigen, a molecule which is antigenic, possesses several unique molecular structures, each of which can elicit an immune response. Thus, antibodies or cells produced against an antigen are not directed against the whole molecule but against different parts of the molecule. These 'antigenic determinants' or 'epitopes' (*Fig. 1*) are the smallest unit of an antigen to which an antibody or cell can bind. For a protein, an antibody binds to a unit which is about three to six amino acids whilst for a carbohydrate it is about five to six sugar residues. Therefore, most large molecules possess many antigenic determinants per molecule i.e. they are 'multideterminant'. However, these determinants may be identical or different from each other on the same molecule. For example, a carbohydrate with repeating sugar units will have several identical determinants, whilst a large single chain protein

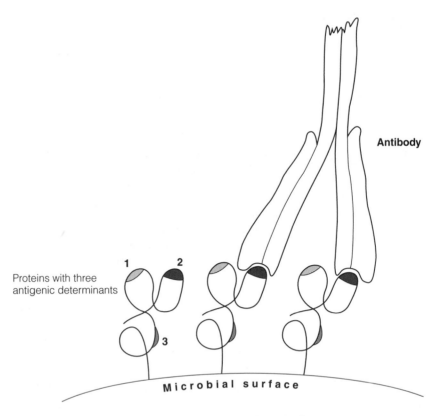

Fig. 1.   Antigenic determinants (epitopes) recognized by antibodies.

will have many units each with a different amino acid sequence and thus many different antigenic determinants. Although the linear sequence of the residues in a molecule have been equated with an antigenic determinant, the physical structure to which antibodies bind are primarily the result of the conformation of the molecule. As a result of folding, residues at different parts of the molecule may be close together and may be recognized by a B cell or an antibody as part of the same determinant (*Fig. 1*). Thus, antibodies made against the native (natural) conformation of a molecule will not, in most instances, react with the denatured molecule even though the primary sequence has not changed. This is in contrast to the

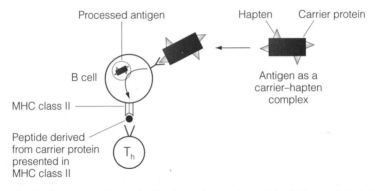

Fig. 2.   Response to hapten by B cells requires carrier protein which permits help from T cells.

way in which T cell receptors recognize antigens in the form of linear amino acid sequences of antigenic determinants (Topic H3). In practical terms, microbes have a large number of different molecules and therefore potentially many different antigenic determinants to stimulate the immune response. However, all antigenic determinants are not equal, some may elicit strong and others weak responses. This is determined by the health, age and genetics of the individual (Topic N1).

Very small molecules which can be viewed as single antigenic determinants are also incapable of eliciting an antibody response. These **haptens**, as they are called, can be attached covalently to larger molecules (**carriers**) and in this physical form are able to induce the formation of antibodies with the help of T cells (*Fig. 2*). Therefore, one should distinguish between molecules which can stimulate an immune response (called **immunogens**) and those which react with antibodies but cannot initiate an immune response (haptens or individual antigenic determinants).

B1 PHAGOCYTES

Key Notes

Mobile phagocytes

The most abundant mobile phagocyte (or eating cell) is the neutrophil (also called a polymorphonuclear cell: PMN). This granular leukocyte comprises the majority of white blood cells. It patrols the blood stream in search of invading microbes.

The mononuclear phagocyte system

This is a system of phagocytes located mainly in the organs and tissues. Monocytes are present in the blood stream and settle in the tissues as macrophages. Macrophage-like cells in the liver are called Kupffer cells and in the brain are called microglial cells.

The phagocytic process

The process of microbe ingestion has several stages which include the phagocyte being attracted to the site of infection, making contact with the microbe, ingestion (endocytosis) and killing of the ingested microbe by means of oxygen and oxygen-independent mechanisms.

Opsonization

This is a way of making microbes more palatable to the phagocyte. Molecules coating a microbe, such as complement or antibody, facilitate contact and ingestion of the microbe.

Related topics

Complement (C2)
Development of the immune
   system (E)

Antibodies (F)
The acute inflammatory response (I)
The microbial cosmos (O1)

Mobile phagocytes Phagocytes are specialized 'eating' cells (phago – I eat, *Latin*) of which there are two main types, neutrophils and macrophages. Neutrophils, often called polymorphonuclear cells (PMNs) because of the multilobed nature of their nuclei (*Fig. 1*), are mobile phagocytes that comprise the majority of blood leukocytes (about 8×10^6 ml^{-1} of blood). They have a very short half-life (days) and die in the blood stream by apoptosis (programmed cell death). They are granular leukocytes which stain with neutral dyes and have a different function from those granulocytes which stain with eosin (eosinophils), or basic dyes (basophils). Their granules contain peroxidase, alkaline and acid phosphatases, and defensins (small antibiotic peptides) which are involved in microbial killing. They have receptors for chemoattractive factors released from microbes, e.g. muramyl dipeptide (MDP), and for complement components activated by microbes. Their main function is to patrol the body via the blood stream in search of invading microbes. As such they are pivotal cells in acute inflammation (Section I). Like the majority of cells involved in the immune system, these phagocytes are produced in the bone marrow (Topic E1).

Table 1.   Cells of the mononuclear phagocyte system

Cells	Location
Monocytes	Blood stream
Kupffer cells	Liver
Mesangial cells	Kidney
Alveolar macrophages	Lungs
Microglial cells	Brain
Sinus macrophages	Spleen, lymph nodes
Serosal macrophages	Peritoneal cavity

The mononuclear phagocyte system

The mononuclear phagocyte system (previously called the reticuloendothelial system), is the name given to the widely distributed tissue bound phagocytic system, whose major function is to dispose of microbes and dead body cells through the process of phagocytosis. Monocytes are blood borne precursors of the major tissue phagocytes, macrophages (*Fig.* 2). Different organs/tissues each have their versions of monocyte-derived phagocytic cells (*Table 1*).

Table 2.   Stages in phagocytosis

Stage	Event	Mechanism
1	Movement of phagocyte towards the microbe	Chemotactic signals e.g. MDP complement
2	Attachment to the phagocyte surface	Sugar e.g. mannose, complement and Fc receptors
3	Endocytosis of microbe resulting in a phagosome	Invagination of surface membrane
4	Fusion of the phagosome with a lysosome	Microtubules involved
5	Killing of microbe	Oxygen dependent killing e.g. O_2-radicals; oxygen independent e.g. myeloperoxidase, nitric oxide

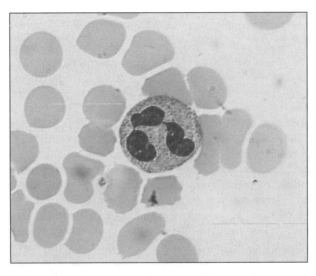

Fig. 1.   A polymorphonuclear cell (neutrophil) in the blood. Reproduced from Immunology 5th edn., 1998, Roitt, Brostoff and Male, with permission from Mosby.

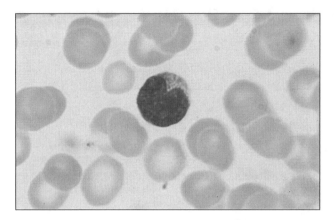

Fig. 2.   A monocyte in the blood. Reproduced from Immunology 5th edn., 1998, Roitt, Brostoff and Male, with permission from Mosby.

The phagocytic process

This is a multistep process which ultimately concludes with the demise of a microbe. The stages in this process are listed in *Table 2*. Phagocytosis is the major mechanism by which microbes are removed from the body and is especially important for defence against extracellular microbes (Topic O1).

Opsonization

This is the process of making a microbe easier to phagocytose. A number of molecules called 'opsonins' (to 'make more tasty' – *Greek*) do this by coating the microbes. They aid attachment of the microbe to the phagocyte and also trigger activation of phagocytosis. Opsonins include the complement component C3b and antibody itself, the latter acting as a bridge between the innate and adaptive immune systems (Topics C2 and F5). Phagocytes use their surface receptors which bind to C3b, or which bind to the Fc region of IgG antibody (Fc receptors, FcR) to attach to C3b or IgG coating the microbes, respectively (*Fig. 2*: Topic C2 and Section I).

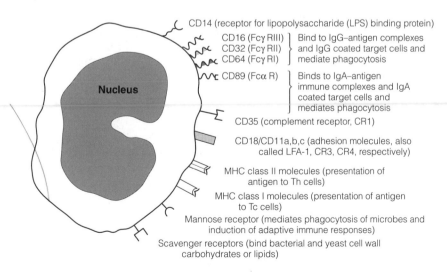

Fig. 3.   Surface molecules on monocytes.

B2 NATURAL KILLER CELLS

Key Notes

Localization and characteristics	Natural killer (NK) cells (large granular lymphocytes) are found throughout the tissues of the body but mainly in the circulation. They contain cytotoxic substances which are important for protection against viruses and some tumors.
NK cells kill virus infected cells	Changes in the surface molecules of cells as the result of virus infection allow NK cells to bind to infected cells. They kill the infected cells by releasing perforins and inducing apoptosis.
NK cells secrete IFNγ	On binding to virus-infected cells, NK cells secrete interferon gamma (IFNγ) which protects adjacent cells from infection by viruses released following cell death, and helps to activate T cell mediated immunity.
Related topics	Complement (C2) Cell recognition of self and non self Interferons (C4) discrimination (M1) Lymphocytes (D1) Transplantation antigens (Q2)

Localization and characteristics

Natural killer (NK) cells are also termed 'large granular lymphocytes' (or LGLs). They differ from classical lymphocytes in that they are larger, contain more cytoplasm, and have (electron) dense granules (*Fig. 1*). They are produced in the bone marrow and are found throughout the tissues of the body, but mainly in the circulation where they comprise 5–15% of the total lymphocyte fraction (Topic D1). They have surface Fc receptors for IgG (FcRγRIII), but also have receptors for certain cell surface molecules called killer activation receptors (KARs) and killer inhibitory receptors (KIRs: *Fig. 2*).

NK cells kill virus infected cells

The main function of NK cells is to kill self cells which contain viruses, as well as some tumor cells. When NK cells bind to uninfected self cells, NK receptors, KIRs, provide a negative signal to the NK cell, preventing it from killing the self cell. These molecules include MHC class I molecules encoded by genes of the HLA A, B and C regions (Topic Q2). However, infection of cells by some viruses reduces the expression of the inhibitory MHC molecules, thus allowing the activation through KAR to induce killing of the infected cell by the NK cell. This is an important mechanism, allowing NK cells to recognize which cells are self and ignore them, whilst killing those self cells which have been infected with a microbe (Topic M1). This results in the delivery of a death signal causing apoptosis of the infected cell.

The mechanism of killing is identical to that used by cytotoxic T cells (Topic K2) and is mediated through release of its granule contents (perforins and granzymes) onto the surface of the infected cell. Perforin has a structure similar to that of C9, a component of complement which can 'punch a hole' in the cell membrane

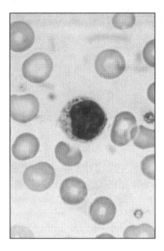

Fig. 1. An NK cell in the blood. Reproduced from Immunology 4th edn, Roitt, Brostoff and Male, with permission from Mosby.

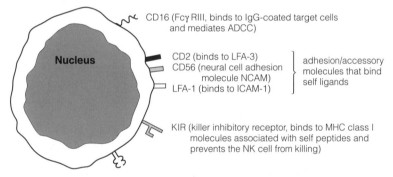

Fig. 2. Surface molecules on NK cells.

(Topics C2 and F5), allowing the passage of the granzymes (proteolytic enzymes) into the cell to induce apoptosis. NK cells, like cytotoxic T cells, are also able to induce target cell apoptosis through surface FasL molecules ligating Fas molecules on the surface of the virus infected cell (Topic K2).

NK cells can be activated by IL-2 (Topic G2) to become lymphokine activated killer (LAK) cells which have been used in clinical trials to treat tumors (Topic P5).

NK cells secrete gamma interferon (IFNγ)

When NK cells are 'activated' by recognizing a virus infected cell they secrete IFNγ. This helps to protect surrounding cells from virus infection. It should be noted that IFNα and IFNβ are probably more important in this role (Topic C4). In addition, IFNγ acts to enhance the development of specific T cell responses directed to virus infected cells (Topic K2).

B3 MAST CELLS AND BASOPHILS

Key Notes

Localization

Mast cells and basophils are produced in the bone marrow and have similar morphology and functions. Basophils are found in low numbers in the circulation whilst mast cells are found in connective tissues and close to mucosal surfaces.

Granule release and function

When activated, these cells degranulate releasing pharmacological mediators which cause vasodilation, increase vascular permeability and attract leukocytes to the site of degranulation.

Related topics

The acute inflammatory response (I)

IgE-mediated type 1 hypersensitivity: allergy (T2)

Localization

Mast cells are found in connective tissues throughout the body, close to blood vessels and particularly in the sub-epithelial areas of the respiratory, urogenital and gastrointestinal tracts. Basophils are granulocytes which stain with basic dyes and are present in very low numbers in the circulation (<0.2% of the granular leukocytes). Basophils and mast cells are very similar in morphology. Both have large characteristic electron-dense granules in their cytoplasm (*Fig. 1*) which are very important for their function. Like all the granulocytes, basophils are produced from stem cells in the bone marrow. The origin of mast cells is uncertain but they probably also originate in the bone marrow.

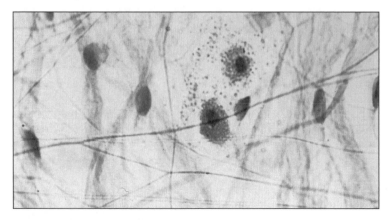

Fig. 1. Mast cells. Note the large granules in the cytoplasm which contain pharmacological mediators.Reproduced from A Photographic Atlas for the Microbiology Laboratory, 1996, Leboffe and Pierce, with permission from Morton Publishing.

Granule release and function

Mast cells/basophils (*Fig. 1*) can be stimulated to release their granules as a result of:

- binding to C3a and C5a (anaphylatoxins),
- crosslinking by IgE antibody and allergens of FcεR on their cell surface,
- binding to lectins (molecules that bind carbohydrates and are found in some fruits).

The activation process results in the fusion of the intracellular granules with the surface membrane and the release of their contents to the exterior by the process of exocytosis. This release is almost instantaneous and is essential in the development of the acute inflammatory response (Section I). The granule contents include a variety of pre-formed pharmacological mediators. Other pharmacological mediators are produced *de novo* when the cells are stimulated. *Table 1* shows some of the important mediators produced and some of their functions. When large numbers of mast cells/basophils are stimulated to degranulate, severe anaphylactic responses can occur, which in their mildest form give rise to the allergic symptoms seen in Type 1 hypersensitivity (Topic T2).

Table 1.   Main mediators released and their effects

Mediators		Effect
Histamine		Vasodilation, vascular permeability
Cytokines	TNFα, IL-8, IL-5	Attracts neutrophils and eosinophils
	PAF	Attracts basophils

* TNFα, tumor necrosis factor; PAF, platelet activating factor.

B4 DENDRITIC CELLS

Key Notes

Localization	There are three main kinds of dendritic cells which are found in skin and in T cell and B cell areas of lymphoid tissues.
The interface of innate and adaptive immunity	Most dendritic cells possess high levels of surface MHC class II molecules and process and present peptide antigens to T cells (Section D). Their role is to recognize microbial antigens through innate receptors and process and present them to T cells of the adaptive immune system. Follicular dendritic cells hold intact antigens in specialized areas of lymphoid tissues.
Related topics	Lymphoid organs and tissues (D2) The major histocompatibility T cell recognition of antigen, the complex and antigen processing T cell receptor complex (H3) and presentation (H4)

Localization Dendritic cells are so called because of their many surface membrane folds, similar in appearance to dendrites of the nervous system (*Fig. 1*). These folds allow maximum interaction with other cells of the immune system. There are three main kinds of dendritic cells (*Table 1*): Langerhans cells (LH); interdigitating cells (IDC); follicular dendritic cells (FDC).

The interface of innate and adaptive immunity The function of dendritic cells is to present antigens to the lymphocytes (Section D). LH and IDC present antigens to T cells. The T cell antigen receptor has to recognize 'pieces' of proteins and therefore the proteins need to be 'processed' (cut up into short peptides), before attachment to the MHC molecules (Topic H4). LH and IDC have large amounts of surface MHC class II to present foreign peptides to CD4 T cells. Although macrophages can process and present antigen to CD4 T cells, the LH and IDC are much more efficient in carrying out this function. These cells are at the interface of innate and adaptive immune systems in that they recognize microbial antigens through innate receptors, and through the endogenous processing pathway are able to present peptide antigens to the T cells. It is likely that both LH cells and IDC are derived from blood borne progenitors produced in the bone marrow. FDC are present within the B cell follicles of lymphoid tissues and hold intact antigens on their surfaces with which B cells can interact. It is thought that this interaction is important in B cell survival within the primary follicles (Topic D2)

Table 1. Dendritic cells

Dendritic cell type	Localization
Langerhans cells (LH)	Skin
Interdigitating cells (IDC)	Lymph node T cell areas
Follicular dendritic cells (FDC)	B cell follicles of the lymphoid tissues

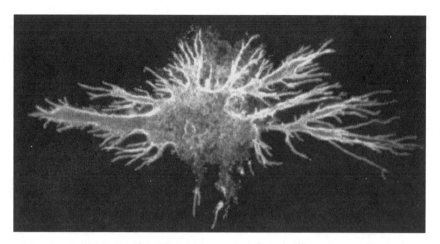

Fig. 1.   Dendritic cell. Note the many membrane processes to allow interactions with lymphocytes. Surface stained with anti CD44 (shown white, see Topic V3). CD44 is an adhesion molecule which allows the dendritic cell to attach to connective tissue and other cells. (Figure courtesy of Dr M. Binks.)

B5 OTHER CELLS OF THE INNATE IMMUNE SYSTEM

Key Notes

Eosinophils	These granular leukocytes are present in low numbers in the circulation. They attack parasites too large to be phagocytosed and kill them by releasing a toxin, major basic protein.
Platelets	Platelets release mediators when activated. The mediators activate complement leading to attraction of leukocytes.
Erythrocytes	Erythrocytes bind small immune complexes and help to remove them from the circulation.
Related topics	The acute inflammatory response (I) Immunity to different organisms (O2)

Eosinophils

These are granular leukocytes which stain with eosin. They are present at low levels in the circulation (2–5% of blood leukocytes). Eosinophils have some phagocytic activity but are primarily responsible for extracellular killing of large parasites (e.g. schistosome worms) which cannot be phagocytosed (Topic O2). They usually bind to an antibody-coated parasite through surface Fc receptors and release the contents of their granules (degranulate) onto the parasite surface. The granules contain peroxides and a toxin, major basic protein, which kill the parasite. Histaminase is also present in the granules. This anti-inflammatory substance dampens the effects of histamine released by mast cells earlier in the response.

Platelets

As well as having a major role in blood clotting, platelets contain important mediators which are released when they are activated at the site of a damaged blood vessel. Parasites coated with IgG and/or IgE antibodies are also thought to activate platelets through surface Fc receptors for these antibody classes. Released mediators activate complement, which in turn attracts leukocytes to the site of tissue damage caused by trauma or infection by a parasite (Section I).

Erythrocytes

Erythrocytes have surface complement receptors which bind to complement attached to small circulating immune complexes. They carry these complexes to the liver where they are released to Kupffer cells which phagocytose them. Thus, erythrocytes have an important immunological role in clearing immune complexes from the circulation in persistent infections and in some autoimmune diseases (Topic B5).

C1 INNATE MOLECULAR DEFENSE AGAINST MICROBES

Key Note

Innate molecular immune defense	A variety of molecules mediate protection against microbes during the period before adaptive immunity develops. Because these molecules react with particular structures that are common to a variety of microbes, they react with many different microbes that express these structures. The molecules of the innate immune system include complement, acute phase proteins, and cytokines, particularly the interferons. Some of these, especially those of the complement system are also vital for the adaptive immune system.

Related topics	External defenses (A2)	The acute inflammatory response (I)

Innate molecular immune defense

There are many molecules of the innate immune system which are important in mediating protection against microbes during the period before the development of adaptive immunity. Although these molecules react with particular structures associated with microbes, they are nonspecific in that they can react with many different microbes that express these structures. The major molecules are those of the complement system, acute phase proteins and cytokines, especially the interferons (Section C). Most of the molecules which play a role in the innate immune system also have functions associated with the adaptive immune system. The complement system can be activated by antibodies, and cytokines are involved in activation of antigen presenting cells critical to triggering T lymphocyte responses. Cytokines released by macrophages also play a role in acute inflammation (Section I). Thus, the immune response to microbes is continuous with both systems being intimately involved and synergistic. A variety of other molecules are also important to the innate immune system, including the antibiotic peptides (Topic C5).

C2 COMPLEMENT

Key Notes

The complement system

The complement system consists of a large number of interdependent proteins, which on sequential activation may mediate protection against microbial infection and contribute to the inflammatory response. Synthesized by hepatocytes and monocytes, these proteins help (complement) antibody responses and have a wide spectrum of activities including a pivotal role in innate defense mechanisms. Complement may be activated by either the classical pathway (through antibody) or the alternative pathway (innate).

Activation

Complement can be activated directly by microbes (**alternative pathway**), or by antibodies bound to a microbe or any other antigen (**classical pathway**). The most important single event in activation is cleavage of C3 into C3a and C3b by C3 convertase. In the absence of antibody mediated immunity, this enzymatic activity can be induced by microbes alone (alternative pathway). C5 is then cleaved into C5a and C5b. C5a is important in chemotaxis and activation of cells of the immune system, whilst C5b is crucial to formation of the complex which mediates lysis of the microbe.

Functions

The major functions of the complement system are: (a) Initiation of (acute) inflammation as a result of the stimulation of degranulation of mast cells by C3a and C5a (anaphylatoxins); (b) Attraction, by C5a, of neutrophils to the site of microbial attack (chemotaxis); (c) Enhancement of the attachment of the microbe to the phagocyte – PMNs attracted to a site of complement activation by C5a bind to C3b enhancing their internalization of the microbe (opsonization); (d) killing of the microbe by the 'membrane attack complex', which through C9 produces 'pores' in the target cell membrane leading to lysis of the microbe.

Regulation

Complement components rapidly lose binding capacity after activation, limiting their membrane-damaging ability to the immediate vicinity of the activation site. The complement system is also tightly regulated by inhibitor/regulatory proteins which include C1 inhibitor, Factor I, C4b binding protein, Factor H, decay-accelerating factor (DAF), membrane cofactor protein (MCP), and CD59 (protectin). These molecules protect host cells from destruction or damage at different stages of the complement cascade.

Related topics

Phagocytes (B1)
The acute inflammatory response (I)

Cell recognition of self and
  non self (M1)

The complement system

The complement system is a protective system common to all vertebrates. In man it consists of a set of over 20 soluble glycoproteins, many of which are produced by hepatocytes and monocytes. They are constitutively present in blood and other body fluids and may be present in quite large amounts. For example C3, the pivotal molecule of the complement system, is present at about $1\,g\,l^{-1}$ in serum. The component molecules (C) include C1 (C1q, C1r, C1s), C2, C3, C4, C5, C6, C7, C8, C9 as well as a set of molecules which are primarily associated with the alternative pathway, including Factor B and Factor D. On appropriate triggering, these components interact sequentially with each other (i.e. in a domino like fashion). This 'cascade' of molecular events involves cleavage of some complement components into active fragments (e.g. C3 is cleaved to C3a and C3b) which contribute to activation of the next component, ultimately leading to lysis of, and/or protection against, a variety of microbes.

Activation

Complement can be 'activated' (*Fig. 1*) directly by certain molecules associated with microbes (**alternative pathway**), or by antibodies bound to a microbe or any other antigen (**classical pathway**). C3, present at high concentrations in the serum, is critical to both of these pathways and its cleavage into C3a and C3b is the single

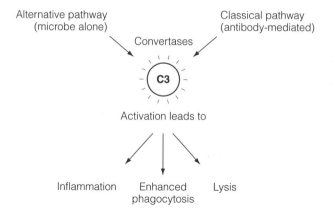

Fig. 1.   The complement system.

most important event in the activation of the complement system. This may be achieved by two different cleavage enzymes, C3 convertases – one as a component of the alternative pathway, the other a part of the classical pathway. The latter is described in more detail in Topic F5. The sequence of activation by the alternative pathway is summarized in *Table 1*.

In the absence of antibody mediated immunity, the alternative pathway is activated by interaction of C3 with certain types of molecules on microbes or by self-molecules (e.g. CRP, Topic C3) which react with these microbes. More specifically, the alternative pathway depends on the normal continuous low level breakdown of C3. One of the fragments, C3b, is very reactive and can covalently bind to virtually any molecule or cell. If C3b binds to a self cell, regulatory molecules associated with this cell (see below) inactivate it, protecting the cell from complement mediated damage. However, if C3b binds to a microbe, factor B is usually activated and its cleavage product Bb binds to C3b on the microbe. This C3bBb complex (C3 convertase) is enzymatically active and amplifies the breakdown of additional C3 to C3b. Equally important, the resulting enzyme cleaves C5 into C5a

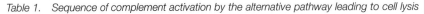

Table 1.   Sequence of complement activation by the alternative pathway leading to cell lysis

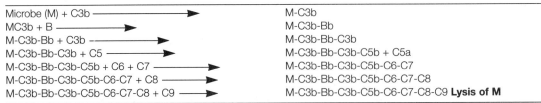

Microbe (M) + C3b ⟶	M-C3b
MC3b + B ⟶	M-C3b-Bb
M-C3b-Bb + C3b ⟶	M-C3b-Bb-C3b
M-C3b-Bb-C3b + C5 ⟶	M-C3b-Bb-C3b-C5b + C5a
M-C3b-Bb-C3b-C5b + C6 + C7 ⟶	M-C3b-Bb-C3b-C5b-C6-C7
M-C3b-Bb-C3b-C5b-C6-C7 + C8 ⟶	M-C3b-Bb-C3b-C5b-C6-C7-C8
M-C3b-Bb-C3b-C5b-C6-C7-C8 + C9 ⟶	M-C3b-Bb-C3b-C5b-C6-C7-C8-C9 **Lysis of M**

and C5b, both of which have critical protective functions. C5b is crucial to formation of the 'membrane attack complex' (MAC), C5b-C6-C7-C8-C9 which mediates lysis of the microbe. This alternative pathway is important for control of infection in the absence of specific immunity. Thus, many different organisms are handled and eliminated as a result of their activation of the alternative pathway.

Functions

The major functions of the complement system are:

- Initiation of (acute) inflammation by direct activation of mast cells.
- Attraction of neutrophils to the site of microbial attack (chemotaxis).
- Enhancement of the attachment of the microbe to the phagocyte (opsonization).
- Killing of the microbe activating the membrane attack complex (lysis).

The components of the complement system most important to its three main functions are:

- The inflammatory peptides C3a and C5a (anaphylatoxins) derived from C3 and C5, respectively. C3a and C5a bind to receptors on mast cells causing them to release pharmacological mediators (degranulate) such as histamine, which result in smooth muscle contraction and increased vascular permeability (Topic I2). C5a is also chemotactic and attracts neutrophils (PMNs) to the site of its generation (e.g. by microbial attack). It also causes PMN adhesion, degranulation and activation of the respiratory burst.
- C3b and its split products (and C4b) act as opsonins, marking a target for recognition by receptors on phagocytic cells. These receptors (complement receptor, CR1 = CD35) are expressed on monocytes/macrophages, PMNs and erythrocytes. PMNs attracted to a site of complement activation by C5a find and bind to C3b through their cell surface CR and this interaction greatly enhances internalization of the microbe by these cells. Therefore, complement can not only lead to lysis of an organism, but attracts cells, and with C3b tells phagocytes what to phagocytose. Even organisms resistant to direct lysis by complement may be phagocytosed and killed. Binding of C3b containing complexes to CR1 on erythrocytes shuttles immune complexes to the mononuclear phagocytes of the liver and spleen, facilitating their removal.
- C5b through C9, the MAC, and especially C9 produce 'pores' in the target cell membrane. These pores have diameters of about 10 nm and permit leakage of intracellular components and influx of water which result in disintegration (lysis) of the cell.

Regulation

The complement system is a powerful mediator of inflammation and destruction and could cause extensive damage to host cells if uncontrolled. However, complement components rapidly lose binding capacity after activation, limiting their membrane-damaging ability to the immediate vicinity of the activation site. This system is also tightly regulated by inhibitory/regulatory proteins. These regulatory proteins (*Table 2*) include C1 inhibitor, Factor I, C4b binding protein, Factor H, decay-accelerating factor (DAF), membrane co-factor protein (MCP), and CD59 (protectin) and protect host cells from destruction or damage at different stages of the complement cascade. Because regulatory proteins are expressed on the surface of many host cells but not on microbes, they limit damage to the site of activation and usually to the invading microbe which initiated complement activation (Topic M1).

It is important to note that, since the activated complement components are unstable, activation of complement is equivalent to its inactivation. That is, depressed complement levels in an individual may indicate that complement is being used up faster than it is being produced, suggesting chronic activation of complement perhaps resulting from continuous *in vivo* formation of antigen–antibody complexes.

Table 2. Regulatory proteins of the complement system

Protein	Function
C1 inhibitor	Binds to C1r and C1s and prevents further activation of C4 and C2
Factor I	Enzymatically inactivates C4b and C3b
C4b binding protein	Binds to C4b displacing C2b
DAF	Inactivates C3b and C4b
CD59	Prevents binding of C5b,6,7 complexes to host cells

C3 ACUTE PHASE PROTEINS

Key Notes

The proteins	Acute phase proteins are a heterogeneous group of plasma proteins important in innate defense against microbes (mostly bacteria) and in limiting tissue damage caused by infection, trauma, malignancy and other diseases. They include C-reactive protein (CRP), serum amyloid protein A (SAA), and mannose binding protein (MBP).
Production	Acute phase proteins are mainly produced in the liver, usually as the result of a microbial stimulus. Production is normally at a low level, but on stimulation increases rapidly within a few hours. These proteins are also produced in response to the cytokines IL-1, IL-6, TNFα and IFNγ that are released by activated macrophages and NK cells.
Functions	Acute phase proteins maximize activation of the complement system and opsonization of invading microbes. They also limit tissue damage caused by microbes, trauma, malignancy and other diseases e.g. rheumatoid arthritis. In particular, CRP and MBP act as opsonins; complement components enhance microbial killing; metal binding proteins inhibit microbial growth; fibrinogen aids blood clotting and protease inhibitors neutralize lysosomal enzymes released from phagocytes.

Related topics	Molecules with multiple functions (G1)	The acute inflammatory response (I)

The proteins

Acute phase proteins are important in innate defense against microbes (mostly bacteria and protozoa) and in limiting tissue damage caused by microbial infection, trauma, malignancy and other diseases e.g. rheumatoid arthritis. They are also important in tissue repair. These molecules include C-reactive protein (CRP), complement components, opsonic proteins such as mannose binding protein (MBP), metal binding proteins and protease inhibitors. The major acute phase proteins CRP and serum amyloid protein A (SAA) have similar structures and are termed pentraxins, based on the pentagonal association of their subunits. CRP, which was named based on its ability to react with the C-protein of pneumococcus, is composed of five identical polypeptides associated by noncovalent interactions. MBP binds residues of mannose on glycoproteins or glycolipids expressed by microbes in a form different from that on mammalian cells. Its binding properties permit it to interact with a variety of pathogens.

Production

These proteins, mainly produced by the liver, can either be produced *de novo* (e.g. CRP is increased by as much as 1000-fold within a few hours), or are present at low levels and rapidly increase following infection (fibrinogen). They are produced by hepatocytes in the liver in response to the cytokines IL-1, IL-6, TNFα and IFNγ released by activated macrophages and NK cells. IL-6 appears to be the major cytokine of importance in enhancing production of acute phase proteins.

Functions

Acute phase proteins have several functions, the most important being to maximize activation of the complement system and opsonization of invading microbes, and to limit tissue damage caused by these microbes. CRP binds to a wide variety of microbes and on binding activates complement through the alternative pathway, causing C3b deposition on the microbe (opsonization) and thus ultimately its phagocytosis by phagocytes expressing receptors for C3b. MBP binding to microbes also initiates complement activation and subsequent opsonization mediated by C3b, but in addition it directly opsonizes these organisms for phagocytosis. In addition, metal binding proteins inhibit microbial growth, and protease inhibitors limit tissue damage by neutralizing lysosomal enzymes released from phagocytes (*Table 1*).

Both CRP and SAA, as well as having complement activation properties, bind to DNA and other nuclear material from cells, helping in their clearance from the host. Quantitation of CRP in the serum of patients with inflammatory diseases, e.g. rheumatoid arthritis, is used as a way to assess the current inflammatory activity of the disease. High levels of CRP signify a high level of disease activity (Topic U5).

Table 1.   Acute phase proteins and their functions

Protein	Function
C-reactive protein (CRP)	Binds to bacterial phosphoryl choline, activates complement (binds to C1q), acts as an opsonin
Serum amyloid A (SAA)	Activates complement (binds to C1q), acts as an opsonin
Mannose binding protein (MBP)	Binds to mannose on bacterial surfaces, attaches to phagocyte MBP receptors (opsonization), activates complement via classical pathway (Section F)
Complement components e.g. C2, C3, C4, C5 and C9	Chemotaxis, opsonization and lysis (Section C)
Metal binding proteins	Removal of essential metal ions required for bacterial growth
Fibrinogen	Coagulation factor
α1 anti trypsin, α1 anti chymotrypsin	Protease inhibitors

C4 INTERFERONS

Key Notes

Protection against virus infection

Interferons (IFNs) are proteins involved in protection against viral infections. The two kinds of interferons, type I and type II, have different cellular origins and mediate a range of different activities. These molecules interfere with viral replication but also are signaling molecules between cells.

Type I interferons

Type I IFNs consist of IFN-alpha (IFNα) and beta (IFNβ), are produced by many different cells in the body and interfere with viral replication. Both IFNα and IFNβ inhibit protein synthesis in virally infected cells by preventing mRNA translation and DNA replication.

Type II interferons

Type II, immune interferon, IFNγ, has no structural homology with type I IFNs, is mainly produced by Th1 cells and NK cells and functions to regulate Th1 responses, increase phagocytic mechanisms and increase antigen presentation.

Related topics

Functions (F5)
Molecules with multiple
    functions (G1)

The major histocompatibility
    complex and antigen processing
    and presentation (H4)
Immunity to different
    organisms (O2)

Protection against virus infection

Interferons are important molecules which can mediate protection against virus infection, and are thus particularly important in limiting infection during the period when specific humoral and cellular immunity is developing. However, they do not simply function by interfering with virus replication but also act as communication molecules between cells. Type I interferons, α and β, are cytokines produced by many different cells in response to a virus and protect adjacent cells from viral infection. Type II IFN, IFNγ, is produced by specialist cells of the immune system (Th1 cells and NK cells) and is important not only for antiviral activity but also for activation of phagocytes. Interferons are pro-inflammatory cytokines (Topic G2).

Type I interferons (IFNα and β)

Type I IFNs have a common ancestral gene and bind to the same cell surface receptor. Their synthesis is induced by viral or bacterial infections and in particular by intracellular microbes. At least 12 different, highly homologous species of IFNα are produced, primarily by infected leukocytes as well as by epithelial cells and fibroblasts. In contrast, a single species of IFNβ is produced, normally by fibroblasts and epithelial cells. The proinflammatory cytokines IL-1 and TNFα are potent inducers of IFN-α/β secretion, as are endotoxins derived from the cell wall

Table 1.   The interferons

	IFN-α/β	IFNγ
Chromosomal location	9	12
Origin	All nucleated cells, especially fibroblasts, macrophages and dendritic cells	NK cells and Th1, γδ and CD8 T cells
Induced by	Viruses, other cytokines, some intracellular bacteria and protozoans	Antigen stimulated T cells
Functions	Antiviral, increases MHC class I expression, inhibits cell proliferation	Antiviral, increases MHC I and II expression, activates macrophages

of gram negative bacteria. These IFNs play an important role in innate defense against viral infections. Both IFNα and IFNβ inhibit protein synthesis in virally infected cells preventing mRNA translation and DNA replication. The importance of IFN-α/β in preventing viral infections has been shown in animal studies in which treatment with antibodies to IFN-α/β resulted in death of mice previously protected. Type I IFNs also activate NK cells and increase MHC class I expression (Topic G1).

Type II interferon (IFNγ)

IFNγ is a multi-functional cytokine produced by Th1 cells and NK cells (*Table 1*). IFNγ increases the expression of Fc receptors for IgG on macrophages and PMNs (Topic F5) as well as increasing MHC Class II expression on a wide variety of cells. This enhances the phagocytic function of these cells as well as increasing the antigen presenting capabilities of professional antigen presenting cells. IFNγ, which is crucial for macrophage function, enhances macrophage killing of intracellular bacteria and parasites probably as a result of its stimulation of their production of reactive oxygen and reactive nitrogen intermediates.

C5 OTHER MOLECULES

Key Notes

Collectins

Collectins are a group of carbohydrate-binding proteins structurally related to C1q that act as opsonins and are probably important in the nonadaptive immune response to infection. Receptors for collectins on macrophages facilitate the removal and destruction of the collectin bound microbe.

Peptide antibiotics

Peptide antibiotics are produced by a wide variety of cells including epithelial and phagocytic cells. They appear to play an important role in the eradication of bacterial infections as part of the body's innate defense system, with different peptides mediating antibacterial effects by different mechanisms.

Related topics

Acute phase proteins (C3)   Functions (F5)

Collectins

Collectins are a group of carbohydrate binding proteins structurally related to the complement component C1q. These molecules act as opsonins and are probably important in the innate immune response to infections. They include mannose binding protein, an acute phase protein, and conglutinin. Receptors for collectins are present on macrophages which therefore facilitate the removal and destruction of the microbe, and on epithelial cells in the lung and gastro-intestinal tract. Mannose binding protein is also able to activate complement via the classical pathway (Topic F5) and thus to engage host inflammatory, lytic and phagocytic responses.

Peptide antibiotics

A family of small peptides, peptide antibiotics, have potent antibacterial activities. These molecules include cecropins, magainins and defensins and are part of the body's innate defense mechanisms against microbial infection. In general, they are basic peptides with molecular weights of 3–5 kDa and are effective against both gram positive and gram negative bacteria. These peptide antibiotics are produced by a wide variety of cells including epithelial and phagocytic cells and appear to be highly conserved, as they are found in a wide variety of species. Different peptides have different antibacterial mechanisms of action. Whereas cecropins and magainins cause lysis, others interfere with ion transport. Peptide antibiotics probably represent the earliest defense mechanism in ontogeny. They are upregulated as a result of bacterial infection and dependent on transcription by NF-kB.

D1 LYMPHOCYTES

Key Notes

Specificity and memory	Lymphocytes provide both the specificity and memory which are characteristic of the adaptive immune response. The two types of lymphocytes involved in the adaptive response are T cells and B cells, both of which have similar morphology. They have specific but different antigen receptors and other surface molecules necessary for interaction with other cells. B cells mature into plasma cells which produce and secrete antibodies.
T lymphocytes	T cells function in the secondary lymphoid organs and tissues of the body to control intracellular microbes and to provide help for B cell (antibody) responses. Two different kinds of T cells are involved in these functions. T helper (Th) cells of which there are two types, Th1 and Th2, express CD4 and provide help for B cell growth and differentiation. T cytotoxic (Tc) cells express CD8 and recognize viral antigens presented on the surface of infected cells and kill these cells.
B lymphocytes and plasma cells	B cells are produced in the bone marrow and like T cells migrate to the secondary lymphoid tissues where they respond to foreign antigens. They have surface antibodies as their antigen receptor. When activated by antigen, in most cases with T cell help, they proliferate and mature into memory cells which remain able to respond to antigen if it is reintroduced, or into plasma cells (factories producing and secreting large amounts of antibody of the same specificity as the antigen receptor on the parent B cell). There are two kinds of B cells, B1 and B2, which have different properties.
Related topics	Hemopoiesis – development of blood cells (E1) B cell recognition of antigen, the B cell receptor complex and co-receptors (H2) T cell recognition of antigen, the T cell receptor complex (H3) Cell mediated immunity (K1) Receptors, co-receptors and signaling (L1)

Specificity and memory

Lymphocytes are responsible for the specificity and memory in adaptive immune responses. They are produced in the primary lymphoid organs (Topic D2) and function in the secondary lymphoid organs/tissues where they recognize and respond to foreign antigens. There are three types of lymphocytes – NK cells, T cells and B cells, although only T and B cells have true antigen specificity and memory. NK cells were considered earlier (Section B) and function in innate protection against viruses and some tumors.

T cells and B cells mature in the thymus and bone marrow, respectively. In the resting state both T and B lymphocytes have a similar morphology with a small

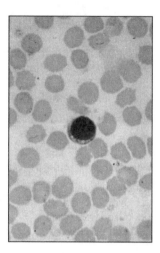

Fig. 1. A blood lymphocyte. Reproduced from Immunology 4th edn, Roitt, Brostoff and Male, with permission from Mosby.

amount of cytoplasm (*Fig. 1*). They have specific but different antigen receptors and a variety of other surface molecules necessary for interaction with other cells. These include molecules required for their activation and for movement into and out of the tissues of the body. This ability to migrate into the tissues and return via the lymphatic vessels to the blood stream (recirculation) is a unique feature of lymphocytes.

There are two classes of T lymphocytes, T helper cells and T cytotoxic cells. All T lymphocytes have antigen receptors (TcR) (Topic H3) which provide their specificity and CD3 which is essential for their activation (Topics L1 and L2). These molecules also serve as 'markers' to identify T cells. B lymphocytes make and use antibodies as their specific antigen receptor. They have molecules similar to CD3, i.e. CD79 which are important in their activation. B lymphocytes can mature into plasma cells which produce and secrete large amounts of antibody. The characteristics of T and B cells are shown in Table 1.

T lymphocytes

T cell precursors migrate from the bone marrow to the thymus, where some mature into antigen specific T cells. These cells then migrate to the secondary lymphoid organs and tissues of the body. Some T cells reside, at least temporarily, in T-cell dependent areas of tissues. T cells can be identified using monoclonal antibodies specific for characteristic molecules such as the T cell receptor (TcR) or CD3 (*Fig. 2* and Topic V5). These cells function to control intracellular microbes and to provide help for B cell (antibody) responses. Two different kinds of T cells are involved in these functions.

T helper (Th) cells provide help for B cells through direct cell surface signaling and by producing cytokines which are critical to B cell growth and differentiation. Th cells, in addition to TcR and CD3, also express cell surface CD4 molecules which can bind to MHC class II molecules (an interaction required for these cells to be activated by antigen) (Section H). Th cells are further subdivided into Th1 and Th2 cells depending on their ability to help in the development of different

Table 1.   Characteristics of human B and T cells

	T cells	B cells
Site of maturation	Thymus	Bone marrow
Antigen receptor	TcR	Antibody
Requirement of MHC for recognition	Yes	No
Characteristic 'markers'	All have TcR/CD3 Th – CD4 Tc – CD8	surface Ig, CD19/CD20/CD21 CD79
Main location in lymph nodes	Paracortical area	Follicles
Memory cells	Yes	Yes
Function	Protects against intracellular microbes	Protects against extra-cellular microbes
Products	Th1 – IFNγ/TNFα Th2 – IL4, IL5, IL6 Tc – Perforins	Antibodies (B cells mature into plasma cells)

immune responses (Topic K3) which is in turn related to their cytokine profiles (*Fig. 3*). The percentages of these cells in the peripheral blood is shown in *Table 2*.

T cytotoxic (Tc) cells mediate killing of infected cells, primarily those infected with virus. These cells express, in addition to TcR and CD3, a cell surface molecule, CD8, that binds to MHC class I and is important for these cells to interact effectively with virally infected cells.

B lymphocytes and plasma cells

B cells are produced in the bone marrow and like T cells migrate to the secondary lymphoid organs and tissues where they respond to foreign antigens. There are two kinds of B cells.

- *B1 cells*: These cells arise early in ontogeny, express mainly IgM antibodies encoded by germ-line antibody genes, mature independently of the bone-marrow, generally recognize multimeric sugar/lipid antigens of microbes and are T cell independent (Section L).
- *B2 cells (conventional B cells)*: These cells are the B cells primarily responsible for the development of humoral (antibody) mediated immunity. They are produced in the bone marrow, and with the help of T cells produce IgG, IgA and IgE antibodies.

Table 2.   Human peripheral blood lymphocyte populations

	T cells		B cells	NK cells
	T helper	T cytotoxic		
Percentage of lymphocytes	55	25	10	10
Functional properties	Antigen specific, produce cytokines, memory cells, effector cells		Antigen specific, produce cytokines, memory cells, plasma cells (antibody factories)	Mediate ADCC, tumor surveillance, no memory, lyze virus infected cells, tumor cells lacking self peptide in MHC class I molecules

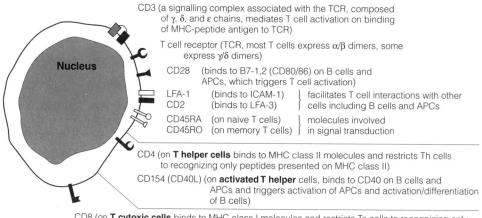

CD3 (a signalling complex associated with the TCR, composed of γ, δ, and ε chains, mediates T cell activation on binding of MHC-peptide antigen to TCR)

T cell receptor (TCR, most T cells express α/β dimers, some express γ/δ dimers)

CD28   (binds to B7-1,2 (CD80/86) on B cells and APCs, which triggers T cell activation)

LFA-1   (binds to ICAM-1)   facilitates T cell interactions with other
CD2   (binds to LFA-3)   cells including B cells and APCs

CD45RA   (on naive T cells)   molecules involved
CD45RO   (on memory T cells)   in signal transduction

Nucleus

CD4 (on **T helper cells** binds to MHC class II molecules and restricts Th cells to recognizing only peptides presented on MHC class II)

CD154 (CD40L) (on **activated T helper** cells, binds to CD40 on B cells and APCs and triggers activation of APCs and activation/differentiation of B cells)

CD8 (on **T cytoxic cells** binds to MHC class I molecules and restricts Tc cells to recognizing only peptides presented on MHC class I)

Fig. 2.   T cell surface molecules.

B cells are mainly found in loose aggregates (primary follicles) in lymphoid tissues or in well-defined proliferating foci (germinal centers) (Topics D2 and E3). Antibodies are the antigen receptor on these cells and are associated with several other molecules which form the B cell receptor complex (Topic H2). The characteristic molecules of human B cells are shown in *Fig. 4*.

When activated by antigen and, in most cases, with T cell help, B cells (*Fig. 4*) proliferate and mature into memory cells or plasma cells. Memory cells only produce antibody for expression on their cell surface and remain able to respond to antigen if it is reintroduced. In contrast, plasma cells do not have cell surface antibody receptors. Rather these cells, which are derived from activated B cells, function as factories producing and secreting large amounts of antibody of the same specificity as the antigen receptor on the stimulated parent B cell. The morphology of a plasma cell (*Fig. 5*) shows the high degree of adaptation of this cell type to high rate glycoprotein (antibody) synthesis. This includes extensive endoplasmic reticulum, mitochondria and Golgi apparatus. It should be noted that a plasma cell only produces antibodies of one specificity and class/subclass (Topic J2).

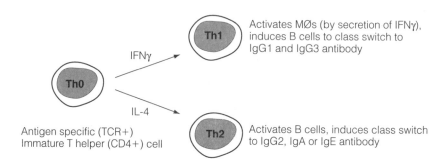

Fig. 3.   Two types of T helper cells. In the presence of Th1 inducing cytokines (e.g. IFNγ, TNFα) Th0 cells differentiate to become Th1 cells whereas in the presence of Th2 inducing cytokines (e.g. IL-4, IL-13, IL-5, IL-10) Th0 cells differentiate into Th2 cells.

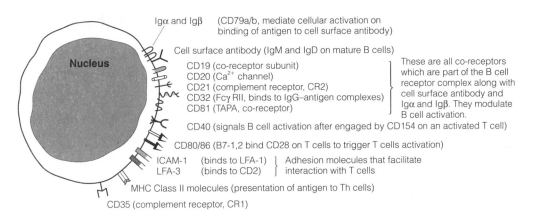

Igα and Igβ (CD79a/b, mediate cellular activation on binding of antigen to cell surface antibody)

Cell surface antibody (IgM and IgD on mature B cells)

CD19 (co-receptor subunit)
CD20 (Ca^{2+} channel)
CD21 (complement receptor, CR2)
CD32 (Fcγ RII, binds to IgG–antigen complexes)
CD81 (TAPA, co-receptor)

These are all co-receptors which are part of the B cell receptor complex along with cell surface antibody and Igα and Igβ. They modulate B cell activation.

CD40 (signals B cell activation after engaged by CD154 on an activated T cell)

CD80/86 (B7-1,2 bind CD28 on T cells to trigger T cells activation)

ICAM-1 (binds to LFA-1) Adhesion molecules that facilitate
LFA-3 (binds to CD2) interaction with T cells

MHC Class II molecules (presentation of antigen to Th cells)

CD35 (complement receptor, CR1)

Fig. 4. B cell surface molecules.

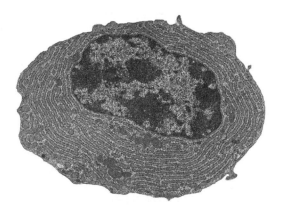

Fig. 5. Ultrastructure of a plasma cell. Note the extensive rough endoplasmic reticulum for antibody production. Reproduced from Immunology 5th edn., 1998, Roitt, Brostoff and Male, with permission from Mosby.

D2 LYMPHOID ORGANS AND TISSUES

Key Notes

Primary and secondary lymphoid organs	The primary lymphoid organs are the thymus and the bone marrow. These are called primary lymphoid organs because T and B cells must first undergo maturation in these tissues before migrating to the secondary lymphoid tissues, such as the spleen, lymph nodes and mucosa associated lymphoid tissues (MALT).
Bone marrow	Bone marrow is the primary source of pluripotent stem cells that give rise to all hematopoietic cells including lymphocytes. The bone marrow is the major organ for B cell maturation and gives rise to the precursor cells of the thymic lymphocytes.
Thymus	The thymus is the major organ for T cell maturation and development. Immature T cell precursors migrate from the bone marrow to the thymus (to become thymocytes) where they are selected through a process of thymic education before being released into the peripheral lymphoid tissues as mature lymphocytes.
Spleen	The spleen contains many phagocytes as well as T and B lymphocytes and is a major component of the mononuclear phagocyte system. Its primary function is to protect the body against blood borne infections and is particularly important in making B cell responses to polysaccharide antigens.
Lymph nodes	Lymph nodes are situated along lymphatic vessels and filter the lymph. They help to generate immune responses to foreign antigens entering the tissues. Like the spleen they contain both T and B lymphocytes as well as accessory cells needed to mount immune responses.
Related topics	T cells are produced in the thymus (E2) The cellular basis of the antibody response (J1)
	B cells are produced in the bone marrow (E3) Central tolerance (M2)

Primary and secondary lymphoid organs

The thymus and bone marrow are the primary lymphoid organs in mammals. T and B lymphocytes with diverse antigen receptors are produced in these organs. Following selection processes (Topics E2 and E3), they migrate to the secondary lymphoid tissues – the lymph nodes, spleen, and the mucosa associated lymphoid tissues (MALT) (*Fig. 1*).

Bone marrow

During early fetal development blood cells are produced in the mesenchyme of the yolk sac. As the development of the fetus progresses the liver and spleen take over

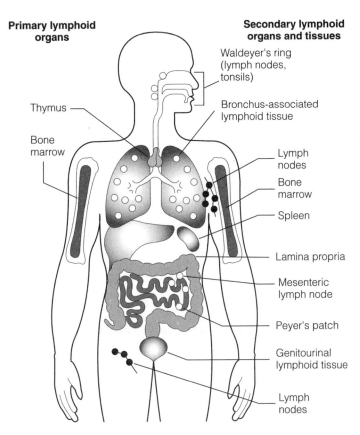

Primary lymphoid organs

- Thymus
- Bone marrow

Secondary lymphoid organs and tissues

- Waldeyer's ring (lymph nodes, tonsils)
- Bronchus-associated lymphoid tissue
- Lymph nodes
- Bone marrow
- Spleen
- Lamina propria
- Mesenteric lymph node
- Peyer's patch
- Genitourinal lymphoid tissue
- Lymph nodes

Fig. 1. Lymphoid organs and tissues. Lymphocytes produced in the primary lymphoid organs (thymus and bone marrow) migrate to the secondary organs and tissues where they respond to microbial infections. The mucosa-associated lymphoid tissue (MALT) together with other lymphoid cells in sub-epithelial sites (lamina propria) of the respiratory, gastro-intestinal and genitourinary tracts comprise the majority of lymphoid tissue in the body.

this role. It is only in the last months of fetal development that the bone marrow becomes the dominant site of hematopoiesis (blood cell formation). Bone marrow is composed of hematopoietic cells of various lineage and maturity packed between fat cells, thin bands of bony tissue (trabeculae), collagen fibers, fibroblasts and dendritic cells. All of the hematopoietic cells are derived from multipotential stem cells which give rise not only to all of the lymphoid cells found in the lymphoid tissue, but also to all of the cells found in the blood. Ultra-structural studies show hematopoietic cells cluster around the vascular sinuses where they mature, before they eventually discharge into the blood. Lymphocytes are found surrounding the small radial arteries, whereas most immature myeloid precursors are found deep in the parenchyma. The bone marrow gives rise to all of the lymphoid cells that migrate to the thymus for T cell maturation as well as to the major population of conventional B cells. B cells mature in the bone marrow and undergo selection for nonself before making their way to the peripheral lymphoid tissues: there they help form primary and secondary follicles and undergo further selection processes in germinal centers to eliminate self-reactive B cells (Topic M3).

Thymus

The thymus is a lymphocyte rich, bilobed encapsulated organ located behind the sternum, above and in front of the heart. It is essential for the maturation of T cells and the development of cell mediated immunity. In fact, the term 'T cell' means thymus derived cell and should only be used to describe mature T cells. The activity of the thymus is maximal in the fetus and in early childhood and then undergoes atrophy at puberty although never totally disappearing. It is composed of cortical and medullary epithelial cells, stromal cells, interdigitating cells and macrophages. These 'accessory' cells are important in the differentiation of the immigrating T cell precursors and their 'education' (positive and negative selection) prior to their migration into the secondary lymphoid tissues (Topics E2 and E3).

The thymus has an interactive role with the endocrine system as thymectomy leads to a reduction in pituitary hormone levels as well as atrophy of the gonads. Conversely, neonatal hypophysectomy results in thymic atrophy. Thymic epithelial cells produce the hormones thymosin and thymopoietin and in concert with cytokines (such as IL-7) are probably important for the development and maturation of thymocytes into mature T cells.

Spleen

The spleen is a large, encapsulated, bean shaped organ with a spongy interior (splenic pulp) and is situated on the left side of the body below the diaphragm. The large splenic artery pervades the spleen and branches of this artery are surrounded by highly organized lymphoid tissue (white pulp: *Fig. 2*). The white pulp forms 'islands' within a meshwork of reticular fibers containing red cells (red pulp). Closely associated with the central arteriole is the 'periarteriolar lymphatic sheath' an area containing mainly T cells and interdigitating cells (IDC). Lymphoid follicles (primary) are contained within the sheath and are composed mainly of follicular dendritic cells (FDC) and B cells. During an immune response these follicles develop germinal centers (i.e. become secondary follicles). The periarteriolar lymphoid sheath is separated from the 'red pulp' by a marginal zone containing macrophages (MØ) and B cells (*Fig. 2*). The central arterioles in

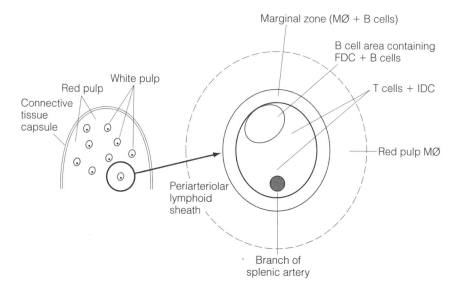

Fig. 2. Structure of lymphoid tissue in the spleen.

the periarteriolar sheath subdivide like the branches of a tree. The space between the branches is filled with 'red pulp' which is composed of splenic cords containing plasma cells and macrophages in addition to vascular channels called splenic sinuses. The spleen is a major component of the mononuclear phagocyte system, containing vast numbers of phagocytes. Unlike lymph nodes, it does not contain either afferent or efferent lymphatics.

The main immunological function of the spleen is to filter the blood by trapping blood borne micro-organisms and producing an immune response to them. It also removes damaged red blood cells and immune complexes. Those individuals who have had their spleens removed (splenectomized) have a greater susceptibility to infection with encapsulated bacteria, and are at increased risk of severe malarial infections, which indicates its major importance in immunity. In addition to its role in immunity, the spleen acts as a reservoir of erythrocytes.

Lymph nodes

Lymph nodes are small solid structures found at varying points along the lymphatic system e.g. groin, armpit and mesentery. They range in size from 2 to 10 mm, are spherical in shape and possess an enveloping capsule. Beneath the capsule is the subcapsular sinus, the cortex, a paracortical region and a medulla. The cortex contains many follicles and on antigenic stimulation becomes enlarged with germinal centers. The follicles are comprised mainly of B cells and follicular dendritic cells. The paracortical (thymus dependent) region contains masses of T

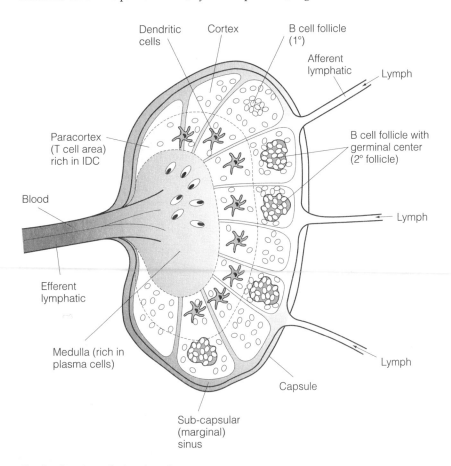

Fig. 3. Structure of a lymph node.

cells interspersed with interdigitating cells (*Fig. 3*). The primary role of the lymph node is to filter lymph and then produce an immune response against any microbe they trap. Lymph arriving from the tissues or from a preceding lymph node in the chain, passes via the afferent lymphatics into the subcapsular sinus and then into the cortex, around the follicles, into the paracortical area and then into the medulla. Lymph in the medullary sinuses then drains into efferent lymphatics and hence through larger lymphatic vessels back into the blood stream. Lymphocytes enter the lymph nodes from the tissues via the afferent lymphatics and from the blood stream through specialized post capillary venules called high endothelial venules which are found in the paracortical region of the node. B cells entering the blood migrate to the cortex where they are found in follicles (B cell areas).

D3 MUCOSA-ASSOCIATED LYMPHOID TISSUES

Key Notes

Mucosa-associated lymphoid tissues (MALT)	The majority (50%) of lymphoid tissue in the human body is located within the lining of the major tracts, including respiratory, digestive and genito-urinary tracts. This is because these are the main sites of entry for microbes into the body.
Nasal-associated lymphoid tissue (NALT)	The lymphoid tissue associated with the throat and nasal passages are the tonsils and come under the collective term NALT. The architecture of these lymphoid tissues, although not encapsulated, is similar to that of the lymph nodes and consists of B cell follicles.
Gut-associated lymphoid tissue (GALT)	The gut-associated lymphoid tissue is composed of lymphoid complexes (also called Peyer's patches in the ileum) which consist of specialized epithelium, antigen processing cells and intraepithelial lymphocytes. These structures occur strategically at specific areas in the digestive tract.
Bronchus-associated lymphocyte tissue (BALT)	The lymphoid tissue associated with the bronchus is structurally similar to Peyer's patches and other lymphoid tissues of the gut. It consists of lymphoid aggregates and follicles and is found along the main bronchi in the lobes of the lungs.
Related topics	Lymphocyte traffic and recirculation (D4) Peripheral tolerance (M3) The microbial cosmos (O1)

Mucosa-associated lymphoid tissues (MALT)

The main sites of entry for microbes into the body is through the epithelial surfaces containing mucosal epithelial cells. It is therefore not surprising that 50% of the lymphoid mass is associated with these surfaces. These are collectively called the mucosa-associated lymphoid tissues (MALT) and include NALT, BALT, GALT and lymphoid tissue associated with the genitourinary system.

Nasal-associated lymphoid tissue (NALT)

The nasal-associated lymphoid system is composed of the lymphoid tissue at the back of the nose (pharyngeal tonsil and other tissue) and that associated with the Waldeyer's ring (palatine and lingual tonsils). The strategic location of the lymphoid tissues suggests that they are directly involved in handling airborne microbes. Their composition is similar to that of lymph nodes, and encapsulated but do not possess afferent lymphatics. Antigens and foreign particles are trapped within the deep crypts of their lympho-epithelium from where they are transported to the lymphoid follicles (*Fig. 1*). The follicles are composed mainly of B cells surrounded by T cells and the germinal center within the follicle is the site of antigen-dependent B cell proliferation.

Gut-associated lymphoid tissue (GALT)

The primary role of GALT is to protect the body against microbes entering the body via the intestinal tract. It is mainly made up of Peyer's patches, lymphoid follicles and lymphoid cells between (intraepithelial lymphocytes) and below (within the lamina propria). In order to distinguish between harmful invaders or harmless food, the gut has a 'sampling' mechanism with which everything that has been ingested (or inhaled in the case of BALT and NALT) is subjected to analysis. The analytical, or antigen-sampling machinery of the gut, consists of specialized epithelial cells the M cells (microfold) and intimately associated 'antigen processing' cells (*Fig. 2*). These take up foreign molecules and pass them to cells beneath which present them in the context of class I and class II MHC molecules expressed on their surface so that the immune competent cells (lymphocytes) can recognize or 'see' them. This determines whether or not immunity or tolerance is induced to the sampled antigen. The combination of specialized epithelium and antigen processing cells plus lymphocytes constitute what has

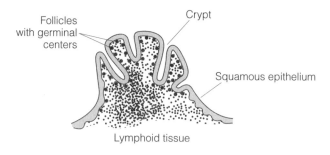

Fig. 1.   *Antigens trapped in the crypts are transported by M cells into the sub-epithelial areas where lymphocytes are stimulated via antigen presenting cells.*

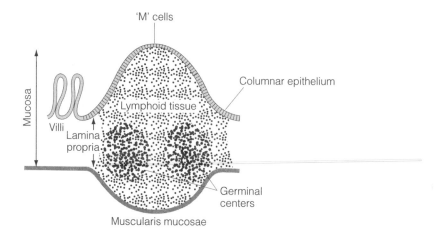

Fig. 2.   *Intestinal 'M' cells in Peyer's patches. Peyer's patches found in the terminal ileum 'sample' antigens transported via M cells. Lymphocytes stimulated here migrate to other sub-epithelial sites (lamina propria) in the intestine, respiratory and urogenital tracts.*

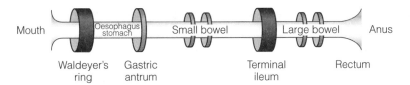

Mouth   Oesophagus   Small bowel   Large bowel   Anus
               stomach

     Waldeyer's   Gastric   Terminal   Rectum
       ring   antrum   ileum

Fig. 3.   Lymphoid complexes along the gastrointestinal tract; volume of the rings indicates
the relative amount of lymphoid tissue.

been called lymphoid complexes. These are localized structures that occur regularly at specific areas in the digestive tract and are exemplified by Peyer's patches in the terminal ileum. Lymphoid complexes are not distributed uniformly throughout the gut as one might initially expect, but are congregated in several zones (*Fig. 3*). Lymphocytes stimulated in the GALT can migrate to other MALT sites (in particular lactating mammary glands, salivary glands and other parts of the GI tract), and thus protect these surfaces from invasion with the same microbes.

Bronchus-associated tissue (BALT)   Bronchus-associated lymphoid tissue is similar to Peyers patches. It is composed mainly of aggregates of lymphocytes organized into follicles which are found in all lobes of the lung and are situated under the epithelium mainly along the bronchi. The majority of lymphocytes in the follicles are B cells. Antigen sampling is carried out by the epithelial cells that line the surface of the mucosa and by way of antigen presenting cells and M cells which transport antigens to the underlying lymphocytes.

D4 LYMPHOCYTE TRAFFIC AND RECIRCULATION

Key Notes

Lymphocyte traffic and recirculation

Lymphocytes produced in the primary lymphoid organs (thymus-T and bone marrow-B) migrate via the bloodstream to the secondary lymphoid organs/tissues where they carry out their function. They do not stay in one site but continually recirculate through the body in search of antigens.

Trafficking in the MALT

Lymphocytes stimulated in the GALT can migrate to the lamina propria at other sites of the mucosal immune system (e.g. lactating mammary glands and salivary glands), and protect these surfaces from invasion with the same microbes.

Mechanisms of lymphocyte trafficking

Lymphocytes have surface structures (adhesion molecules) which they use to attach to endothelial cells of blood vessels to exit the blood system.

Related topics

Lymphoid organs and tissues (D2)

Mucosa-associated lymphoid tissues (D3)

Lymphocyte traffic and recirculation

Lymphocytes produced in the primary lymphoid organs, thymus (T) and bone marrow (B)), migrate via the blood stream to the secondary lymphoid organs or tissues where they carry out their function. Since these cells have not yet encountered antigen they are called 'naive cells' and do not remain in one secondary lymphoid organ, but continue to recirculate around the body until they recognize their specific antigen. The overall recirculation pathway is shown in *Fig. 1*. They enter the lymph nodes via the high endothelial venules (HEV) and if they are not activated there, they pass via efferent lymphatic vessels into the thoracic duct and hence back into the blood stream. Both memory and naive cells may recirculate through the lymphoid tissues. T and B cells migrate to different sites within the lymph nodes. T cells reside in the paracortical region whereas the B cell domain is the lymphoid follicle. B cells must traverse through the T cell area to reach the follicle. Lymphocytes enter the PALS by way of the marginal zone (MZ) and leave through the splenic veins (SV) in the red pulp (RP). The lymphoid tissues are dynamic structures, wherein both T and B lymphocytes are continuously trafficking through each other's territories as well as being challenged by antigen on antigen presenting cells. Lymphocytes also traffic to the MALT.

Trafficking and the MALT

One of the unique features of MALT is that lymphocytes stimulated in one site can migrate to other sites of the mucosal immune system to protect them from invasion with the same microbes (*Fig. 1*). Thus, lymphocytes stimulated in the GALT can migrate via the blood to distant sites including the salivary glands and lactating mammary glands. For this the lymphocytes have specialized 'homing' molecules which determine where they exit the blood stream into the MALT sites around the body.

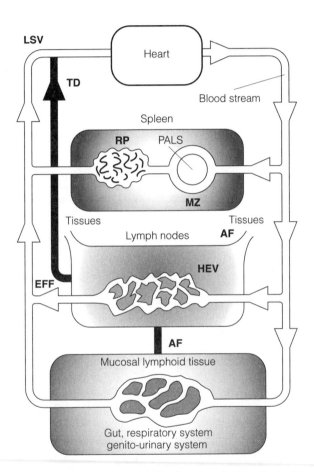

Fig. 1. Lymphocyte recirculation. Lymphocytes travel in the blood stream to the spleen where they enter the periarteriolar lymphoid sheath (PALS) via the marginal zone (MZ) and re-enter the blood stream via the red pulp (RP). Lymphocytes enter the lymph nodes via high endothelial veins (HEV) in the paracortical regions and pass via the efferent lymphatics (EFF) into the lymphatic system and via the thoracic duct (TD) into the left subclavian vein (LSV). Lymphocytes pass into the mucosal tissues through the HEV and return via the afferent lymphatics (AF) of the draining lymph nodes. Lymphocytes stimulated by microbes in the MALT migrate back to the mucosal tissues where they have been stimulated. Thus lymphocytes stimulated in the intestine will migrate back to sites in the lamina propria along the intestine to protect the body against the specific microbial attack via this route. Arrows indicate the direction of flow.

Mechanisms of lymphocyte trafficking

Lymphocytes have surface structures (adhesion molecules) which they use to attach to the endothelial cell walls of blood vessels to exit the blood system. These allow lymphocytes to enter lymph nodes via the HEV (*Fig. 2*). Other lymphocytes have specific adhesion molecules ('homing' molecules) which attach to specific surface molecules on endothelial cells of blood vessels ('addressins') in particular sites of the body. Thus, mucosal lymphocytes have specific homing molecules which allow them to migrate into the MALT areas of the body (*Fig. 3*).

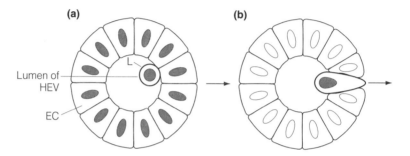

Fig. 2. Traffic of lymphocytes from the blood stream via HEV. (a) Lymphocytes (L) attach to the endothelial cells (EC) in the HEV by adhesion molecules. (b) Lymphocytes pass between endothelial cells to exit the HEV into lymph nodes or the MALT.

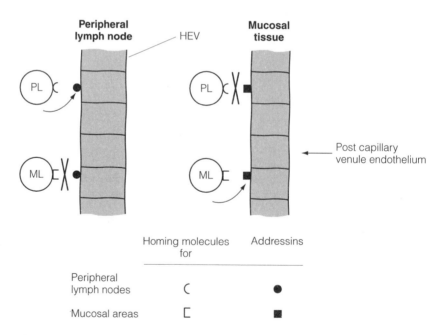

Fig. 3. Homing molecules allow trafficking of lymphocytes into specific anatomical locations. Lymphocytes entering peripheral lymph nodes (PL) have specific homing molecules for 'addressins' on endothelial cells of the HEV. These are absent from endothelial cells in the MALT. Lymphocytes primed in the MALT (ML) have their own homing molecules which allow them to bind to addressins on endothelial post capillary venules at distant mucosal sites.

E1 HEMOPOIESIS – DEVELOPMENT OF BLOOD CELLS

Key Notes

A common stem cell	The majority of the cell types involved in the immune system are produced from a common hemopoietic stem cell (HSC). HSC are found in the fetal liver, fetal spleen and neonate and adult bone marrow. They differentiate into functionally mature cells of all blood lineages.
Stromal cells	Direct contact with stromal cells (including epithelial cells, fibroblasts and macrophages) is required for the differentiation of a particular lineage. Adhesion molecules and cytokines are involved in this process.
The role of cytokines	Stromal cells produce many cytokines, including stem cell factor (SCF), monocyte colony stimulating factor (M-CSF) and granulocyte colony stimulating factor (G-CSF). Interaction of stem cells with stromal cells and M-CSF or G-CSF results in the development of monocytes and granulocytes, respectively.
Related topic	Cytokine families (G2)

A common stem cell

The majority of the cell types involved in the immune system are produced from a common hemopoietic stem cell (HSC) and develop through the process of differentiation into functionally mature blood cells of all different lineages, e.g. monocytes, platelets, lymphocytes, etc. (hemopoiesis: *Fig. 1*). These stem cells are replicating self-renewing cells, which in early embryonic life are found in the yolk sac and then in the fetal liver, spleen and bone marrow. After birth the bone marrow contains the HSCs.

The lineage of cells differentiating from the HSC is determined by the micro-environment of the HSC and requires contact with stromal cells and interaction with particular cytokines. These interactions are responsible for switching on specific genes coding for molecules required for the function of the different cell types, e.g. those used for phagocytosis in macrophages and neutrophils, and the receptors on lymphocytes which determine specificity for foreign molecules (antigens). This is, broadly speaking, the process of differentiation.

Stromal cells

Stromal cells, including epithelial cells and macrophages, are necessary for the differentiation of stem cells to cells of a particular lineage, e.g. lymphocytes, and involves direct contact of the stromal cell with the stem cell. Within the fetal liver, and in the thymus and bone marrow, a variety of stromal cells (including

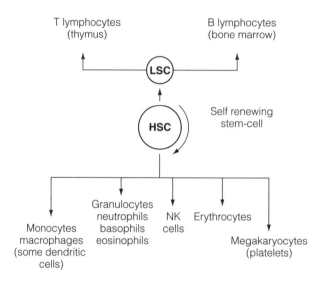

Fig. 1.   Origin of blood cells (hemopoiesis); LSC, lymphoid stem cell; HSC, hemopoietic stem cell.

macrophages, endothelial cells, epithelial cells, fibroblasts and adipocytes) each kind of which create discrete foci where different cell types develop. Thus, different foci will contain developing granulocytes, monocytes or B cells. Cytokines are essential for this process, and it is thought that adhesion molecules also play an important role (*Fig. 2*).

The role of cytokines

Different cytokines are important for renewal of HSC and their differentiation into the different functionally mature blood cell types. Although an oversimplification, the processes related to HSC regeneration depend largely on SCF, IL-1 and IL-3, whereas the development of granulocytes and monocytes, for example, involve production of monocyte colony stimulating factor (M-CSF) and granulocyte colony stimulating factor (G-CSF), among others, by the stromal cells. Interaction of the stem cells with stromal cells and with M-CSF or G-CSF results in the development of monocytes and granulocytes, respectively (*Fig. 3*). Other cytokines are important for the early differentiation of T cells in the thymus and B cells in particular locations within the bone marrow.

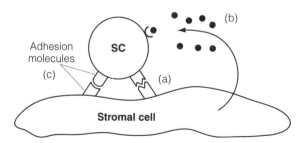

Fig. 2.   Role of stromal cells in hemopoiesis. (a) Stromal cell bound cytokine (e.g. stem cell factor) and (b) released cytokines (e.g. IL 7) determine the differentiation pathway of the stem cell (SC) attached through (c) specific adhesion molecules (e.g. CD44) on the SC attached to hyaluronic acid molecules on the stromal cell.

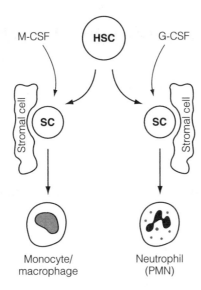

Fig. 3.   Different cytokines and stromal cells induce different pathways of differentiation.

E2 T CELLS ARE PRODUCED IN THE THYMUS

Key Notes

Overview	T lymphocytes are produced in the thymus from circulating T cell precursors derived from HSC in the bone marrow. These T cell precursors differentiate within the thymus into mature T cells expressing molecules important to T cell function, such as the T cell receptor, CD4 and CD8. The thymus thus generates large numbers of functionally mature antigen-specific T cells which then migrate to the peripheral lymphoid tissues to mediate protection against invading microbes.
Generation of T cell diversity	Very large numbers of different T cells are produced in the thymus, each having only one specificity. These different T cells each have receptors specific for a different antigen. The T cell receptors for antigen are generated in each T cell by gene rearrangement from multiple, inherited germ-line genes.
Positive and negative selection	T cells undergo selection using their newly produced receptors. T cells with receptors which bind weakly to MHC molecules are selected to survive, whilst those with receptors which bind strongly to MHC and self antigens die through apoptosis.
Related topics	Generation of diversity (F3) cell receptor complex (H3)
	T cell recognition of antigen, the T Central tolerance (M2)

Overview

The thymus is derived from the third and fourth pharyngeal pouches during embryonic life and attracts (by chemoattractive molecules) circulating T cell precursors derived from HSC in the bone marrow. These precursors differentiate into functional T lymphocytes under the influence of thymic stromal cells and cytokines. In the thymus, the precursors (now thymocytes) associate with cortical epithelial nurse cells which are important in their development. The thymic cortex is the major site of activity and thymocyte proliferation, with a complete turnover of cells approximately every 72 hours. These thymocytes then move into the medulla, where they undergo further differentiation and selection and finally migrate via the circulation to the secondary lymphoid organs/tissues where they are able to respond to microbial antigens.

Most of the thymocytes generated each day in the thymus die by apoptosis with less than 5% surviving. Molecules important to T cell function such as CD4, CD8 and the T cell receptor develop at different stages during the differentiation process (*Fig. 1*). The main functions of the thymus as a primary lymphoid organ are: (a) To produce sufficient numbers (millions) of different T cells each express-

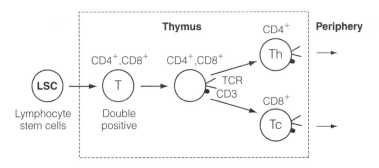

Fig. 1. *Development of CD4⁺ and CD8⁺ T cells in the thymus.*

ing unique T cell receptors such that, within this group, there are at least some cells potentially specific for the huge number of microbial antigens in our environment (generation of diversity); (b) To select for survival those T cells which bind weakly to self MHC molecules (positive selection), but then to eliminate those which bind too strongly to these same self MHC molecules (negative selection) so that the chance for an auto-immune response is minimized. This process is described in more detail in Sections H and M.

Although dependent on self antigens (MHC molecules), T cell development within the thymus is *independent* of exogenous (foreign) antigens. T cells which survive the selection process migrate to the peripheral lymphoid tissues where they complete their maturation and function to protect against invading microbes. Some extrathymic development of T cells may possibly occur as a result of differentiation of bone marrow precursors in mucosal tissues.

Generation of T cell diversity

Each of the very large numbers of T cells produced in the thymus has only one specificity, coded for by its antigen receptor. Millions of T cells, each with receptors specific for different antigens, are generated by gene rearrangement from multiple (inherited) germ-line genes. The T cell receptor consists of two polypeptide chains, α and β or γ and δ (*Fig. 2*). Each chain is a member of the immunoglobulin superfamily and thus has a uniform domain structure produced by intrachain disulfide bonding. Unlike most proteins produced in the body, each polypeptide chain of the T cell receptor is coded for by several different genes (Topic H3).

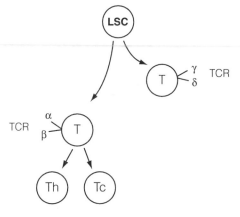

Fig. 2. *Development of αβ and γδ T cells. Two types of T cells are produced in the thymus with different TCRs (αβ and γδ): the classical T cells (Th and Tc) utilize αβ for their TCR.*

Positive and   Once produced in the thymus, T cells undergo selection using their newly
negative selection produced receptors. T cells with receptors which bind weakly to MHC molecules
are selected whilst those with receptors which bind strongly to MHC and self
antigens die through apoptosis (central tolerance to self) and are removed by
phagocytic macrophages (Topics H3 and M2).

E3 B CELLS ARE PRODUCED IN THE BONE MARROW

Key Notes

Overview

The microenvironment for HSC differentiation into B cells is provided within the fetal liver and after birth, the bone marrow. Germinal centers of the secondary lymphoid organs are also sites of B cell maturation. The main functions of the bone marrow as a primary lymphoid organ are to produce B cells with diverse antigen receptors (antibodies) and to eliminate B cells with antigen receptors that react with self. The early stages of B cell development (like that of T cells) is independent of exogenous antigen.

Generation of antigen receptor diversity

Antibodies are coded for by multiple genes which rearrange early in B cell development to create many different B cells each with a unique specificity of antigen receptor (antibody). These antigen receptors are expressed on the B cell surface and those B cells which bind self antigen are eliminated.

Development of immunoglobulin class diversity

IgM is the first antibody expressed on B cells followed by co-expression of IgD. These IgM/IgD expressing *mature* B cells may also express other classes of antibody, all having the same specificity, but this requires their activation by antigens and T cell help. The first antibodies to be produced and found in the fetal circulation and at birth are IgM antibodies followed by IgG and IgA.

Development of other functional B cell molecules

Molecules associated with B cell function also appear on the cell surface during differentiation. These include MHC class II and CD19.

Germinal centers as sites of B cell maturation

B cells in the peripheral lymphoid tissues are activated by antigen to proliferate and mature into either plasma cells or memory cells. Germinal centers are important in the generation of memory cells and the maturation of antibody affinity, due to hypermutation of variable region genes. This may result in modified receptors being expressed on the B cell surface which may bind with higher affinity than the original receptor and survive as memory cells.

Related topics

Lymphocytes (D1)
Antibody classes (F2)
Generation of diversity (F3)
B cell recognition of antigen, the
  B cell receptor complex and

co-receptors (H2)
Affinity maturation and class
  switching (J2)
Central tolerance (M2)

Overview

Birds have a specialized organ in which B cells develop (the Bursa of Fabricius) after which *B cells* were named. However, mammals do not have a discrete specialized organ for B cell development and the microenvironment for HSC differentiation is provided within the fetal liver and after birth, the bone marrow. B cells produce both cell surface and secreted antibodies; the former are their antigen receptors. Antibodies first appear in the cytoplasm of pre-B cells during early B cell differentiation and are then expressed on the cell surface where they function to bind antigen. Two main functions of the bone marrow as a primary lymphoid organ are to: (a) produce large numbers of B cells, each with unique antigen receptors (antibodies) such that, overall, there is sufficient B cell diversity to recognize the millions of microbial antigens in our environment (Generation of Diversity); (b) eliminate B cells with antigen receptors having high affinity for self molecules (negative selection: central tolerance). The early stages of B cell development (like that of T cells) is independent of exogenous antigens. Mature B cells leave the bone marrow and migrate via the blood stream to the secondary lymphoid organs/tissues where, following antigen stimulation, they become plasma cells and memory cells. The germinal centers of the secondary lymphoid organs and tissues are also sites of maturation of B cells.

Generation of antigen receptor diversity

Antibodies, like T cell receptors, are coded for by multiple genes (Topic F3) which rearrange during the pro-B cell stage (*Fig. 1*). Since rearrangement occurs in millions of different ways in these developing cells, many B cells, each with a different specificity, are generated. This generation of diversity occurs in the absence of foreign protein and thus yields large numbers of mature B cells, of which at least some have specificity for virtually any foreign substance or microbe. The first genes to rearrange code for the variable part of the H chain of the antibody molecule which together with the genes of the constant part of the molecule (and in particular genes which code for the μ H chain) are transcribed first in the differentiation process and appear in the cytoplasm. At this stage, the genes in these Pre-B cells which code for the variable region of the L chains rearrange. The transcribed H and L chains combine, giving rise to a functional IgM antigen receptor which is then expressed on the surface of the cell (immature B cell). It is during this stage that B cells with high affinity for self antigens are induced to die by apoptosis (negative selection). As in the thymus, the majority of the B cells die during development from production of antigen receptors which cannot be assembled or those directed against self antigens.

Development of immunoglobulin class diversity

IgM is the first antibody expressed on a B cell and is initially its antigen receptor. Another class of antibody, IgD, with the same antigen specificity is then expressed on the B cell surface. The variable regions of the IgD and IgM antibodies on the same cell are identical. The function of the IgD is probably that of regulating B cell function when it encounters antigen (Topic N2). Some B cells, in addition to IgM and IgD, may also express other classes of antibody including IgA, IgG or IgE, but all antibodies produced by the same B cell have the same specificity for antigen regardless of their class. The expression of these other classes of antigen receptor generally requires their activation by antigens and the involvement of T cells and cytokines (*Fig. 2*). The generation of class diversity is achieved through movement (translocation) of variable region genes next to the different heavy chain constant region genes. The first antibodies to be produced and found in the fetal circulation and at birth, are IgM antibodies, followed after birth by IgG and IgA antibodies (see Topic G5, *Fig. 1*).

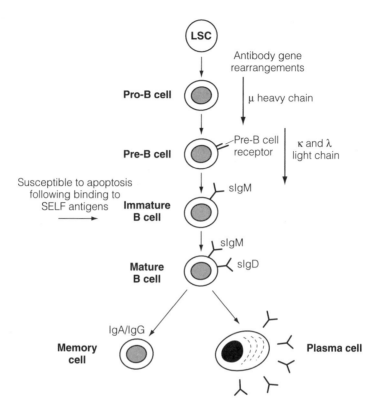

Fig. 1.　*Life history of a B cell. Lymphoid stem cells (LSC) develop into pro-B cells which begin to re-arrange their μ H chain V genes. During the pre-B cell stage the H chain peptide assembles with surrogate L chain (sLch) to form the pre-B cell receptor. This is thought to stimulate further development of the B cell. During this time, κ or λ L chain V genes rearrange with one class of L chain being transcribed and translated into protein. This appears with the μ chain on the cell surface of the immature B cell as IgM, the cell's antigen receptor. This B cell is susceptible to apoptosis/anergy on contact with self-antigen. Mature B cells acquire surface IgD in addition to IgM and migrate to the secondary lymphoid organs where they respond to foreign antigens by proliferation and development into memory and plasma cells.*

Development of other functional B cell molecules

Molecules associated with the B cell receptor complex are expressed early in development to enable assembly of a functional antigen receptor on the B cell surface (Topic H2). Other molecules important for B cell functions, including their ability to present antigen, e.g. MHC class II molecules, also develop early in the life of a B cell.

Germinal centers as sites of B cell maturation

Germinal centers are unique structures within the secondary lymphoid tissues where two important processes in B cell development occur – the generation of memory cells and the maturation of antibody affinity (*Fig. 3*). Primary B cell follicles in secondary lymphoid tissues, e.g. lymph nodes and spleen, are made up of aggregates of B cells. When B cells in the primary follicle are stimulated by antigen and also receive T cell help (Topic J1), they proliferate, associate with dendritic cells in the follicle (FDC), and begin to form the germinal center. These B cells begin to lose their surface IgM and IgD, and switch to IgG or to IgA (usually in mucosal tissues). During this time, there is hypermutation of the variable region genes, and receptors with slightly different amino acid sequences appear on the surface of these B cells (Topic J2). Many of these modified receptors are unable to bind the same antigen that triggered them and will not be restimulated by this antigen. However, some will be able to bind more strongly to this same antigen, which is often found bound to the surface of the FDC in the form of

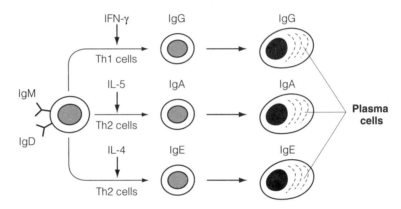

Fig. 2.   Generation of antibody class diversity.

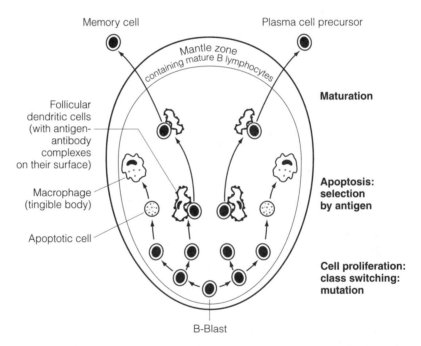

Fig. 3.   B cell maturation in the germinal center. One or two B cells, stimulated in a primary follicle, begin to proliferate and initiate germinal center formation. The B cells undergo class switching and mutation of their antibody V genes. B cells with receptors for antigen on follicular dendritic cells (bound in the form of antigen/antibody complexes) are selected to proceed through maturation, those not binding through their mutated V gene products die by apoptosis and are taken up by tingible body macrophages. T cells in the germinal center probably help B cells which have taken up and processed antigen. B cells leave the germinal center either as memory cells or plasma cell precursors which either mature locally into plasma cells or leave via the blood stream to mature in the bone marrow, lymph nodes, spleen or mucosal tissue dependent on the Ig class of the plasma cell precursor cell.

antibody/antigen complexes. Thus, B cells with higher affinity receptors for the antigen are selected, survive, proliferate and some mature into memory cells which stay in the mantle of the germinal center or join the recirculating lymphocyte pool. Others mature into plasma cells each of which can only synthesize and secrete one class of specific antibody (Topic D1).

E4 IMMUNITY IN THE NEWBORN

Key Notes

Lymphocytes in the newborn

Slightly higher than normal numbers of T and B lymphocytes are present in the blood of newborns and many are fully functional, but their ability to mount an immune response to certain antigens (e.g. polysaccharides of pneumococcus) may be deficient. This sequential appearance of specific immunity may be due to immaturity of B cells, of T helper cells, or of antigen presenting cells, to the sequential expression of genes coding for receptors for each antigen, and/or to the passive immunity (IgG or IgA) acquired from the mother.

Antibodies in the newborn

Maternal IgG crosses the placenta (mediated by Fc receptors) and is present in high levels at birth. IgG is not synthesized *de novo* until birth and IgA not for 1–2 months after birth, whereas IgM is produced during fetal development. Maternal IgA obtained by the infant from colostrum and milk during nursing, coats the infant's gastrointestinal tract and supplies passive mucosal immunity.

Related topics   The role of antigen (N2)   Primary/congenital (inherited)
                                                         immunodeficiency (S2)

Lymphocytes in the newborn

Slightly higher than normal numbers of apparently mature T and B lymphocyte populations (as well as NK cells) are present in the blood of newborn individuals. Even so, the ability to mount an immune response to certain antigens may be lacking. Thus, children under 2 years do not usually make antibody to the polysaccharides of pneumococcus or *Haemophilus influenzae*. In general, the ability to respond to a specific antigen depends on the age at which the individual is exposed to the antigen. There are a variety of explanations for this sequential appearance of specific immunity, including: (a) Sequential expression of genes coding for receptors for each antigen; (b) Immaturity of B or helper T cell populations; (c) Requirement for further maturation of antigen presenting cells (e.g. macrophages).

Since hemophilus polysaccharide conjugated to tetanus toxoid evokes protective anti-polysaccharide antibodies during the first year of life, the neonatal deficiency is likely to be in the Th cell population. Delayed maturation of the CD4$^+$ Th population may contribute to the generally low levels of IgG leading to immunodeficiency in transient hypogammaglobulinemia (Topic S2).

Antibodies in the newborn

Normally, IgG crosses the placenta (mediated by Fc receptors) and is present in high levels at birth. IgM is produced during fetal development but IgG is not synthesized *de novo*, until birth (*Fig. 1*). IgA begins to appear in the blood stream at 1–2 months of age. This partly compensates for the deficiencies in the ability of the infant to initially synthesize antibody through an immature immune system. Furthermore, maternal IgA obtained by the infant from colostrum and milk during nursing coats the infant's gastrointestinal tract and supplies passive mucosal immunity. Unresponsiveness to certain antigens may be related to this passive immunity acquired from the mother since until maternal antibodies are degraded or used up, they may bind antigen and remove it, thereby interfering with development of active immunity (Topic N2).

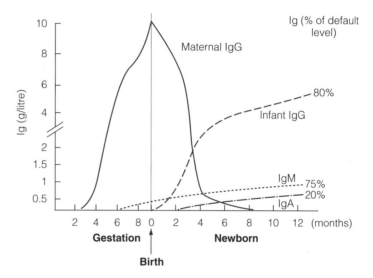

Fig. 1.   *Maternal IgG is actively transported across the placenta and accumulates in the baby's blood until birth. This protective IgG then decreases due to catabolism and disappears completely by about 6–8 months of age. De novo synthesis of IgM by the baby occurs first at 6–8 months of gestation and this is followed around birth by IgG and later IgA. At one year of age, the levels of the baby's IgG, IgM and IgA are about 80, 75 and 20% of adult levels respectively.*

F1 BASIC STRUCTURE

Key Notes

Molecular components

Antibodies, often termed 'immunoglobulins', are glycoproteins that bind antigens with high specificity and affinity. In humans there are five chemically and physically distinct classes of antibodies (IgG, IgA, IgM, IgD, IgE).

Antibody units

Antibodies have a basic unit of four polypeptide chains – two identical pairs of light (L) chains and heavy (H) chains – bound together by covalent disulfide bridges as well as by noncovalent interactions. These molecules can be proteolytically cleaved to yield two Fab fragments (the antigen binding part of the molecules) and an Fc fragment (the part of the molecule responsible for effector functions, e.g. complement activation). Both H- and L-chains are divided into V and C regions – the V regions containing the antigen binding site and the C region determining the fate of the antigen.

Affinity

Affinity is the tightness of binding of an antibody binding site to an antigenic determinant – the tighter the binding, the less likely the antibody is to dissociate from antigen. Different antibodies to an antigenic determinant vary considerably in their affinity for that determinant. Antibodies produced by a memory response have higher affinity than those in a primary response.

Antibody valence and avidity

The valence of an antibody is the number of antigenic determinants with which it can react. Having multiple binding sites for an antigen dramatically increases its binding (avidity) to antigens on particles such as bacteria or virus. For example, two binding sites on IgG are 100 times more effective at neutralizing virus than two unlinked binding sites.

Related topics

Antibody classes (F2)
B cell recognition of antigen, the
  B cell receptor complex and

co-receptors (H2)
Affinity maturation and class
  switching (J2)

Molecular components

Antibodies are glycoproteins that bind antigens with high specificity and affinity (they hold on tightly). They are molecules, originally identified in the serum, which are also referred to as 'immunoglobulins,' a term often used interchangeably with antibodies. In humans there are five chemically and physically distinct classes of antibodies (IgG, IgA, IgM, IgD, IgE).

Antibody units

All antibodies have the same basic four polypeptide chain unit: two light (L) chains and two heavy (H) chains (*Fig. 1*). In this basic unit, one L-chain is bound, by disulfide bridges and noncovalent interactions, to one H-chain. Similarly, the two H-chains are bound together by covalent disulfide bridges as well as by noncovalent hydrophilic and hydrophobic interactions. There are five different

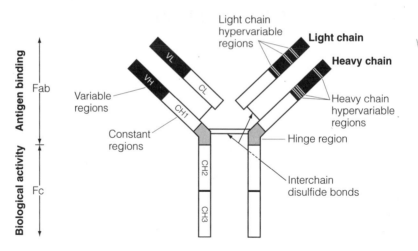

Fig. 1. IgG immunoglobulin: basic 4 chain structure representative of all immunoglobulins.

kinds of H-chains (referred to as μ, δ, γ, ε and α chains), which determine the class of antibody (IgM, IgD, IgG, IgE and IgA, respectively). There are also two different kinds of L-chains – κ and λ, each with a MW of 23 kD. Each antibody unit can have only κ or λ L-chains but not both. The properties of the different antibody classes are shown in *Table 1*.

Both H- and L-chains have intrachain disulfide bridges every 90 amino acid residues, which create polypeptide loops, domains, of 110 amino acids. These domains are referred to as VH, VL, CH1, CH2, etc. (*Fig. 1*) and have particular functional properties (e.g. VH and VL together form the binding site for antigen). This type of structure is characteristic of many other molecules, which are thus said to belong to the *Immunoglobulin gene superfamily*.

The N terminal half of the H-chain and all of the L-chain together make up what is called an Fab fragment (*Fig. 1*) and contains the antigen binding site. The actual binding site of the antibody is composed of the N-terminal quarter of the H-chain combined with the N terminal half of the L-chain. The amino acid sequence of these regions differ from one antibody to another and are thus called variable (V) regions and contain the amino acid residues involved in binding an antigenic determinant. Most of the antibody molecule (the C terminal three-quarters of the

Table 1. Properties of the human immunoglobulins

	IgG	IgA	IgM	IgD	IgE
Physical properties					
Molecular weight, kD	150	170–420	900	180	190
H-chain MW, kD	50–55	62	65	70	75
Physiologic properties					
Normal adult serum (mg/ml)	8–16	1.4–4.0	0.4–2.0	0.03	ngs
Half-life in days	23	6	5	3	<3
Biologic properties					
Complement-fixing capacity	+	–	++++	–	–
Anaphylactic hypersensitivity	–	–	–	–	++++
Placental transport to fetus	+	–	–	–	–

There are four IgG (IgG1, IgG2, IgG3, IgG4), two IgA subclasses and two L chain types (κ and λ).

H-chain and the C terminal half of the L-chain) are constant (C) regions of the antibody molecule and are the same for all antibodies of the same class and subclass. These C regions do not bind antigen, but rather determine the fate of antigen bound by the antigen binding site. In particular, the C terminal half of the H-chain, the Fc region (**F**ragment that **c**rystallized), serves others functions, i.e., combines with complement, is cytophilic (binds to certain types of cells, such as macrophages), etc. Carbohydrates are also present on antibodies, primarily on the Fc portion of H-chains.

Affinity

Different antibody molecules produced in response to a particular antigenic determinant may vary considerably in their tightness of binding to that determinant (i.e., in their **affinity** for the antigenic determinant). The higher the binding constant the less likely the antibody is to dissociate from the antigen. Clearly, the affinity of an antibody population is critical when the antigen is a toxin or virus and must be neutralized by rapid and firm combination with antibody. Antibodies formed soon after the injection of an antigen are generally of lower affinity for that antigen whereas antibodies produced later have dramatically greater affinities (association constants 1000 times higher).

Antibody valence and avidity

The valence of an antibody is the maximum number of antigenic determinants with which it can react. For example, IgG antibodies contain two Fab regions and can bind two molecules of antigen or two identical sites on the same particle, and thus have a valence of two. Valence is important for binding affinity, as having two or more binding sites for an antigen can dramatically increase the tightness of binding of the antibody to antigens on a bacteria or virus. This combined effect, avidity, results from synergy of the binding strengths of each binding site. Avidity is the firmness of association between a multideterminant antigen and the antibodies produced against it.

Determining the avidity of an antibody population is very difficult since it involves evaluating some function of the group interactions of a large number of different antibodies, with a large number of different antigenic determinants.

	Fab	IgG	IgM
Binding sites	1	2	up to 10
Relative binding avidity	1	100	1 000 000

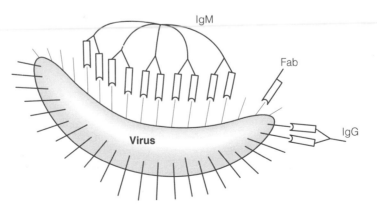

Fig. 2. Avidity and antibody valence in viral neutralization.

Even so, the importance of avidity can be demonstrated both mathematically and biologically. For example, as a result of working together (being on the same molecule) two IgG binding sites are 10–100 fold more effective at neutralizing a virus than two unassociated binding sites, and if the antibody has more binding sites, as in the case of IgM (Topic F2), it may be a million times more effective (*Fig. 2*). This can be visualized by considering antibodies with one or two binding sites for a particular antigenic determinant on a microorganism. The antibody with one site can bind to, but can also dissociate from, a determinant on the organism. When it comes off, it can diffuse away. However, the antibody with two sites can bind two identical determinants on the organism (each organism has many copies of each protein or carbohydrate). If one binding site dissociates, the other is probably still attached and permits the first site to reform its association with the organism. It therefore follows that the larger the number of binding sites per antibody molecule, the larger the number of bonds formed with an organism, and the less likely it will be to dissociate. Thus, an antibody with a poor intrinsic affinity for an antigenic determinant can, as a result of a large number of combining sites per molecule, be extremely effective in neutralizing a virus or complexing with a microorganism.

F2 ANTIBODY CLASSES

Key Notes

Functional diversity

Different antibody classes with different biological activities have evolved to deal with antigens (e.g. microbes) with different properties and which enter the body at different sites – through the skin, the gastrointestinal or the genitourinary tracts.

IgG

IgG immunoglobulins, of which there are four different subclasses (IgG1, IgG2, IgG3, IgG4) provide the bulk of immunity to most blood borne infectious agents, and are the only antibody class to cross the placenta to provide humoral immunity to the infant.

IgA

IgA is a first line of defense against microbes entering through mucosal surfaces (the respiratory, gastrointestinal and genitourinary tracts). Secretory (dimeric) IgA is synthesized locally by plasma cells, binds to the poly-Ig receptor on epithelial cells and is transported through these cells to the lumenal surface where it is released with a portion of the poly-Ig receptor (secretory component, SC). This antibody prevents colonization of mucosal surfaces by pathogens and mediates their phagocytosis.

IgM

IgM is an antigen receptor on B cells and the first antibody produced in an immune response. In the circulation, IgM is composed of five four-chain units with 10 combining sites. It thus has high avidity for antigens and is very efficient per molecule in dealing with pathogens especially early in the immune response before sufficient quantities of IgG have been produced.

IgD

This immunoglobulin functions primarily as an antigen receptor on B cells.

IgE

Allergic reactions are predominantly associated with IgE. Antigen reintroduced into a previously sensitized individual binds to antigen specific IgE on 'armed' mast cells and triggers release of the pharmacologically active agents (e.g., histamine) involved in immediate hypersensitivity syndromes such as hay fever and asthma.

Related topics

Mucosa-associated lymphoid
   tissues (D3)
Immunity in the newborn (E4)

Antibody responses in different
   tissues (J3)
IgE-mediated type 1
   hypersensitivity: allergy (T2)

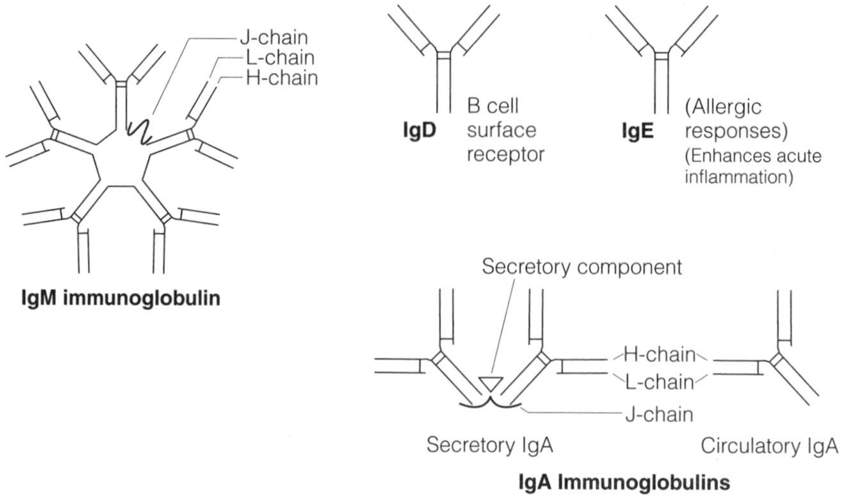

Fig. 1.   Chain structures of different classes of immunoglobulins.

Functional diversity

Different antigens, in particular microbes, have different biological properties and can enter the body through different routes (the skin, the gastrointestinal tract, the respiratory tract or the genitourinary tract). It is likely that the five different antibody classes (IgM, IgD, IgG, IgE and IgA; *Fig. 1*) and their subclasses have evolved at least partly to facilitate protection against microbes entering at the different sites and with different properties. There is some overlap in their function and in where they are produced, but generally there is a division of labor among the different antibody classes, e.g. IgA is the most common antibody in mucosal secretions while IgM is mainly found in the plasma, and both are most effective at those locations.

IgG

Immunoglobulins of the IgG class have a MW of 150 kD and are found both in vascular and extravascular spaces as well as in secretions. IgG is the most abundant immunoglobulin in the blood (Section F1, *Table 1*), provides the bulk of immunity to most blood borne infectious agents and is the only antibody class to cross the placenta to provide passive humoral immunity to the developing fetus and thus to the infant on its birth. IgG has two H-chains (referred to as γ chains) with either two κ or two λ L-chains. Furthermore, there are four different subclasses of IgG (designated IgG1, IgG2, IgG3, IgG4) which have slightly different sequences in their H-chains and corresponding differences in their functional activities.

IgA

This immunoglobulin is present in the serum as a 170 kD, four polypeptide (two L and two H) chain protein. More important, it is the major immunoglobulin present in external secretions such as colostrum, milk, and saliva where it exists as a 420 kD dimer (*Fig. 1*). In addition to the κ or λ L-chains and the IgA heavy chain (designated α), which distinguishes it from IgG or other antibody classes, secreted IgA also contains two other polypeptide chains – secretory component (SC) and J-chain (joining chain). SC is part of the molecule (poly-Ig receptor) involved in the transepithelial transport of exocrine IgA and stabilizes IgA against proteolytic degradation. The two four-chain units composing secretory IgA are held together by the J-chain through disulfide bridges. Most IgA is synthesized locally by plasma cells in mammary and salivary glands, and along the respiratory, gastrointestinal and genitourinary tracts (Topic J3). It is then transported through epithelial cells to the lumen. This antibody is a first line of defense against microbial invaders at mucosal surfaces.

IgM

IgM is the first antibody produced by, and expressed on the surface of, a B cell. It acts as an antigen receptor for these cells, and is also present as a soluble molecule in the blood. On the B cell surface this molecule is expressed as a four-chain unit – two μ H-chains and two L-chains (Topic H2). In the blood, IgM is composed of five four-chain units held together by disulfide bridges at the carboxy-terminal end of the μ chains (*Fig. 1*). J-chain is also associated with IgM in the blood and initiates the polymerization of its subunits at the time of its secretion from a plasma cell. Because of its size (900 kD), IgM is found primarily in the intravascular space. As IgM is the first antibody produced in an immune response, its efficiency in combining with antigen is of particular importance until sufficient quantities of IgG antibody have been synthesized. Although IgM antibodies usually have low affinity binding sites for antigen, they have 10 combining sites per molecule which can synergize with each other on the same molecule when it binds to a microbe. Thus, the overall tightness of binding of an IgM molecule (avidity) to a microbe is quite high, making antibodies of this class very effective in removal of the microbe.

IgD

IgD is present in low quantities in the circulation (0.3 mg/ml in adult serum). Its primary function is that of an antigen receptor on B lymphocytes (*Fig. 1*). B cells thus can express both IgM and IgD and both are specific for the same antigen. When IgM and IgD expressed on a B cell interact with an antigen for which they are specific, the antigen is internalized, and processed and presented to helper T cells which trigger the B cells to proliferate and differentiate into plasma cells, thus initiating the development of a humoral immune response.

IgE

IgE is present in the serum at very low levels (nanograms per milliliter), but plays a significant role in enhancing acute inflammation, in protection from infection by worms, and in allergic reactions (Topics I1, T2, O2). Antibody mediated allergy is predominantly associated with IgE. After stimulation of the development of IgE producing plasma cells by an antigen, the IgE produced binds to receptors on mast cells which are specific for the Fc region of IgE. When antigen is *reintroduced* into an individual with such 'armed' mast cells, it binds to the antigen binding site of the IgE molecule on the mast cell, and as a result of this interaction, the mast cell is triggered to release pharmacologically active agents (e.g., histamine). IgE antibodies are thus important components of immediate hypersensitivity syndromes such as hay fever and asthma (Topic T2, *Fig. 1*).

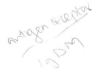

F3 GENERATION OF DIVERSITY

Key Notes

Antibody genes

The DNA encoding immunoglobulins is found in three unlinked gene groups – one group encodes κ L-chains, one λ L-chains, and one H-chains. Each L-chain gene group has multiple different copies of V gene segments and J gene segments. In addition, in the κ chain group there is one gene segment encoding the constant region of κ chains, while in the λ group there are four λ chain C region gene segments. The H-chain gene group has multiple different copies of V, D and J gene segments and one gene segment for each of the constant regions for the different antibody classes and subclasses.

Gene rearrangement

During its development, a single B cell randomly selects from its H-chain gene group, one V, one D and one J gene segment for rearrangement (translocation). It then selects from the κ or λ gene group one V and one J gene segment for translocation. These gene segments then recombine to create a gene (VJ) encoding a binding site for an L chain and a gene (VDJ) encoding a binding site for an H-chain.

Allelic exclusion

After successful rearrangement of the Ig DNA segments, the cell is committed to the expression of a particular V region for its H-chain and a particular V region for its L-chain and there is active suppression, allelic exclusion, of other H- and L-chain V region rearrangements. Each B cell and all of its progeny will therefore express and produce antibodies, all of which have exactly the same specificity.

Synthesis and assembly of chains

After successful rearrangement of L- and H-chain DNA, primary L- and H-chain mRNAs are transcribed and the RNA between the newly constructed V region gene and the constant region gene spliced out. After translation, the L and H polypeptide chains combine in the ER to form an antibody molecule, which then becomes the antigen specific receptor for that B cell. In plasma cells, the part of the mRNA encoding the H-chain transmembrane domain, which is important for its membrane expression on B cells, is spliced out and the antibody produced is secreted.

Differential splicing and class switching

A mature B cell expresses both IgM and IgD with the same specificity. This results from differential cleavage and splicing of the primary transcript to yield two mRNAs – one for an IgM H-chain and the other for an IgD H-chain – both of which are translated and expressed on the B cell surface with L-chain. Properly stimulated, a B cell can undergo class switching that involves translocation of the VDJ gene segment next to another C region gene with the loss of intervening DNA. The primary transcript is then spliced to give an mRNA for the new H-chain.

Ways of creating diversity	Antibody diversity, i.e. the generation of antibodies with different specificities, is created at the DNA level by multiple germ line V, D and J, and V and J genes, by their random combination, by imprecise joining, and by subsequent somatic mutations in the resulting V regions. At the protein level, diversity is created by random selection and pairing of L- and H-chains.
Antigen selection of B cells for stimulation	During an immune response, the overall affinity of antibodies for an antigen increases with time. This is partly a result of the fact that B cells expressing higher affinity antibody compete more successfully for antigen and contribute a higher proportion to the antibody pool. In addition, mutations in VH and VL genes of activated B cells generate higher affinity antibodies (affinity maturation) allowing these cells to compete most successfully for antigen, clonally expand and contribute to the antibody pool.
Related topics	B cells are produced in the bone marrow (E3) The cellular basis of the antibody response (J1) B cell recognition of antigen, the B cell receptor complex and co-receptors (H2) Affinity maturation and class switching (J2)

Antibody genes

There are three unlinked gene groups encoding immunoglobulins – one for κ chains, one for λ chains and one for H-chains, each on a different chromosome (*Table 1*). Within each of these gene groups on the chromosome there are multiple coding regions (**exons**) which recombine at the level of DNA to yield a binding site. In a mature B cell or plasma cell, the DNA encoding the V region for the H-chain of a specific antibody, consists of a continuous uninterrupted nucleotide sequence. In contrast, the DNA in a germ line cell (or non B cell) for this V region exists in distinct DNA segments, exons, separated from each other by regions of noncoding DNA (*Fig. 1*). The exons found in the area encoding the V region of the H-chain are: V segment (encoding approximately the first 102 amino acids), D segment (encoding 2–4 amino acids), and J segment (encoding the remaining 14 or so amino acids in the V region). For L-chains there are only V (encoding the first approximately 95 amino acids) and J segment (encoding the remaining 13 or so amino acids) exons. In each gene group, there are from 30–65 functional V segment genes. The D and J regions are between the V and C regions on the chromosome and there are multiple different genes for each. Thus, DNA segments that ultimately encode the binding site of antibodies have to be moved over distances (translocated) on the chromosome to form a DNA sequence encoding the V region.

The DNA sequences encoding the C region of the L- and H-chains are 3' to the V genes, but separated from them by unused J segment genes and noncoding DNA. Furthermore, each gene group usually has one functional gene segment for each class and subclass. Thus, the H-chain gene group has nine functional C region genes, one each encoding μ, δ, γ1, γ2, γ3, γ4, ε, α1, α2. For the L-chain gene groups, there is one gene segment encoding the C region of κ L-chains, but for encoding λ L-chain C regions.

Table 1.   Genes for human immunoglobulins

Ig polypeptide	Chromosome
H-chain	14
κ-chain	2
λ-chain	22

Gene rearrangement

During its development, a single B cell randomly selects one V, one D and one J (for H-chains), and one V and one J (for L-chains) for rearrangement (transloca-tion). Gene segments encoding a portion of the V region are moved adjacent to other gene segments encoding the rest of the V region to create a gene segment encoding the entire V region, with the intervening DNA removed. More specifi-cally, the H-chain gene group is the first to rearrange, initially moving one of sev-eral D segment genes adjacent to one of several J segment genes. This creates a DJ combination, which encodes the C terminal part of the H-chain V region. A V seg-ment gene then rearranges to become contiguous with the DJ segment, creating a DNA sequence (VDJ) encoding a complete H-chain V region (*Fig. 1*). This VDJ combination is 5' to the group of H-chain C region genes, of which the closest one encodes the μ chain. A primary mRNA transcript is then made from VDJ through the μ C region gene, after which the intervening message between VDJ and the μ C region gene is spliced out to create an mRNA for a complete μ H-chain.

After the H-chain has successfully completed its rearrangement, one of the V region gene segments in either the λ or κ gene groups (but not both) translocates next to a J segment gene to create a gene (VJ) encoding a complete L-chain V region (*Fig. 2*). For κ chains, the DNA sequences encoding the C region of the L-chains are 3' to the V genes, but separated from them by unused J segment genes and noncoding DNA (*Fig. 2(a)*). For λ chains, since the J segment genes are each associated with a different Cλ gene, translocation of a V gene segment to a J gene segment results in a V region next to a particular Cλ gene (e.g. Cλ2 as shown in *Fig. 2(b)*). It is important to repeat that in each B cell, only one of two L-chain gene groups will be used. A primary mRNA transcript is then made from VJ

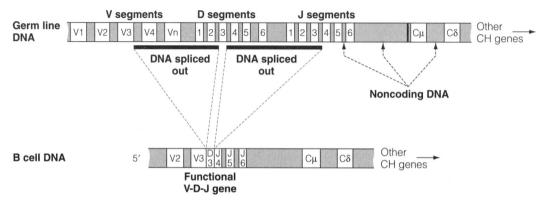

Fig. 1.   *H-chain genes and translocation. In the germ line, and therefore in a cell destined to become a B cell, the H-chain gene loci contains many V segment genes. In a developing B cell, one of these V segments recombines with one of many D segments, which has already recombined with one of several J segments, to produce a functional VDJ gene. In each B cell, the rearranged gene is transcribed, spliced and translated into an H-chain protein.*

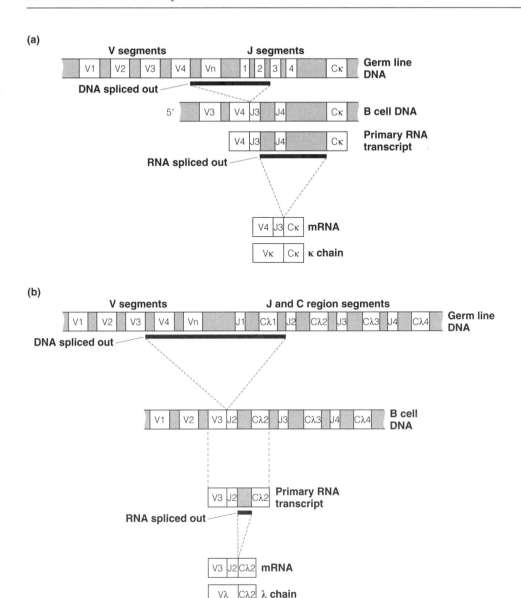

Fig. 2. L-chain genes and translocation. During differentiation of a B cell, and after rearrangement of the H-chain genes, one of the two L-chain groups rearrange. In particular, either (a) a germ line Vκ gene combines with a J segment gene to form a VJ combination; or (b) a germ line Vλ gene combines with one of the J segment Cλ gene combinations to form a VJ Cλ combination. The rearranged gene is then transcribed into a primary RNA transcript which then has the intervening noncoding sequences spliced out to form mRNA. This is then translated into light chain protein.

through the L-chain C region gene, after which the intervening message between VJ and the C region gene is spliced out to create an mRNA for a complete L-chain.

Gene rearrangement in B cells requires the products of two recombination-activating genes, RAG-1 and RAG -2, which appear to be only expressed together in developing lymphocytes. These enzymes break and rejoin the DNA during translocation and are thus critical to the generation of diversity.

Allelic exclusion   After successful rearrangement of the Ig DNA segments, the cell is committed to the expression of a particular V region for its H-chain and a particular V region for its L-chain and *excludes* other H- and L-chain V region rearrangements. This process is referred to as **allelic exclusion** and is unique to B and T cell antigen receptors. If an aberrant rearrangement occurs on the first chromosome the process will continue, i.e., the process does not stop if the cell does not get it right the first time. The process stops, however, if the cell gets it right or runs out of chromosomes to rearrange. In fact, following successful VH gene rearrangement on one chromosome there is active suppression of further rearrangement of the other VH gene segments. Similarly, following successful VL gene rearrangement there is active suppression of further rearrangement of other V and J gene segments.

Thus, each B cell makes L-chains all of which contain a V region encoded by the same VJ region sequence and H-chains all of which contain a V region encoded by the same VDJ sequence. Each B cell will therefore express antibodies on its surface, all of which have exactly the same specificity. This cell and all of its progeny are committed to express and produce antibodies with these V regions.

Synthesis and assembly of H and L chains   After successful rearrangement of both L- and H-chain DNA, L- and H-chain mRNA is produced and translated into L- and H-polypeptide chains that combine in the ER to form an antibody molecule, which is transported to the plasma membrane as the antigen specific receptor for that B cell. Since the gene encoding the

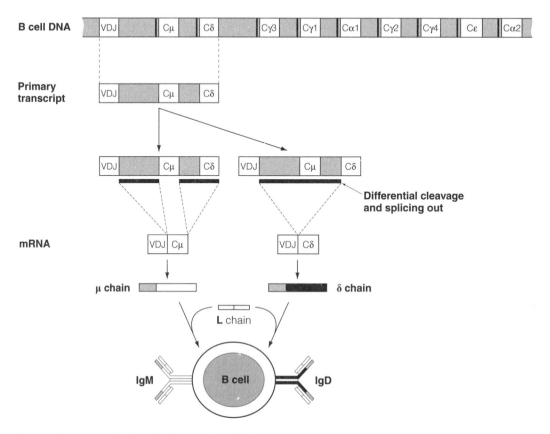

Fig. 3. Expression of IgM and IgD on a mature B cell.

H-chain also contains coding sequences for a transmembrane domain, the H-chain produced contains a C terminal amino acid sequence which anchors the antibody in the plasma membrane. In plasma cells, the part of the mRNA encoding the H-chain transmembrane domain important for its membrane expression on B cells is spliced out. Thus, the antibody produced by a plasma cell does not become associated with the membrane, but rather is secreted.

Differential splicing and class switching

As indicated above, the first antibody produced by a B cell is of the IgM class. Soon thereafter the B cell produces both an IgM and an IgD antibody, each having the same V regions and thus the same specificity. This is the result of the differential cleavage and splicing of the primary transcript. In particular, a primary transcript is made which includes information from the VDJ region through the Cδ region (*Fig. 3*). This transcript is differentially spliced to yield two mRNAs – one for an IgM H-chain and the other for an IgD H-chain. In a mature B cell both are translated and expressed on the B cell surface with L-chain.

B cells expressing IgM and IgD on their surface are capable of switching to other H-chain classes. This isotype (class) switching requires stimulation of the B cell by T cells and cytokines. These signals induce translocation of VDJ and its insertion 5′ to another constant region gene (*Fig. 4*). Class switch is guided by repetitive DNA sequences 5′ to the C region genes and occurs when these **switch regions** recombine. The intervening DNA is cut out and the resulting DNA in the B cell which has class switched, and in plasma cells derived from this B cell, no longer contains Cμ, Cδ or other intervening H-chain C region genes. A primary transcript

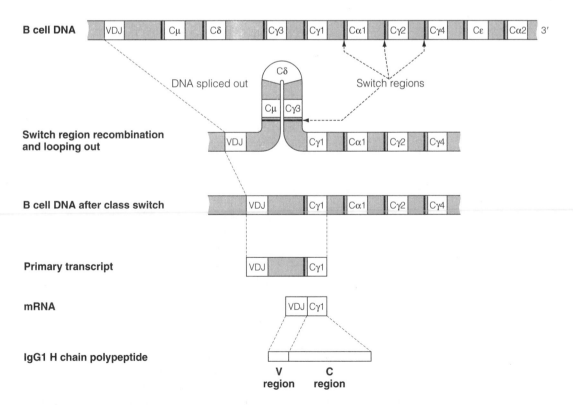

Fig. 4.   Class switching.

is made and the RNA between the VDJ coding region and the new H-chain coding region is spliced out to give an mRNA for the new H-chain.

Ways of creating diversity

Ig diversity (the generation of antibodies with different specificities) is created by several antigen independent mechanisms. In addition, in B cells that have been stimulated by antigen and received T cell help, Ig genes undergo mutational events that may increase the affinity of the antibody produced by the B cell. Overall, diversity is generated by:

Antigen independent events

- at the DNA level as a result of multiple germ line V, D and J and V and J genes,
- at the DNA level as a result of random combination of V, D and J segments or V and J segments,
- at the DNA level as a result of imprecise joining of V, D and J segments,
- at the protein level as a result of random selection and pairing of different combinations of L- and H-chain V regions in different B cells.

Antigen dependent events

- at the DNA level as a result of somatic mutation in the V region, which may create higher affinity antibody binding sites.

Although rearrangement of the gene segments that will make up the V region genes occurs in an ordered fashion, they are chosen at random in each B cell. As these events occur in a vast number of cells, the result is that millions of B cells, each with a different antigen specificity, are generated. Additional diversity is created during recombination of V and J (L-chain) and V, D and J (H-chain) gene segments due to imprecise joining of the different gene segments making up the V region. That is, for example, although translocation of a V gene segment to a J gene segment could occur with all three nucleotides of the last codon of the V segment joining with all three nucleotides of the first codon of the J segment, it is also possible that one or two nucleotides at the 3' end of the V segment could replace the first one or two nucleotides of the J segment. Such a difference in the position at which recombination occurs can change the amino acid sequence in the antigen binding area of the resulting V region of the antibody, and thus change its specificity.

Furthermore, after antigen stimulation of the B cell, the DNA of its L- and H-chain V regions becomes particularly susceptible to somatic mutation. This results in changes in the nucleotides of the DNA and thus corresponding changes in the amino acid sequence of the V regions of the antibody expressed by the B cell. As a result, the B cell may have a different specificity and not bind to or be stimulated by the original antigen. However, it often happens that at least some mutations result in amino acid changes which increase the tightness of binding of the antibody on the B cell to its antigen. These B cells will compete more efficiently for antigen than the original B cell, and will differentiate into plasma cells producing a higher affinity antibody (**affinity maturation**).

Diversity is also generated as a result of the fact that any L-chain can interact with any H-chain to create a unique binding site. Thus, for example, an L-chain with a particular VJ combination for its binding site could be produced by many different B cells and interact with the different H-chains (i.e. different in their VH region) generated in each of these B cells to create many different specificities.

In sum, almost unlimited diversity is created from a limited number of V regions. The diversity almost certainly exceeds the amount of diversity needed to bind the immunogens of microbes. Moreover, the vast majority of the different B cells generated will never encounter antigen to which they can bind, and thus will not be stimulated to further development. And yet, such apparent wastefulness is justified by the fact that this mechanism of creation of diversity ensures that there are B cells and thus antibodies reactive with virtually all antigens that will be encountered. When an antigen to which this antibody binds is encountered, the B cell is triggered to divide and to give rise to a clone of cells, each one of which makes, at least initially, the originally displayed antibody molecule (clonal selection: Topics A3 and J1).

Antigen selection of B cells for stimulation

During an antibody response to an antigen, the overall affinity of the antibodies produced increases with time. This is partly because, as the B cell numbers increase during an immune response, antigen becomes limiting and there is competition for antigen among B cells. Those expressing higher affinity antibody compete more successfully for antigen and clonally expand, contributing a higher proportion to the antibody pool. Thus, the affinity of antibody produced in the secondary immune response is higher and thus more efficient at effector functions than that produced in the primary response.

In addition and of particular importance (see above), B cells already stimulated by antigen and T cells undergo somatic mutation in the V regions of their H and L genes, which results in affinity maturation – the generation of B cells expressing antibody with higher affinity for the antigen (see Topic J2). These B cells contribute significantly to the pool of antibodies in the circulation. Typical antibodies have binding constants of 10^{6-7} M^{-1}. After successive immunization with limiting antigen they are usually 10^{8-9} M^{-1} but may be as high as 10^{12} M^{-1}.

F4 ALLOTYPES AND IDIOTYPES

Key Notes

Allotypes	These are genetic markers on immunoglobulins (Ig) that segregate within the species. If Ig expressing a particular allotype is injected into an individual whose Igs do not express that allotype, an immune response will develop against the allotype. Like blood types, they are inherited in Mendelian fashion but are usually of no functional consequence.
Idiotypes	These are unique antigenic determinants associated with antigen binding sites of antibodies and are the result of the different amino acid sequences which determine their specificities.
Related topics	Other control mechanisms (N5) Transplantation antigens (Q2)

Allotypes

In addition to class and subclass categories, an immunoglobulin (Ig) can be defined by the presence of genetic markers termed allotypes. These markers are different in different individuals and are thus immunogenic when injected into individuals whose Ig lacks the allotype. Like the blood group antigens (ABO), they are determinants which segregate within a species (the Ig of some members of the species have them, others do not). Allotypes are normally the result of small amino acid differences in Ig L- or H-chains. For example, the Km (*Inv*) marker is an allotype of human κ L-chains and is the result of a leucine vs valine difference at position 191. The *Gm* markers are allotypes associated with the IgG H-chains. Allotypes are inherited in a strictly Mendelian fashion, and usually have no significance to the function of the antibody molecule.

Idiotypes

Antigenic determinants associated with the binding site of an antibody molecule are called idiotypes and are unique to all antibodies produced by the same clone of B cells. That is, although all antibodies have idiotypic determinants, these determinants are different for all antibodies not derived from the same clone of B cells. Thus, the number of different idiotypes in an individual is at least as numerous as the number of specificities. Antibodies are produced against these idiotypic determinants when they are injected into other animals. In fact, one's own idiotypes may be recognized by one's own immune system. That is, the amino acid sequence associated with the combining site of an antibody (the idiotype, D) is immunogenic even in the individual in which it is produced (*Fig. 1*). An immune response (IR) produced against this idiotype (anti-D) can eliminate the B cells producing the antibody with this idiotype and thus decrease the antibody response to the antigen which initially triggered production of this idiotype. Furthermore, an anti-idiotype IR (antibody or T cell mediated) expresses its own idiotype (call it E) which in turn can be recognized as foreign and an anti-

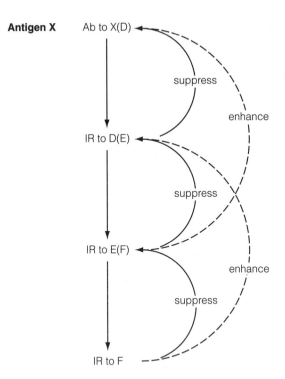

Fig. 1.   Idiotypes and anti-idiotypes. An antigen X initiates the production of antibodies reactive to X (with combining site = idiotype = D). This new antigen D is recognized as foreign and an immune response (IR) is produced against it (IR to D). The IR to D on cells suppresses production of D. However, the IR to D has its own idiotype = E which may be viewed as foreign, and to which an IR may be produced. Such an anti-E IR could suppress E production. In the absence of E, D would not be suppressed. Thus, an IR to E would have the effect of enhancing the production of antibodies to X (D).

idiotype IR made against this idiotype. Jerne (who shared the Nobel prize with Kohler and Milstein in 1984) described a *Network Theory* which proposes that a series of idiotype–anti-idiotype reactions are partially responsible for regulation of the immune response (Topic N5). *Fig. 1* diagrams the inter-relationships involved and the potential enhancing or suppressing effects of the various interactions.

F5 FUNCTIONS

Key Notes

Role of antibody alone	Antibody alone can neutralize viruses and toxins if it binds tightly to, and blocks, a part of the toxin or virus critical to its biological activity. Similarly, antibodies can inhibit microbes from colonizing mucosal areas and in some cases may induce programed cell death (apoptosis).
Role of antibody in complement activation	IgG or IgM antibodies can, on binding to antigen, activate the classical pathway of complement leading to lysis of the cell on which the antigen is located, and/or to attraction of immune cells (chemotaxis) which phagocytose the antigen expressing cells.
Role of antibody with effector cells	Phagocytes (PMNs and macrophages) have various receptors including those for complement component C3b, for the Fc region of IgG (FcγR) and for the Fc region of IgA (FcαR). These receptors enhance binding to, and phagocytosis or ADCC of, antibody and/or complement opsonized microbes. Binding of antigens (e.g. allergens) to IgE already bound to Fc receptors for IgE on mast cells results in degranulation and subsequent enhancement of the acute inflammatory response.
Related topics	Phagocytes (B1) Immunity to different organisms Complement (C2) (O2) The acute inflammatory response (I1)

Role of antibody alone

Antibody alone can, in some instances, neutralize, and thus protect against, viruses and toxins. However, its effectiveness depends greatly on the specificity and affinity of the antibody. That is, it must react with the part of the toxin or virus critical to its biological activity, and it must bind tightly enough to prevent interaction of the toxin or virus with the cell surface receptor through which it gains entry. Similarly, antibodies, primarily of the IgA class, can bind to bacteria and inhibit their attachment to mucosal epithelial cells. They can also cause their agglutination and thus prevent colonization of mucosal areas. In addition, antibodies specific for certain molecules on the surface of cells can induce programed cell death (apoptosis).

Role of antibody in complement activation

The ability of antibody to protect against infection is, in many instances, greatly enhanced by or dependent on the complement system. When an antibody of the IgG or IgM class (Topic F1, *Table 1*) attaches to an antigen, the classical pathway of complement is activated leading to complement mediated lysis of the microbe (or other cell) on which the antigen is located. In addition, complement activation can also lead to attraction of immune cells (chemotaxis), and to opsonization and phagocytosis of the cell on which complement is being activated (Topic C2).

Table 1.   Sequence of complement activation by the classical pathway leading to cell lysis.

T (target cell) + A (antibody) ────────▶	TA complex
TA + C1q,r,s ────────▶	TAC1
TAC1 + C4 ────────▶	TAC1,4b **+ C4a**
TAC1,4b + C2 ────────▶	TAC1,4b,2a **+ C2b**
TAC1,4b,2a + C3 ────────▶	TAC1,4b,2a,3b **+ C3a**
TAC1,4b,2a,3b + C5 ────────▶	TAC1,4b,2a,3b,5b **+ C5a**
TAC1,4b,2a,3b,5b + C6 + C7 ────────▶	TAC1,4b,2a,3b,5b,6,7
TAC1,4b,2a,3b,5b,6,7 + C8 ────────▶	TAC1,4b,2a,3b,5b,6,7,8
TAC1,4b,2a,3b,5b,6,7,8 + C9 ────────▶	TAC1,4b,2a,3b,5b,6,7,8,9 **Lysis of T**

T refers to target cell, A refers to antibody

The **classical** pathway of complement mediated cytotoxicity begins with the attachment of antibody (*IgM* or *IgG*) to antigens on the surface of the target cell. This pathway can also be activated by an Ag-Ab lattice, but of course this lattice would not be lysed.

Formation of a site to which the first component of complement (C1) can bind requires a single bound antibody of IgM, or two IgG molecules bound in close proximity to each other. The Clq component of the C1 complex (C1q, C1r, C1s) then binds to the Fc regions of the cell-bound antibodies (*Fig. 1*). This results in activation of C1 which then catalyzes the cleavage of C4 and C2, pieces of which (C4b and C2a) then bind to the cell surface forming a new cell-bound enzyme, C3 convertase (C4b+C2a). C3 convertase then cleaves C3 into C3a and C3b. C3b binds to the cell surface, forming a C4b, 2a, 3b complex which then governs the reaction and binding of the next complement components, C5, C6, C7, C8 and C9 to the cell surface (*Table 1*).

The sequence of activation of the C5–9 components (the membrane attack complex) is the same as that described for the alternative pathway (Topic C2), and leads to functional and structural damage to the membrane as a result of the formation of pores created by insertion of C9 complexes into the membrane.

The classical pathway has the same biological activities as the alternative

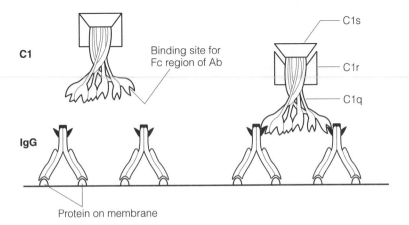

Fig. 1.   Initiation of complement activation by binding of C1 to antibody. The CH2 domains of the Fc regions of adjacent IgG molecules, bound to repeating antigenic determinants on a membrane, interact with the C1q subunit of C1. This results in the activation of C1r and C1s subunits, exposing an enzymatic active site.

pathway, including: (a) induction by C3a and C5a of mast cell degranulation and release of mediators; (b) stimulation by C3a and C5a of contraction of smooth muscle and increased vascular permeability; (c) directed migration (chemotaxis) of neutrophils by C5a; (d) enhancement of phagocytosis, opsonization, by C3b.

Role of antibody with effector cells

A variety of effector cells have receptors for the Fc region of antibodies. Phagocytes (PMNs, macrophages and eosinophils) utilize their Fc receptors (FcR) for IgG (FcγR) or IgA (FcαR) to enhance phagocytosis of antibody opsonized microbes. In addition, these FcR can mediate killing of cells through antibody dependent cellular cytotoxicity (ADCC). PMNs, monocytes, macrophages, eosinophils and NK cells can kill antibody coated target cells directly (*Fig. 2*). That is, in ADCC, lysis of the target cell does not require internalization (although that may also happen) and involves release of toxic molecules (e.g. TNFα, Topic G2) at the surface of the target.

Enhanced phagocytosis can also be mediated by phagocyte receptors for the complement component C3b, which is generated by antibody mediated activation of the complement sequence (classical pathway) or on activation by certain microbes of the alternative pathway of complement. Mast cells and basophils have FcR for IgE (FcεR), which on binding of IgE coated antigens or cells can trigger degranulation and subsequent enhancement of the acute inflammatory response. Over-stimulation of mast cells/basophils by this mechanism leads to pathology (Topic T2).

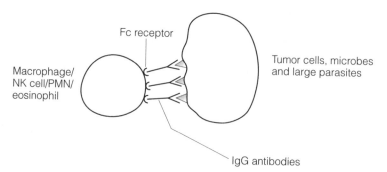

Fc receptor

Macrophage/
NK cell/PMN/
eosinophil

Tumor cells, microbes
and large parasites

IgG antibodies

Fig. 2. Antibody dependent cellular cytotoxicity (ADCC) of an antibody coated target cell. Several effector cell populations have Fc receptors (FcR) for IgG. Antibody coated microbes attach to macrophages or PMNs through these receptors, and their resulting crosslinking leads to release of toxic substances. This extracellular killing probably occurs prior to phagocytosis of opsonized microbes through FcR or complement receptors. This also occurs when the antibody coated target is too large to be phagocytosed, e.g. a worm. Eosinophils are particularly important in killing worms by this mechanism (Topic O2). Macrophages, PMNs, and eosinophils can also use IgA FcR for ADCC. NK cell mediated death of virus-infected cells and tumor cells can be enhanced through ADCC.

F6 MONOCLONAL ANTIBODIES

Key Notes

Monoclonal antibodies	Standardized procedures involving fusion of an immortal cell (a myeloma tumor cell) with a specific predetermined antibody-producing B cell have been used to create hybridoma cells producing monospecific and monoclonal antibodies (mAb). These mAb are standard research reagents and many have significant clinical utility.
Fv libraries	By randomly fusing H- and L-chain V region genes from B cells, Fv libraries containing a vast number of binding specificities can be generated and used as a source for creation of specific mAbs.

Related topics
Lymphocytes (D1)
Immunodiagnosis (P4)
Immunotherapy of tumors with
    antibodies (P6)

Monoclonal and recombinant
    antibodies (V5)

Monoclonal antibodies

In 1975, Kohler and Milstein developed a procedure to create cell lines producing predetermined, monospecific and monoclonal antibodies (mAb). This procedure has been standardized and applied on a massive scale to the preparation of antibodies useful to many research and clinical efforts. The basic technology involves fusion of an immortal cell (a myeloma tumor cell) with a specific predetermined antibody-producing B cell from immunized animals or humans. The resulting hybridoma cell is immortal and synthesizes homogeneous, specific, mAb which can be made in large quantities. MAbs have become standard research reagents and have extensive clinical applications (Section V5).

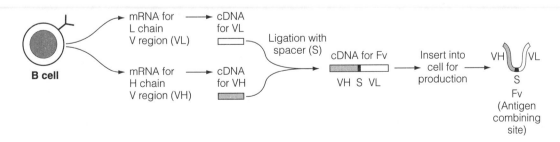

Fig. 1. Fv preparation. mRNA for the V regions of L- and H-chains is prepared from B cell mRNA using the polymerase chain reaction. From this mRNA, cDNA for each H chain V region is prepared and joined to the cDNA for each L chain V region, with a spacer between. This yields a gene encoding the antigen binding region of the antibody, which is inserted into a cell for production of a protein, Fv, that is the combining site of an antibody.

Fv libraries   Another way of preparing mAbs involves Fv libraries. This approach initially involves obtaining message for the VH and VL regions from a large number of B cells. From this mRNA, cDNA for each H chain V region is prepared and joined to the cDNA for each L-chain V region (*Fig. 1*) to create all combinations, and thus genes encoding a vast number of different antigen combining sites (**Fv** regions). These are cloned into cells for production of the protein they encode and then selected for their specificity. These Fvs can be used as a source from which specific mAbs can be created.

G1 MOLECULES WITH MULTIPLE FUNCTIONS

Key Notes

Functions of cytokines	Cytokines are small molecules that signal between cells, inducing growth, differentiation, chemotaxis, activation, enhanced cytotoxicity and/or regulation of immunity.
Cytokine nomenclature	They are referred to as interleukins if produced primarily by leukocytes, monokines if produced by myeloid cells, lymphokines if produced by lymphocytes. Chemokines are cytokines which direct cell migration and/or activate cells, and interferons are involved in defense against viral infection and in activation and modulation of immunity.
The same cytokine: different cell origin and different functions	The same cytokine can be made by different cell types (e.g. IFNγ produced by T cells and NK cells) and may have different effects on different cell populations (i.e. activate macrophages to kill intracellular microbes and B cells to undergo antibody class switching).
Related topics	Phagocytes (B1) Lymphocytes (D1)

Functions of cytokines

Cytokines are small molecules, secreted by cells in response to a stimulus. They may have an effect on the cell that produces them and are critical to signaling between cells, with each cytokine often inducing several different biological effects. Many different cells release cytokines, but each cell type releases only certain of these molecules. As a group, cytokines induce growth, differentiation, chemotaxis, activation, and/or enhanced cytotoxicity. Moreover, it is not uncommon for some cytokines to have similar activities and for many cytokines, some with opposing activities, to be released by a particular stimulus. Thus, the resulting biological effect is a factor of the sum of all of these activities.

Cytokine nomenclature

To some extent cytokines can be grouped by the cell populations that secrete them. **Monokines** are cytokines secreted by cells of the myeloid series (monocytes, macrophages) and **lymphokines** are cytokines secreted primarily by lymphocytes, although some cytokines are produced by both lymphocytes and myeloid cells. The term **interleukin** (IL) is often used to describe cytokines produced by leukocytes although some cytokines labeled as IL are also produced by other cell populations. A group of small heparin binding cytokines, **chemokines**, has recently been recognized which direct cell migration, and may also activate cells in response to infectious agents or tissue damage. **Interferons** are produced by a variety of cells in response to viral infection. In addition, a variety of other less easily categorized cytokines exist which have critical immunologic activities.

The same cytokine: different cell origin and different functions

The same cytokine can be made by entirely different cell populations. For example, IFNα is made by all nucleated cells of the body in response to viral infection. IFNγ is produced both by Th1 cells and by NK cells. IL-1 is produced by macrophages, B cells and nonimmune keratinocytes. Many different cell types make IL-6, several make IL-4, etc. In terms of function, the same cytokine can induce different functions in different cell types. For example, TNFα can promote the proliferation of B cells but activate killing mechanisms in other cell populations. IFNγ activates macrophages to kill intracellular microbes, induces B cells to switch their antibody class to IgG and induces endothelial cells to increase expression of MHC class II molecules.

G2 CYTOKINE FAMILIES

Key Notes

Interferons

Type I IFNs, IFNα and IFNβ, are produced in response to viral infection by many different cells. They inhibit viral replication and cell proliferation, increase the NK cell lytic activity and modulate MHC expression. Type II IFN, IFNγ, is produced by Th1 cells and NK cells, activates MØ and PMNs for enhanced killing and induces the development of Th1 cells that are critical to CTL responses and IgG antibody production.

Lymphokines

These cytokines are growth factors for lymphocytes or influence the nature of the immune response. IL-2 is made by T cells as a T cell growth factor for Th0 and Th1 cells and CTL. IL-3 is important in hematopoiesis. IL-4 is produced by Th2 cells and mast cells and is a growth and differentiation factor for Th2 cells and B cells, and for B cell class switch to IgE. IL-4 also induces the development of Th2 cells from Th0 cells. IL-5 is also produced by Th2 cells and mast cells and is important to B cell activation and production of IgA. IL-10, which is produced by Th2 cells and MØ, induces Th2 responses.

Monokines

These cytokines, including IL-1, IL-6, IL-8, IL-12 and tumor necrosis factor α (TNFα), have activities critical to immune defense and inflammation. IL-1, TNFα and IL-6 activate lymphocytes, increase body temperature, activate and mobilize phagocytes and activate vascular endothelium. TNFα also activates MØ and induces their production of nitric oxide. IL-8 increases access for, and chemotaxis of, PMNs. IL-12 activates NK cells to produce IFNγ, which can induce development of Th1 cells.

Chemokines

These small, closely related cytokines are produced by many cell types in response to infection or physical damage. They activate and direct effector cells to sites of tissue damage and regulate leukocyte migration into tissues. CC chemokines are chemotactic for monocytes, CXC chemokines are chemotactic for PMNs. Chemokine receptors are expressed on particular cell populations, permitting different chemokines to have selective activity.

Other cytokines

Colony stimulating factors (CSFs) drive the development, differentiation and expansion of cells of the myeloid series. GM-CSF induces commitment of progenitor cells to the monocyte/granulocyte lineage, G-CSF and M-CSF commitment to the granulocyte or monocyte lineage, respectively. Tumor growth factor β (TGFβ) inhibits activation of MØ and growth of B and T cells. Tumor necrosis factor β (TNFβ, lymphotoxin) is cytotoxic.

Related topics

Interferons (C4)
Hemopoiesis – development
  of blood cells (E1)
T helper cells (K3)

T cell activation (L2)
B cell activation (L3)
Genes, T helper cells and
  cytokines (N3)

Interferons

These molecules can be divided into two groups, type I IFNs (IFNα and IFNβ) and type II IFN (IFNγ) also called immune IFN. IFNα and IFNβ are produced in response to viral infection (and probably to double-stranded viral RNA) by many different cells. They inhibit viral replication in uninfected cells, inhibit cell proliferation, increase the lytic activity of NK cells and modulate the cellular expression of MHC molecules. The receptor for both interferon α and interferon β is the same and found on most nucleated cells. Binding of interferons α or β to this receptor inhibits viral replication in that cell as a result of blocking translation of viral proteins and induction of the synthesis of inhibitory proteins. In addition, these interferons induce increased expression of MHC class I and other components of the class I processing and presentation pathway which leads to induction of antigen specific $CD8^+$ CTL responses against virally infected cells. Induction of MHC class I is also important for protection of uninfected cells from killing by NK cells (Topic B2).

In contrast to the broad and rather nonspecific antiviral activity of IFNs α and β, IFNγ is primarily a cytokine of the adaptive immune response, as it is involved in both regulation of the development of specific immunity and in activation of cells of the immune system, MØ and PMNs. Produced primarily by Th1 cells and NK cells, IFNγ is an activator of monocytes and MØs and plays a critical role in induction of Th1 immune responses. Thus, Th1 cells or CTLs responding to peptides presented in MHC molecules produce IFNγ which acts both locally and systemically to activate MØ, which are then better able to kill intracellular pathogens. In addition, early in the development of a specific immune response, IFNγ (perhaps produced by NK cells) is involved in inducing Th0 cells to differentiate to Th1 cells which make IFNγ and provide help for development of CTL responses and for IgG antibody production.

Lymphokines

A variety of cytokines are produced by lymphocytes and lymphocyte subsets (*Table 1*), many of which are growth factors for lymphocytes or which influence the nature of the immune response (*Table 2*). IL-2 is made by T cells as a critical autocrine growth factor that is required for proliferation of T cells, especially Th0 and Th1 cells and CTL. On activation of these T cells as a result of the interaction of their antigen receptor complexes with antigenic peptide in MHC molecules on APCs, the T cells make IL-2 for secretion and at the same time IL-2 receptors with which to bind and be stimulated by the released IL-2. In the absence of IL-2 and/or its receptor, many antigen specific T cells do not expand, severely compromising immune responses.

IL-3 is a cytokine that appears to be involved in the growth and differentiation of a variety of cell types as a result of its synergistic activity with other cytokines in hematopoiesis. IL-4 is produced by Th2 cells and mast cells. It is a growth and differentiation factor for T (primarily Th2 cells) and B cells, and in particular for B cell class switch to the production of IgE antibodies. Closely related to this activity, IL-4 has an important role in influencing the nature of the immune response, as it can induce the development of Th2 cells from Th0 cells and can inhibit the development of Th1 responses (*Table 2*). Thus, IL-4 not only is involved in B cell growth, but it can also influence the B cell and its subsequent plasma cells to produce IgE antibody (Topics J2 and K3). Like IL-4, IL-5 is also produced by Th2 cells and mast cells and is important to B cell activation and production of IgA antibody. It also has a role in eosinophil growth and differentiation. IL-10, which is produced by Th2 cells and MØ, is involved in B cell activation. It induces Th2 responses and inhibits Th1 responses, perhaps by enhancing IL-4 production and/or by suppressing MØ activity and production of IL-12, a Th1-stimulatory cytokine.

Monokines

This group of cytokines (*Table 1*) has many different local and systemic activities that are critical to immune defense. In addition, these molecules, also called pro-inflammatory cytokines, are important mediators of inflammation. In particular, as a result of an appropriate stimulus, including ingestion of gram negative bacteria and subsequent activation by LPS, MØ secrete IL-1, IL-6, IL-8, IL-12 and TNFα. IL-1, TNFα and IL-6 have activities which include: (a) increasing body temperature and lymphocyte activation, which decrease pathogen replication and

Table 1.   Representative lymphokines and monokines

Cytokine	Produced by	Activity
IL-1	MØ, epithelial cells	Activates vascular endothelium; tissue destruction; increased effector cell access; fever; lymphocyte activation; mobilization of PMNs; induction of acute phase proteins (CRP, MBP)
IL-2	T cells	Proliferation of T and NK cells
IL-3	T cells, thymic cells	Proliferation, differentiation of hematopoietic cells
IL-4	Th2 cells, mast cells	B cell activation, proliferation, IgE response; induces Th2 and inhibits Th1 responses
IL-5	Th2 cells, mast cells	Eosinophil growth, differentiation; B cell activation, IgA response
IL-6	T cells, MØ	Lymphocyte activation; fever
IL-8	Mo, MØ, Fb, Kr	Increases tissue access for, and chemotaxis of PMNs
IL-10	Th2 cells, MØ	B cell activation; suppression of MØ activity; induces Th2 and inhibits Th1 responses
IL-12	B cells, MØ	Induces Th1 and inhibits Th2 responses; activates NK cells
IFNγ	T cells, NK cells	MØ and PMN activation; induces Th1 and inhibits Th2 responses
TNFα	MØ, T cells	Activates vascular endothelium; fever; shock; increases vascular permeability; mobilization of metabolites

Monocytes (Mo), macrophages (MØ), endothelial cells (En), fibroblasts (Fb), keratinocytes (Kr), neutrophils (PMNs), chondrocytes (Co)

Table 2.   Cytokine effects on Th1 and Th2 immune responses

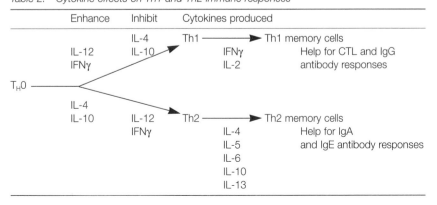

increase specific immune responses; (b) mobilization of neutrophils for phagocytosis; (c) induction of release of acute phase proteins (CRP, MBP) and thus complement activation and opsonization.

IL-1 also activates vascular endothelium (in preparation for neutrophil chemotaxis) and induces systemic production of IL-6. IL-8 increases access for, and chemotaxis of, neutrophils. It also activates binding by integrins, which facilitates neutrophil binding to endothelial cells and migration into tissues. Like IL-1, TNFα also activates vascular endothelium and is able to increase vascular permeability. It activates MØ and induces their production of nitric oxide (NO). Although produced by monocytes and MØ, TNFα is also produced by some T cells. Finally, IL-12, which is also produced by B cells, activates NK cells which then produce IFNγ, a cytokine important to inducing differentiation of Th0 cells to Th1 cells (*Table 2*).

Chemokines

This group of more than 50 small, closely related cytokines (mol. wt 8–10 kDa) are primarily involved in chemoattraction of leukocytes (lymphocytes, monocytes and neutrophils) (*Table 3*). They are made by monocytes/macrophages, but also by other cells including endothelial cells, platelets, neutrophils, T cells, keratinocytes and fibroblasts. Chemokines can be divided into four different groups based on unique aspects of their amino acid sequence, and in particular the position of conserved cysteine residues. One group has two adjacent cysteines (CC), a second has two cysteines separated by another amino acid (CXC), another has one cysteine, and the last has two cysteines separated by three other amino acids. For the most part, CC chemokines such as monocyte chemotactic protein (MCP-1) are chemotactic for monocytes, inducing them to migrate into tissues and become macrophages, whereas CXC chemokines such as IL-8 are chemotactic for neutrophils inducing them to leave the blood and migrate into tissues. Some of these chemokines also are chemotactic for T cells. Chemokines can be produced by many cells in response to an infectious process or to physical damage. They not only direct a cell to the source of infection/damage, but may also activate the cell for dealing with the infectious agent or damage.

Receptors for chemokines are all integral membrane proteins with the characteristic feature that they span the membrane seven times (seven transmembrane glycoproteins). These molecules are coupled to G (guanine nucleoside binding) proteins which act as the signaling moiety of the receptor. Although most of these

Table 3. Representative chemokines*

Class	Name	Source	Chemoattractant for	Activation of
CXC (α)	IL-8	Mo, MØ, Fb, Kr	Naive T cells, PMNs	PMNs
	NAP-2	Platelets	Neutrophils	
	MIP-1β	Mo, MØ, En, PMNs	CD8 T cells	
CC (β)	MCP-1	Mo, MØ, Fb, Kr	Memory T cells, Mo	Monocytes
	Rantes	T cells	Memory Th cells	
C (γ)	Lymphotactin		Lymphocytes	
CX₃C (δ)	Fractalkine		Lymphocytes, monocytes, NK cells	

*See footnote Table 1.

receptors can bind more than one type of chemokine, they are usually distributed only on particular cell populations, permitting different chemokines to have selective activity.

Some of these chemokines, for example IL-8 and MCP-1, have been shown to work by first binding to proteoglycan molecules on endothelial cells or on the extracellular matrix. On this solid surface they then bind blood neutrophils or monocytes, slowing their passage and directing them to migrate down a chemokine concentration gradient toward the source of the chemokine. Although the role that each plays in immune defense and pathology is still being clarified, it is evident that these molecules are potent agents for activating and directing effector cell populations to the site of tissue damage as well as for controlling leukocyte migration in tissues.

Other cytokines

Of the many other cytokines which are important to immune defense, several are particularly noteworthy (*Table 4*). A group of CSFs, including granulocyte-monocyte CSF (GM-CSF), granulocyte CSF (G-CSF) and monocyte CSF (M-CSF) are cytokines which drive the development, differentiation and expansion of cells of the myeloid series. GM-CSF induces expansion of myeloid progenitor cells and their commitment to the monocyte/MØ and granulocyte lineage, after which G-CSF and M-CSF induce specific commitment to the granulocyte or monocyte lineage, respectively, and then their subsequent expansion. These factors, and especially G-CSF, are important clinical tools in a number of disease situations as they are used to expand myeloid effector cell populations critical to defense against pathogens (Topic G3).

TGFβ is produced by a variety of cells including monocytes, MØ, T cells and chondrocytes, and plays an important role in suppressing immune responses, as it can inhibit activation of MØ and growth of B and T cells. TNFβ (lymphotoxin) is a molecule which is cytotoxic to a variety of cell types, including ineffectual chronically infected MØ. The released pathogen is then killed by less compromised MØ.

*Table 4.   Other cytokines**

Cytokine	Produced by	Activity
GM-CSF	MØ, T cells	Stimulates growth, differentiation & activation of granulocytes, Mo, MØ
G-CSF	Mo, Fb, En	Stimulates PMN development
M-CSF	Fb	Stimulates Mo, MØ development
TGFβ	Mo, T cells, Co	Inhibits cell growth and inflammation
TNFβ (lymphotoxin)	T cells	cytotoxic to T, B and other cells

* See footnote *Table 1*.

G3 CYTOKINES IN THE CLINIC

Key Notes

Cytokine treatment

Several cytokines which enhance immune responses, including IL-2, IFNγ and IFNα have been approved for treatment of certain tumors. G-CSF is extremely useful in treating cancer patients with low PMN counts resulting from chemotherapy or irradiation.

Cytokine receptor targeting

Antibodies to cytokine receptors or soluble cytokine receptors themselves are used to treat autoimmune diseases where pro-inflammatory cytokines are involved in maintenance of chronic inflammation e.g. TNFα in RA.

Related topics

Cytokine and cellular
  immunotherapy of tumors (P5)
Diagnosis and treatment of
  immunodeficiency (S4)

Diagnosis and treatment of
  autoimmune disease (U5)

Cytokine treatment

Based on an increasing understanding of the mechanisms of action of these cytokines, many have been evaluated for their potential to treat some human diseases. Several cytokines with the ability to enhance immune responses to infectious microbes and tumors, including IL-2, IFNγ and IFNα have been tested and approved for treatment (*Table 1*). Cytokines which have been used in immunodeficient states (Topic S3) include IFNγ for CGD and G-CSF for treating patients with low granulocyte counts resulting from, for example, the use of chemotherapy

Table 1. Cytokines and their inhibitors as tools in the clinic.

Cytokine treatment	Patient group
For infection	
IFNα	Some infections
IFNγ	Treatment of patients with CGD
G-CSF	Treatment of patients with low granulocyte counts (e.g. resulting from chemotherapy or irradiation)
For tumors	
IL-2	Renal cell carcinoma (20% of patients have partial responses). It has been used together with tumor infiltrating lymphocytes for some tumors
IFNα	Hairy cell leukemia
Cytokine inhibitors (anti-inflammatory)	
Anti-TNFα	Some success in treating RA
Soluble cytokine receptors e.g. IL1, TNFα	Some success in treating RA

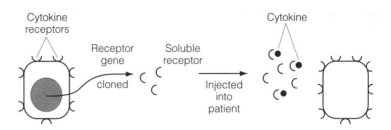

Fig. 1.   Inhibition of cytokine function by blocking with soluble receptor.

or irradiation in cancer therapy. G-CSF induces differentiation of stem cells to mature PMNs, critical in protection against microbial infection (Topic O2). IFNα and IL-2 have been shown to be successful in the treatment of some tumors.

Cytokine receptor targeting

As the pro-inflammatory cytokines, e.g. TNFα and IL-1, have been shown to be important in the maintenance of chronic inflammation in several autoimmune diseases, specific cytokine inhibitors, either antibodies or soluble cytokine receptors (*Fig. 1*) are being used to treat these disorders. In particular, success has been achieved using soluble receptors in therapy of rheumatoid arthritis.

H1 NON SELF RECOGNITION BY THE INNATE IMMUNE SYSTEM

Key Notes

Pattern recognition receptors

Receptors of the innate immune system interact with, and facilitate removal of, groups of organisms with similar structures. These pattern recognition receptors (PRR) recognize molecular patterns associated with certain groups of microbes, and act not only as a first line of defense against infectious organisms, but also to prime the adaptive immune system.

Mannose receptor

The mannose receptor is expressed on macrophages, dendritic cells and endothelial cells and recognizes variations on a Ca^{2+} dependent, mannosyl/fucosyl pattern. It also mediates phagocytosis of microbes and processing and presentation of peptides from the microbe on MHC Class II molecules, thus permitting induction of specific anti-microbial T and B cell responses.

Toll receptors

Toll proteins or Toll-like receptors (TLRs) are a family of germline encoded proteins that recognize and distinguish between molecular patterns of different groups of pathogens. They not only signal the presence of a pathogen, but trigger the expression of co-stimulatory molecules and effector cytokines important in the development of adaptive immune responses.

CD14

This molecule is expressed on macrophages, binds LPS on gram negative bacteria, and facilitates destruction of the microbe and induction of secretion of cytokines involved in triggering adaptive immune responses.

Scavenger receptors

Scavenger receptors on macrophages recognize carbohydrates or lipids in bacterial and yeast cell walls.

Related topics

Phagocytes (B1)
Innate molecular immune
   defense against microbes(C1)

The microbial cosmos (O1)

Pattern recognition receptors

In addition to the soluble molecules of the innate immune system, an increasing number of cell surface receptors have been identified that not only act as a first line of defense against infectious organisms, but also links to and primes, the adaptive immune system. These pattern recognition receptors (PRR) do not have the remarkable specificity of the T and B cell systems, but have developed over evolutionary time to interact with, and facilitate removal of, groups of organisms with similar structures. Moreover, the receptors involved are expressed on a variety of cells some of which are critical to adaptive immunity.

In particular, these PRR have evolved to recognize molecular patterns associated with certain kinds of microbes. These molecules include mannose receptors, CD14 (which binds LPS) and scavenger receptors (which bind carbohydrates/lipids), all expressed on macrophages (*Fig. 1*), as well as a recently identified family of molecules, the Toll receptors (*Table 1*). It seems likely that additional molecules important to innate immunity will also be found.

Table 1. Cell surface receptors recognizing nonself

Name	Specificity	Cellular location
Mannose receptors	Mannosyl/fucosyl structures	Macrophages, endothelial cells, dendritic cells
CD14	LPS	Macrophages
Scavenger receptors	Carbohydrates or lipids	Macrophages
Toll receptors	LPS, peptidoglycan, glucans, teichoic acids, arabinomannans	APCs, B cells macrophages, other

Mannose receptor

The mannose receptor is a 180 kDa transmembrane receptor expressed on macrophages, dendritic cells and subsets of endothelial cells. This receptor has eight carbohydrate recognition domains (CRDs), at least some of which have different pattern recognition motifs, making this one receptor fairly broad in the number and range of ligands it can recognize. Its Ca^{2+} dependent, mannosyl/fucosyl recognition pattern permits it to interact with a variety of pathogens that enter through mucosal surfaces (*Table 2*). Because the mannose receptor is expressed on macrophages throughout the body, it is likely to be one of the first of

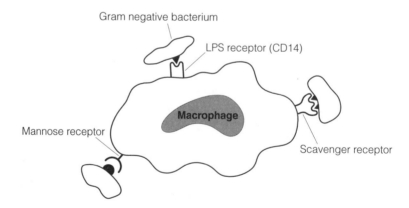

Fig. 1. Macrophage expression of receptors involved in nonself recognition.

Table 2. Microorganisms that express ligands to which the mannose receptor binds

Pseudomonas aeruginosa
Mycobacterium tuberculosis
Candida albicans
Pneumocystis carinii
Klebsiella pneumoniae
Leishmania donovani

the innate receptors to interact with microbes (*Fig. 1*). Furthermore, this receptor mediates phagocytosis and destruction of microbes even before the adaptive immune response is induced.

In addition to its role as a front line receptor mediating destruction of a wide range of organisms, the mannose receptor represents an important direct link to the adaptive immune system. Thus, microbes bound by mannose receptor are internalized and degraded in endosomes. Peptides from the microbe are loaded on MHC class II molecules for display on the surface of these APCs such that the adaptive immune system can now recognize the microbe, permitting induction of specific T and B cell responses to it.

Toll receptors

Toll proteins or Toll-like receptors (TLRs) are a family of closely related proteins of which there are at least five known members. They all have an extracellular leucine-rich repeat (LRR) domain and a cytoplasmic domain that mediates signal transduction of a variety of effector genes. One of these TLRs (TLR4) has been found to induce cytokine and co-stimulatory molecule expression on APCs. Another TLR2 appears to bind LPS and induce intracellular signaling. Furthermore, a molecule very similar to the TLRs, RP105, has been found on human B cells and dendritic cells. Cross-linking of this molecule on B cells induces expression of co-stimulatory molecules and proliferation.

These and other findings indicate that different Toll proteins may be able to recognize molecular patterns of different pathogens and to distinguish between different groups of pathogens. In fact, it has been proposed that different TLRs may discriminate between the major molecular signatures of pathogens, including: peptidoglycan, teichoic acids (Gram-positive bacteria), LPS (Gram-negative bacteria), arabinomannans, and glucans. Of particular importance, these germline encoded molecules of the innate immune system are not only able to signal the presence of a pathogen, but trigger expression of co-stimulatory molecules and effector cytokines, and in so doing prepare the cell for its involvement in the development of the adaptive immune response.

CD14

CD14 is a phosphoinositolglycan linked cell surface receptor on macrophages (*Table 1*) that binds to lipopolysaccharide (LPS), a unique bacterial surface structure found only in the cell walls of gram-negative bacteria, e.g. *E. coli*, *Neisseria*, *Salmonella*. The core carbohydrate and lipid A of LPS are virtually the same for these microbes and are the target for binding by CD14. Binding of LPS on a gram negative bacteria to macrophage CD14 facilitates destruction of the microbe as well as induction of secretion of various cytokines involved in triggering a wide array of immune responses.

Scavenger receptors

Macrophages express a family of proteins called scavenger receptors that recognize carbohydrates or lipids in bacterial and yeast cell walls.

H2 B CELL RECOGNITION OF ANTIGEN, THE B CELL RECEPTOR COMPLEX AND CO-RECEPTORS

Key Notes

The B cell receptor (BCR) complex	The BCR complex consists of the antigen receptor, Ig, in association with two other polypeptides, Igα and Igβ. Igα and Igβ are signaling molecules for the BCR and are also required for assembly and expression of Ig.
B cell co-receptors	These co-receptors, including CD21, CD32, CD19 and CD81, associate with the BCR complex especially when both the BCR and one or more of the co-receptors are linked through an antigen-complement/antibody complex. Depending on which molecules are ligated, signaling by the Ig-Igα/Igβ complex is enhanced or inhibited.
Related topics	Lymphocytes (D1) B cells are produced in the bone marrow (E3) The cellular basis of the antibody response (J1) B cell activation (L3) The role of antibody (N4)

The B cell receptor (BCR) complex

As described in Section H, the receptor for antigen on B cells is Ig. Initially cells make IgM and then IgD, which are both displayed on the surface of a mature B cell. These Igs are transmembrane molecules although the cytoplasmic domain of each is only three amino acids long, too short to signal the cell when antigen binds to the antibody. However, this membrane bound Ig is associated with two other polypeptides on the B cell, Igα and Igβ (*Fig. 1*). These small molecular weight (20 kDa) transmembrane molecules are the signaling molecules for the BCR. When IgM, IgD (or other Ig isotypes on the B cell) are cross linked by binding to antigen, Igα and Igβ transduce signals which begin to prepare the cell for a productive interaction with T helper cells (Topics K3 and N3) Igα and Igβ are also required for assembly and expression of immunoglobulin, and thus of the B cell receptor complex, in the plasma membrane.

B cell co-receptors

There is also a co-receptor complex on the surface of B cells that can, depending on which molecules are ligated, enhance or inhibit signaling by the Ig-Igα/Igβ-complex. This co-receptor complex includes CD21 (complement receptor 2, CR2), CD32 (a receptor for the Fc region of IgG, FcγRIIB), CD19 (a signaling molecule) and CD81. These molecules associate with the BCR complex especially when both

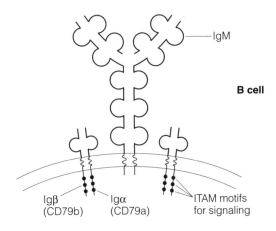

Fig. 1.   *The B cell receptor complex (BCR).*

the BCR and the co-receptor complex interact with the same antigen (Topic L3), i.e., if the BCR binds antigen with which soluble Ab and/or complement have also interacted, CD21 and CD32 will be engaged and, through these signaling molecules, CD19 and CD81 influence signaling by the Igα/Igβ complex (*Fig. 2*).

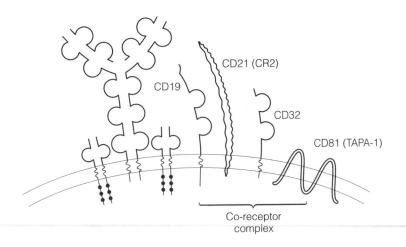

Fig. 2.   *The BCR complex associating with its co-receptor complex.*

H3 T CELL RECOGNITION OF ANTIGEN, THE T CELL RECEPTOR COMPLEX

Key Notes

Overview	As with humoral immunity, clonal selection of antigen specific T cells is followed by proliferation, differentiation and the subsequent development of the effector cells of cellular immunity. Through cell to cell signaling and production of lymphokines, T helper (Th) cells aid B cells, macrophages, and other T cells in their response to antigen. Cytolytic T cells eliminate virus-infected and tumor cells, and reject transplants.
T cell receptor (TCR) for antigen	The TCR for antigen is only found on the T cell membrane and is composed of two polypeptide chains, α and β. Each of these glycoproteins is made up of constant and variable regions, like those of Igs, and together the α and β chain variable regions compose the antigen binding site. Some T cells, whose function is not clear, express a TCR consisting of γ and δ chains.
The T cell receptor complex	The T cell receptor complex consists of the antigen receptor, the αβ or γδ dimer, plus CD3, a signaling complex composed of γ, δ and ε chains. CD4 on T cells binds to the nonpolymorphic region of MHC class II on APCs restricting Th cells to recognizing only peptides presented on MHC class II molecules. CD8 on cytolytic T cells binds the nonpolymorphic region of MHC class I, restricting killing to cells presenting peptide in MHC class I.
Generation of T cell diversity	The genes for the α, β, γ and δ chains, are encoded by three unlinked gene groups each consisting of multiple gene segments which encode V, D, and J gene segments (β and δ genes) or V and J gene segments (α and γ genes), as well as constant region genes. These T cell gene segments rearrange in each developing T cell in the thymus, resulting in a breadth of T cell diversity similar to that for B cells. Allelic exclusion assures that each T cell will have a single specificity.
Selection of the T cell repertoire	In the thymus, those T cells that express a TCR that binds weakly to self MHC are positively selected. Of this group, those that express a TCR that binds strongly to self MHC are negatively selected. Thus, the T cells that survive and mature are those that recognize modified self MHC molecules – self-MHC molecules plus foreign peptide.
Antigen recognition by T cells	Since the function of T cells is to help or kill cells, the TCR must recognize antigens on the surface of cells, but not native antigen. Thus, the TCR recognizes short peptides derived from foreign proteins that are bound to MHC molecules on the surface of cells. As T cells recognize modified self MHC molecules, the recognition of an antigen by a T cell is MHC restricted.

Related topics	Lymphocytes (D1)	The cellular basis of the antibody
	T cells are produced in the thymus (E2)	response (J1)
		T cell activation (L2)
	Major histocompatibility complex and antigen processing and presentation (H4)	

Overview

The mechanisms involved in the development of cellular immunity parallel those outlined for humoral immunity, with the antigens to which this system responds being as varied as for the humoral immune system. Clonal selection of antigen specific T cells is followed by proliferation and differentiation and the subsequent development of the effector cells of cellular immunity.

Cellular immunity is carried out through two major subpopulations of T cells, helper and cytolytic. Helper T cells aid B cells, macrophages, as well as other T cells in their response to antigen, by directly signaling these cells through cell to cell contact and by producing lymphokines (Topic G2) that modulate immune responses. This provides appropriate checks and balances for the development of immunity. Cytolytic T cells eliminate virus-infected and tumor cells, and reject transplants.

T cell receptor (TCR) for antigen

There is as much diversity of TCR as of Ig receptors, but unlike the B cell antigen receptor (Ig), the TCR for antigen is only found on the T cell membrane and not in the serum or other body fluids. The majority of peripheral T cells express a TCR composed of two polypeptide chains, α and β, which in the human have molecular weights of 50 and 39 kDa, respectively. Each of these glycoproteins is made up of constant and variable regions like those of Ig and together the α and β variable regions compose a T cell antigen binding site (*Fig. 1*). The genes coding for TCR polypeptides are members of the Ig super family, as are many similar surface receptor molecules. A subpopulation of thymocytes and a small group of peripheral T cells express a TCR consisting of γ and δ chains, which are similar to the αβ TCR. These γ and δ chains have V and C regions like α and β chains, and have antigen recognizing capabilities. The function of these γδ TCR expressing T cells is not well understood.

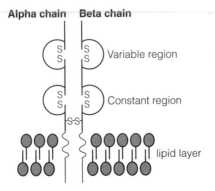

Fig. 1. T cell antigen receptor αβ dimer.

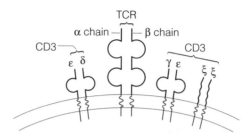

Fig. 2.   The TCR complex consists of the antigen receptor, the αβ or γδ dimer, associated with several other polypeptides important in T cell signaling and recognition. CD3 is the signaling complex for the TCR and consists of γ, δ, ε and ξ chains.

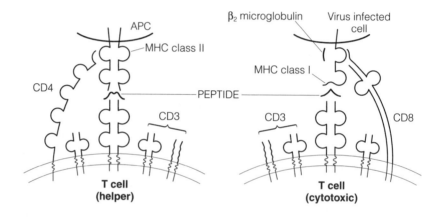

Fig. 3.   CD8 and CD4 recognition of MHC class I and class II molecules, respectively. CD4 on T helper cells bind to the nonpolymorphic region of MHC class II; CD8 on cytolytic T cells binds the nonpolymorphic region of MHC class I.

The T cell receptor complex

The T cell receptor complex consists of the antigen receptor, the αβ or γδ dimer, associated with several other polypeptides important in T cell signaling and recognition. In particular, the TCR is associated with CD3, a signaling complex which is itself composed of several polypeptides including γ, δ and ε chains (*Fig. 2*). Together these molecules form an αβ-CD3 complex. T cells expressing the γδ antigen receptor form a γδ-CD3 complex. Two other molecules on T cells also play a role in T cell recognition of antigen. CD4 is not just a marker on Th cells, but also a molecule that can bind to the non-polymorphic region of MHC class II. This molecule restricts these Th cells to recognizing only peptides presented on MHC class II molecules (*Fig. 3*). Similarly, CD8 on cytolytic T cells binds the nonpolymorphic region of MHC class I, restricting these killer T cells to recognizing only cells presenting peptide in MHC class I molecules.

Generation of T cell diversity

Like B cell diversity, the diversity demonstrated by the cellular immune system results from gene rearrangements in early T cells. The genes for the TCR α, β and γ chains are coded by three unlinked gene groups, whereas the δ chain genes lie within the α chain genes. Each gene group consists of multiple gene segments which code for V, D, and J gene segments (β and δ genes) or V and J gene segments (α and γ genes), as well as constant region genes (*Fig. 4*). In the germ line the V and J (α chain) or V, D, and J (β chain) segments are separated by non-coding DNA.

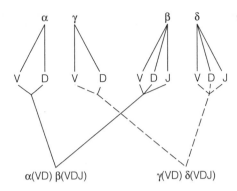

Fig. 4. Gene segments involved in formation of the V region of the different polypeptides of the TCR.

During T cell differentiation these V, D, and J segments are rearranged to form a complete V gene. As in the case of immunoglobulin rearrangements, the expression of a V-C (constant region) gene product by the T cell excludes further rearrangement (allelic exclusion) and the T cell thus becomes committed to the expression of a single V-C α-chain combination and a single V-C β-chain combination, which together constitute an antigenic binding site and determine the specificity of the T cell. Since the rearrangements occur randomly in millions of T cells, considerable diversity of specificity is generated *prior* to antigen stimulation.

Selection of the T cell repertoire

Precursors of T cells migrate from the bone marrow to the thymus where only a small fraction mature and eventually leave as immunocompetent cells, as most die in the thymus. Upon entry into the thymus, T cells initiate TCR rearrangement and this receptor is expressed on thymocytes that bear both CD4 and CD8 markers (double positive thymocytes). T cells that express a TCR that can bind *weakly* to self MHC are spared from death and are *positively selected* to survive. Therefore, the T cell repertoire is first selected for cells that can bind self MHC. Of this group, those that express a TCR that binds *strongly* to self MHC are auto-reactive and may cause problems if they enter the periphery. These cells are induced to die (are *negatively* selected). This positive and negative selection results in survival of T cells that recognize peptides in the context of self-MHC, but cannot react productively with self antigens (Section G).

Antigen recognition by T cells

Since the function of T cells is to help or kill cells, the TCR has to recognize antigens on the surface of those cells and not recognize native antigen. That is, the TCR cannot react with Ag alone or with an antigen on a bacteria or virus. Rather, it recognizes short peptides that are derived from the antigen (e.g. bacteria or viruses) and that are bound to major histocompatibility complex (MHC) molecules on the surface of antigen-presenting cells (APC). There are two ways that foreign proteins can get into APCs: (a) by the whole microbe growing inside of cells (e.g. viruses); or (b) by being endocytosed (engulfed) by phagocytes. These proteins are degraded by cellular proteases, and the resulting peptides are 'loaded' onto MHC molecules. These complexes, after transport to the surface of the cell, are what antigen-specific T cells recognize. Thus, all protein antigens (and in particular peptides derived from them) are recognized by T cells 'in the context of' (physically associated with) self MHC proteins, i.e. the T cell recognizes modified self MHC molecules, and thus the recognition of an antigen by a T cell is *MHC restricted*.

H4 THE MAJOR HISTOCOMPATIBILITY COMPLEX AND ANTIGEN PROCESSING AND PRESENTATION

Key Notes

The structure of MHC molecules

Two classes (Class I and II) of polymorphic MHC genes code for human leukocyte antigens (HLA) which act as peptide receptors and are critical to antigen presentation. *Class I genes* (HLA-A, -B, -C) encode two polypeptide chains, a polymorphic heavy chain and β_2-microglobulin, expressed on the surfaces of all nucleated cells. The heavy chain has a 'binding groove' for peptides to be recognized by T cells. *Class II genes* (HLA-D) encode molecules (HLA-DP, -DR, and -DQ) composed of two dissimilar polymorphic polypeptide chains (an α and β chain), both of which contribute to the peptide binding groove.

Nature of the antigen (peptides) associated with MHC class I and class II molecules

The polymorphic regions of MHC class I and class II are the peptide binding domains of these molecules and bind peptides ranging from 9–10 and 12–20 amino acid residues, respectively. Anchor residues on the peptides bind to residues in the class I and II groves and vary for different MHC alleles. This forms at least one basis for the genetic control of immune responses.

Cellular distribution of class I and class II MHC molecules

MHC class II molecules are expressed on B cells, dendritic cells and macrophages, efficient APCs for the activation of CD4$^+$ helper T cells. MHC class I molecules are expressed on all nucleated cells, permitting cytolytic T cells to recognize cells infected with intracellular pathogens. Cytokines modulate the expression of MHC Class I and/or II molecules.

Class I processing pathways

Peptides that bind to class I MHC molecules are derived from viruses that have infected host cells. Peptides generated in the cytosol (e.g. from viral proteins) become associated with MHC class I molecules which move to the surface (*endogeneous pathway*) and are recognized by CD8$^+$ cytotoxic T lymphocytes (CTL).

Class II processing pathways

Some pathogens replicate in cellular vesicles of macrophages, others are endocytosed from the environment into endocytic vesicles (*exogenous pathway*). In both cases peptides from proteins associated with these microbes are primarily presented on MHC class II molecules to CD4$^+$ helper T cells.

MHC molecules and immune defense against intracellular pathogens	MHC restricted CTL recognition has probably evolved to protect against acute viral infections. Neutralizing antibody is effective against free virus, but much less so against infected cells. Since T cells do not recognize native protein, they directly target the infected cell. Moreover, cytotoxic T cells can directly lyse the infected cell and are restricted by MHC class I molecules which are found essentially on all cells that can harbor viruses.
Related topics	Antigens (A4) Factors predisposing and/or T cytotoxic cells (K2) contributing to the T helper cells (K3) development of autoimmune T cell activation (L2) disease (U2) Transplantation antigens (Q2)

The structure of MHC molecules

Although molecules coded for by the MHC were originally identified based on their role in transplant rejection, they actually evolved to present foreign antigens to T cells. Two classes (Class I and II) of MHC genes, closely linked on chromosome 6 in humans, code for human leukocyte antigens (HLA) which are the molecules critical to antigen presentation. There are many alternative forms of genes for each subregion of the MHC. This high degree of polymorphism in class I MHC and class II MHC molecules is *not* due to generation of diversity within the individual (as is the case for Ig molecules) but rather to the many alternative forms or alleles of MHC that exist in the species (Topic Q2). These different alleles are not inherited entirely randomly as there is a variable distribution of determinants among different ethnic groups. Moreover, these alleles are inherited in groups. The combination of the encoded alleles at each of the loci within the MHC on the same chromosome is referred to as the haplotype (for haploid, as opposed to diploid). Since genes within the MHC are closely linked, haplotypes are usually inherited intact.

Class I genes **(HLA-A, -B, -C)**
These code for molecules (referred to by the same designation) that are expressed on the surfaces of all nucleated cells as two polypeptide chains. Only the H-chain is coded by the MHC, and contains regions of sequence variability thus accounting for the more than 35 million HLA phenotypes. The L-chain, β_2-microglobulin (different from κ and λ Ig L-chains), shows no polymorphism and is coded for on chromosome 15. The H-chain of these molecules has a region that forms a 'binding groove' for peptides, such that when the class I molecule is synthesized it is able to interact with and bind certain kinds of peptides. Only the H-chain is involved in this binding, with β_2-microglobulin stabilizing the molecule and permitting it to be displayed on the cell surface (*Fig. 1*).

Class II genes **(HLA-D, in man)**
These code for structural glycoproteins found on B cells, macrophages and dendritic cells, as well as sperm, and vascular endothelial cells. The HLA-D region can be subdivided into sets of genes which encode different HLA-DP, -DR, and -DQ class II molecules. Class II molecules are composed of two dissimilar polypeptide chains (i.e. an α and β chain heterodimer), but both chains are encoded by the MHC and β_2-microglobulin is *not* involved. As with class I MHC molecules, class II MHC molecules are polymorphic. As with class I molecules, MHC class II

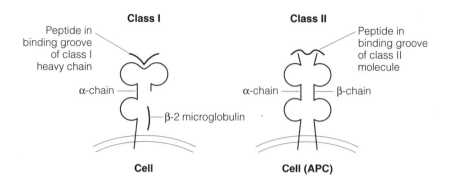

Fig. 1. MHC class I and class II molecules binding peptide.

molecules are also able to bind peptides. In this case both the α and β chains of the class II molecule contribute to the binding groove (*Fig. 1*). Thus, both class I and class II molecules (which are also members of the immunoglobulin superfamily) contribute to the antigen binding groove.

Nature of the antigen (peptides) associated with MHC class I and class II molecules

The peptide binding domains of MHC class I and class II molecules are the portions of these molecules that are polymorphic. That is, there are particular amino acid residues in the 'binding groove' that vary from individual to individual. The residues that are polymorphic represent sites within the peptide binding pocket of each of the molecules that make contact with the antigenic peptide. The peptides that are bound by MHC class I and class II molecules are short, ranging from nine amino acid residues (for MHC class I) to 12–20 amino acid residues (for MHC class II). The sites on the peptides that bind to the MHC molecules are **anchor residues** that anchor the peptide to the MHC molecule. The anchor residues do not vary for a specific MHC molecule, but the other residues in the peptide can vary to some extent. Therefore, each 'type' of MHC molecule is only able to bind peptides bearing specific anchor residues. Thus, depending on the MHC molecules that are inherited, a person might not be able to bind specific peptides from e.g. viruses. If the person's MHC molecules cannot bind the peptides generated from a specific virus, then they will be unable to mount a CD8 response to that virus. This forms at least one basis for the genetic control of immune responses. That is, the MHC molecules inherited by an individual ultimately determine to which peptides that individual can elicit T cell-mediated immune responses, and at the population level, the polymorphism increases the chances of survival of at least some individuals.

Cellular distribution of class I and class II MHC molecules

MHC class I and MHC class II molecules have a distinct distribution on cells (*Table 1*) that directly reflects the different effector functions that those cells play. Furthermore, under some conditions (e.g. cytokine activation) the expression of MHC class I and/or II molecules may be induced or enhanced (e.g. activated T cells become class II positive). Cells that express MHC class II molecules (B cells, dendritic cells, macrophages) are efficient antigen-presenting cells for the activation of CD4$^+$ helper T cells. In contrast, MHC class I molecules are expressed on virtually all cells in humans except for RBC. The expression of MHC class I molecules on all nucleated cells permits the immune system to survey these cells for infection with intracellular pathogens and allows destruction via class I-restricted CTLs. It is interesting to note that the absence of class I MHC molecules on RBC may allow the unchecked growth of *Plasmodium*, the agent responsible for malaria.

Table 1.   Expression of MHC class I and II molecules

Tissue	MHC class I	MHC class II
T cells	+++	–
B cells	+++	+++
Macrophages	+++	++
Dendritic cells	+++	+++
Neutrophils	+++	–
Hepatocytes	+	–
Kidney	++	–
Brain	+	–
Red blood cells	–	–

Class I processing pathways

To a large extent, fragments of peptides that bind to class I MHC molecules are derived from viruses that have infected host cells (*Fig. 2*). Degraded viral proteins (peptides) are transported into the endoplasmic reticulum by specific transporter proteins (transporters associated with antigen processing; TAP). In this intracellular compartment peptides bind to class I MHC molecules (*endogeneous pathway*). The class I MHC-peptide complex is then exported to the cell surface. In general, peptides generated in the cytosol (e.g. from cytosolic microbes) become associated with MHC class I molecules which move to the surface and can be recognized by cytotoxic T lymphocytes (CTL) which are distinguished by expression of CD8 (*Table 2*).

Class II processing pathways

While viruses and some bacteria replicate in the cytosol, several types of pathogens including mycobacteria and *Leishmania* replicate in cellular vesicles of macrophages. In addition, pathogens can be endocytosed from the environment into endocytic vesicles (*Table 2*). Thus, both pathogens in cellular vesicles and

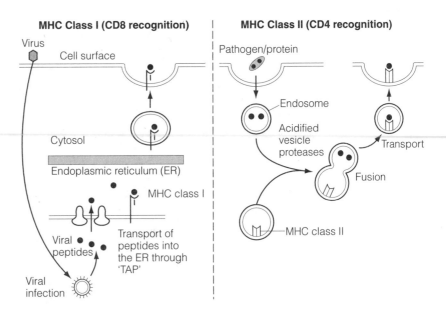

Fig. 2.   Comparison of the pathways used to generate peptides that bind to MHC class I and class II molecules.

Table 2.   MHC class I and II processing pathways.

	Cytosolic pathogens	Intracellular pathogens	Extracellular pathogens
Degraded in:	Cytosol	Acidic vesicles	Acidic vesicles
Peptides presented by:	Class I MHC	Class II MHC	Class II MHC
Peptides presented to:	CD8 T cells (cytotoxic)	CD4 T cells (helper)	CD4 T cells (helper)
Effect on APC:	Cell death	Activation of macrophages to kill intracellular parasites	Activation of B cells to secrete Ig to eliminate extracellular pathogens/toxins

pathogens and antigens that come from outside the cell (*exogenous pathway*) are primarily presented on MHC class II molecules. Class II MHC molecules are present in the endocytic vesicles of macrophages, B cells and other cells that present antigen to CD4$^+$ helper T cells. Upon fusion with the endocytic vesicles, class II MHC molecules become loaded with peptides, and the class II-MHC peptide complex is transported to the cell surface where it can be recognized by CD4$^+$ T cells (*Fig. 2*). CD4 T cells also assist in the destruction of parasites in vesicular compartments e.g. mycobacteria, by activating the cells that harbor these pathogens to kill them. For extracellular parasites, CD4 T cells can activate macrophages to endocytose and destroy the pathogens, as well as instruct B cells to produce antibody to opsonize the pathogens. There are two subsets of CD4$^+$ cells potentially involved in these responses (Topic K3).

MHC molecules and immune defense against intracellular pathogens

Why has an MHC restricted CTL recognition system evolved, when B cells have developed a highly workable Ig receptor system in which native foreign antigen *per se* is recognized without fragmentation of the antigen, or the need for presentation of foreign antigen by self MHC? This is best understood by considering viral infections in which the immune system is simultaneously confronted with large numbers of free infectious virus and a smaller number of infected cells which continue to release virus, both of which need to be eliminated for resolution of the disease. Although neutralizing antibody is effective against free virus, it is much less effective against cells harboring the virus. As a consequence, infected cells continue to release virus and the humoral immune system may never 'catch up' to the growing virus load or cure the infection. However, the cellular immune system ignores free virus (T cells do not recognize native protein) and can directly target the infected cell. MHC restricted T cells, which bind foreign antigen only in the context of self MHC molecules, are uniquely suited for this function. Cytotoxic T cells are especially effective in that they are restricted by class I MHC molecules which are found on essentially all cells of the body (all nucleated cells can potentially harbor viruses), and because they can directly lyse the infected cell. Such a T cell recognition system has therefore probably evolved because of genetic pressure to protect against acute viral infections.

I1 THE ACUTE INFLAMMATORY RESPONSE

Key Notes

Initiation of the acute inflammatory response

Infection, trauma or allergy can initiate acute inflammation through the release of inflammatory mediators into the tissues. These mediators may be derived from microbes, damaged tissue, mast cells, other leukocytes and complement components. Although the initiating events may be different, the final pathway to inflammation is the same in all instances. The activation phase of the acute inflammatory response may also be initiated by autoimmunity.

Vascular changes

Inflammatory mediators, including mast cell and other leukocyte products, cytokines, and complement cleavage products, induce changes in the expression of adhesion molecules on vascular endothelial cells. This results in the further recruitment of inflammatory cells which bind to these adhesion molecules and extravasate into the site of inflammation.

Termination of the response and repair

The acute inflammatory response is brought under control by anti-inflammatory cytokines, soluble receptors for inflammatory cytokines, products of the endocrine system such as corticosteroids, corticotrophin and α-melanocyte-stimulating hormone. Repair is facilitated by collagen producing fibroblasts, protein C and the bradykinin system.

Related topics

Phagocytes (B1)	Cytokine families (G2)
Mast cells and basophils (B3)	IgE-mediated type 1
Complement (C2)	hypersensitivity: allergy (T2)

Initiation of the acute inflammatory response

Acute inflammation is caused by the release of inflammatory mediators from microbes, damaged tissue, mast cells and other leukocytes, and complement cleavage products (*Fig. 1*). Although the initiating events may be different, the overall inflammatory response they trigger is similar, with the exception of inflammation caused by IgE/mast cells interactions, which are more immediate and can be systemic. These mediators cause edema, swelling, redness and pain – the classical indicators of inflammation – and may also cause changes in neurovasculature and neuromusculature.

The main cells involved in the acute inflammatory response are mast cells and neutrophils, although tissue macrophages also play a role. Mast cells are distributed throughout the body (Topic B3) and some of their products such as histamine and heparin cause smooth muscle contraction, capillary dilation and vascular permeability. Other cells involved include eosinophils, basophils and lymphocytes (Topics B1 and T2).

Microbes may release endotoxins and/or exotoxins, both inflammatory mediators. LPS, a component of the cell wall of gram negative bacteria, is a polyclonal

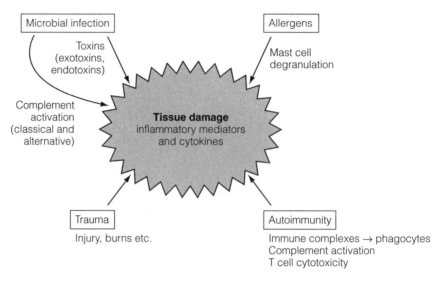

Fig. 1.   Causes of acute inflammation. The activation phase of the acute inflammatory response may be initiated by trauma, infection, allergy and autoimmune reactions, although the latter is more often associated with the chronic form of inflammation. While the initiating events may be different, the overall inflammatory response is similar, with the exception of inflammation caused by IgE/mast cell interactions where the response may be immediate and more systemic.

activator of the immune system that causes the release of a wide variety of pro-inflammatory cytokines including IL-1, IL-6, IL-12, IL-18, TNFα and IFNγ. Bacterial toxins may also cause tissue damage by stimulating release of thrombin, histamine and cytokines and may also damage nerve endings. Microbes may also activate the classical or alternate complement pathways resulting in production of complement cleavage products which have inflammatory and/or chemoattractant properties.

In acute inflammation caused by trauma, tissue substances such as thrombin, histamine and TNFα are released. Reactions to allergens are a major cause of acute inflammation, which occur when IgE fixed to mast cells or basophils is cross-linked by the specific allergen resulting in mast cell degranulation (Topic T2).

Less well characterized components of the acute inflammatory response are those of the nervous system. These include substance P, which affects T cell migration and communication, nerve growth factor (NGF), a powerful mast cell degranulator and T cell mitogen, and neuropeptide Y, a potent mast cell degranulator.

The activation phase of the acute inflammatory response may also be initiated by autoimmunity. This involves T and B cells, immune complex deposition, complement activation through the classical pathway and the release of pro-inflammatory cytokines. These factors cause inflammation and the infiltration of neutrophils and macrophages into the site of injury. Tissue destruction similar to that seen in trauma follows with further amplification of the inflammatory process. In general, because of the persistence of autoantigen, chronic inflammation ensues and it is this process which often leads to the tissue damaging reactions seen in autoimmune diseases.

Vascular changes   Inflammatory mediators increase blood flow and smooth muscle contraction and cause changes in tight junctions in endothelial cells that result in edema. In addition these mediators cause rapid alterations to the blood vessel endothelium and induce increased expression of cellular adhesion molecules. These molecules assist in the transfer of blood leukocytes and serum proteins into the damaged tissues so as to combat the infectious agent and/or help repair the damage. Cells entering the site of injury release cellular products that may further the inflammatory process and in some instances cause collateral damage as a result of the release of reactive oxygen species.

In particular, IL-1 and TNFα cause increased expression of ICAM-1 and VCAM-1 adhesion molecules, central to the progression of acute inflammation. Adhesion molecules expressed on the surface of endothelial cells interact with their counter-receptor (ligand) on leukocytes (e.g. ICAM-1 binds to LFA-1, VCAM-1 binds to VLA-4). This is important in the movement of cells from the blood to the site of injury (*Fig. 2*), and involves the capture and rolling of cells, followed by their activation, flattening, and extravasation.

Mast cells play a pivotal role in this process (*Fig. 3*). Their products include a variety of pro-inflammatory molecules including IL-1, TNFα, vasoactive amines, leukotrienes, PAF and nitric oxide, some of which cause blood vessel dilation and edema and increase adhesion of neutrophils and monocytes to endothelium. Mast cells will also degranulate as a result of nervous system release of neuropeptide Y or NGF. Complement cleavage products C3a, C4a and C5a may also be involved, as they trigger release of histamine from mast cells, which induces vascular changes leading to edema. These three complement cleavage products also increase neutrophil and monocyte adherence to endothelial cells. Thus, while the inflammatory mediators associated with the initiating events of acute inflammation may be different, they share common pathways in the inflammatory process as a result of the intimate involvement of mast cells in this process. TNFα and IL1 produced by macrophages following activation by endotoxins released from microbes also plays a role in altering vascular permeability.

Termination of the response and repair

Once the offending insult has been removed or controlled, inhibitors dampen inflammation and tissue repair mechanisms become activated. Inhibitors of the pro-inflammatory cytokines include soluble receptors (sIL-1 RA, sTNFαR, sIL-6R,

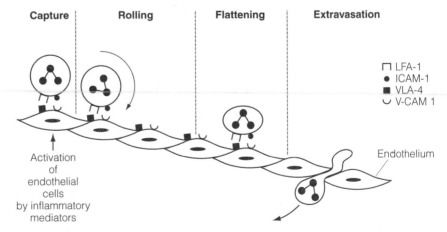

Fig. 2. Adhesion to endothelium and extravasation of neutrophils. Inflammatory mediators activate endothelial cells resulting in expression of adhesion molecules (e.g. ICAM-1 and VCAM-1). These capture leukocytes expressing LFA-1 and VLA-4 (e.g. PMNs) respectively causing them to roll, flatten and squeeze through tight junctions between the endothelial cells (extravasation) and into the tissues where inflammatory mediators are being released.

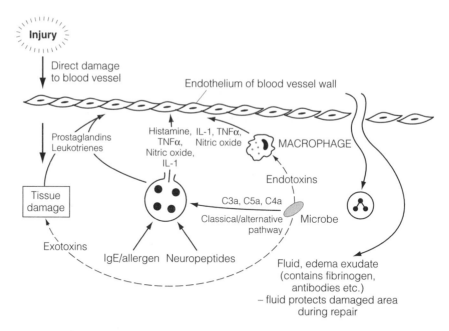

Fig. 3. The mast cell in acute inflammation. Direct tissue damage by injury or via endotoxins produced by microbes leads to release of mediators eg. prostaglandins and leukotrienes which increase vascular permeability. Tissue damage also activates mast cells which can be activated by complement components through microbes (alternative or classical pathways), via IgE/allergen complexes or neuropeptides. The inflammatory mediators released also change vascular permeability and result in vasodilation. Microbial endotoxins also activate macrophages to release TNFa and IL1 which have vasodilatory properties. The outcome of this barrage of mediators is the loosening of the endothelial tight junctions, increased adhesion of neutrophils (and monocytes) and their passage out into the surrounding tissues where they are able to phagocytose microbes. Fluid containing fibrinogen, antibodies etc is released which protects the damaged area during repair.

sIL-12R, etc.), anti-inflammatory cytokines (IL-4, IL-10 and TGFβ), components of the hemostasis and thrombosis system, and glucocorticoids.

The Th2 cytokine IL-4 down-regulates the production of pro-inflammatory cytokines from Th1 cells and TGFβ is a potent inhibitor of many immune functions (Topic N3). Protein C, a component of the hemostasis and thrombosis system, is an anti-inflammatory agent and functions by inhibiting cytokines such as TNFα. Glucocorticoids are well known as anti-inflammatory agents and inhibit production of nearly all pro-inflammatory mediators (Topic N5). Other hormones such as α-melanocyte-stimulating hormone (αMSH) and corticotrophin also have immune inhibitory effects. αMSH reduces fever, IL-2 synthesis and prostaglandin production while corticotrophin inhibits macrophage activation and IFNγ synthesis. The neuropeptides somatostatin and VIP reduce inflammation by inhibiting T cell proliferation and migration.

As the inflammatory phase is neutralized by these anti-inflammatory molecules, repair of the damage begins and involves various cells including myofibroblasts and macrophages, both of which make collagen required to mend tissues.

J1 THE CELLULAR BASIS OF THE ANTIBODY RESPONSE

Key Notes

Selection and activation of B cells	Antigen introduced into an individual binds specifically to B cells with receptors for that antigen. In the presence of T cell help these B cells clonally expand and some differentiate into plasma cells which make antibody specific for the antigen triggering the response.
Primary and memory responses	On first exposure to antigen, a primary immune response develops resulting in production of IgM antibodies. This is usually followed by an IgG immune response within 4–5 days. This response is self limiting and will stop when antigen is no longer available to stimulate B cells. When antigen is reintroduced, there are more antigen specific B cells which have differentiated to more responsive memory B cells, resulting in a more rapid response and usually in IgG antibody production.
Responses are usually multiclonal	Antibodies produced by a single cell are homogeneous, but the response to a given antigen involves many different specific antibody producing cells and thus, overall, is very heterogeneous (i.e. multiclonal). Moreover, the effectiveness of an antibody response to a microorganism may depend on this heterogeneity.
Cross-reactive responses	Similar or identical antigenic determinants are sometimes found in association with widely different molecules or cells. This cross-reactivity is important: (a) in protection against organisms with cross-reactive antigens; and (b) in autoimmune diseases induced by infectious organisms bearing antigens cross-reactive with normal self antigens (e.g. streptococcal infections which predispose to rheumatic fever).
Related topics	Lymphocytes (D1) Antibody classes (F2) Affinity maturation and class switching (J2)	T helper cells (K3) B cell activation (L3) Genes, T helper cells and cytokines (N3)

| **Selection and activation of B cells** | When antigen is introduced into an individual, B cells with receptors for that antigen bind and internalize it into an endosomal compartment, and process and present it on MHC class II molecules to helper T cells (Topics H2 and H4). These B cells are triggered to proliferate, giving rise to clones of large numbers of daughter cells. Some of the cells of these expanding clones serve as memory cells, others differentiate and become plasma cells (Topic E3) which make and secrete |

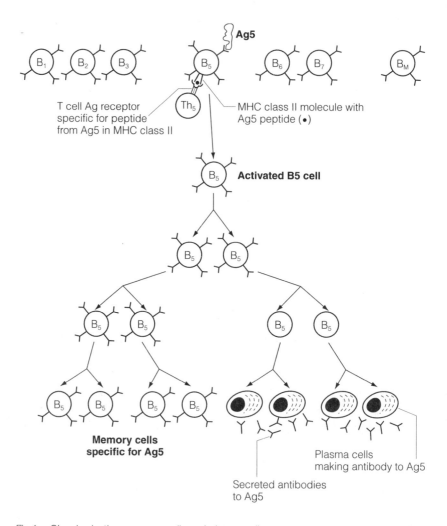

Fig.1. Clonal selection, memory cells and plasma cells.

large quantities of specific antibody. For example, on introduction of antigen 5 (Ag5) into a person (*Fig. 1*), more than 10^6 B cells have the opportunity to interact with it. Only a very few B cells (e.g. B5) have receptors specific for this antigen. B5 binds Ag5, internalizes, and processes and presents it on MHC class II molecules on the surface of this B cell. T helper cells with specific receptors for a peptide from Ag5 in MHC class II bind to this complex and stimulate this B cell to clonally expand and differentiate into memory B cells and plasma cells which produce soluble antibody to Ag5. In addition, direct T cell interaction with the B cell induces class switching, which depending on the type of helper cell (Th1 vs Th2) and the cytokines it secretes, will result in production of antibody of the IgG, IgA or IgE classes (Topic F2).

Primary and memory responses

When introduced into an individual who has not previously encountered the antigen (e.g. microbe), a **primary** immune response will develop within 4–5 days (*Fig. 2*). This response results initially in the production of IgM and then IgG or other antibody isotypes directed toward the antigen, and has a duration and

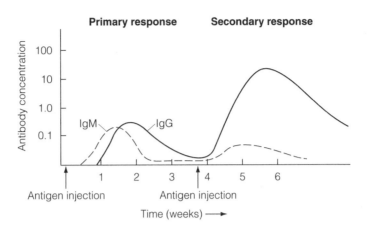

Fig. 2.   Kinetics of the immune response.

antibody isotype profile which depends on the quantity of antigen introduced and its mode of entry. The antibody produced reacts with remaining antigen, forming complexes and/or precipitates which are eliminated by phagocytes. Antibody is continually made by plasma cells during their short life span (3–4 days). If enough antigen is introduced initially, there could be restimulation of antigen specific B cells, subsequent development of more plasma cells and thus increased production of antibody. Eventually, when all of the antigen has been removed and none remains to stimulate B cells, the antibody response will reach its peak and the concentration of antibody in the circulation will begin to decrease as a result of the normal rate of catabolism of the antibody.

At the time antigen is reintroduced, more antigen specific B cells exist in the individual compared with the period before primary introduction of antigen. Moreover, these cells have differentiated to more responsive memory B cells. Thus, a secondary (**memory** or anamnestic) antibody response occurs which is characterized by a much shorter lag period before significant levels of antibody are found in the serum, by the presence of many more plasma cells, by a higher rate of antibody production, and thus a much higher serum concentration of antibody, usually of the IgG class.

Responses are usually multiclonal

Although antibodies produced by a single cell and its daughter cells are identical (homogeneous or monoclonal), the response to a given antigen involves many different clones of cells and thus, overall, is very heterogeneous (multiclonal). Considering the size of an antigenic determinant, the number of determinants on a molecule, and the number of different molecules on a microorganism, the response to a microorganism results in a large number of different antibodies (*Fig. 3*). Even antibodies against a single antigenic determinant are heterogeneous, indicating that the immune system is capable of producing many different antibodies, even to a single well-defined antigenic determinant. This heterogeneity is essential for many of the protective functions of antibodies (Topic F5).

Cross-reactive responses

Occasionally, a similar or identical antigenic determinant is found in association with widely different molecules or cells. This is termed cross-reactivity. Thus, the presence in most individuals of antibodies directed toward blood group carbohydrates other than their own is a result of the presence on certain

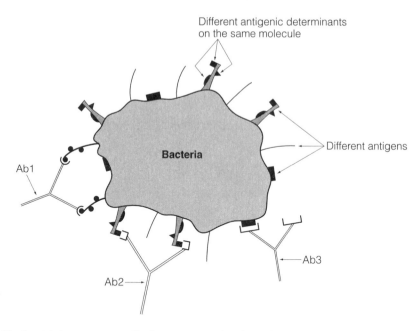

Fig. 3. A heterogeneous antibody response against bacteria.

microorganisms of carbohydrate antigens which are very similar, if not identical, with the blood group antigens. Infection with such an organism causes the production of antibodies directed toward the antigenic determinants of the microorganism including these carbohydrate antigens (*Table 1*).

The development of immunity to one organism could, in some instances, protect against infection by another organism with cross-reactive antigens. Many vaccines are effective because of similar or identical determinants expressed by: (a) both virulent and avirulent strains of the organism; or (b) toxic molecules and their non-toxic derivative (Topic R4). Natural or innate antibody to a wide variety of molecules is probably a result of the same phenomenon. In addition, certain kinds of autoimmune disease may be due to infection by organisms bearing antigens that are cross-reactive with normal self antigens. Group A β-hemolytic streptococcal infections may lead to rheumatic fever as a result of the development of antibodies to the streptococcal determinants. Because of the similarity of the streptococcal antigens to molecules in heart tissue, the antibodies may then react with and damage not only the microorganism but also heart muscle cells (Topic U3).

Table 1. Examples of clinically relevant cross-reactivity

Immunogen	Cross-reactive antigen	Importance
Tetanus toxoid	Tetanus toxin	Protection vs bacterial toxin
Sabin attenuated strain of polio virus	Poliomyelitis	Protection vs pathogenic polio virus
Various microorganisms	Type A and type B RBC carbohydrates	Transfusions
β-hemolytic *Streptococcus*	Heart tissue antigens	Rheumatic fever

J2 AFFINITY MATURATION AND CLASS SWITCHING

Key Notes

Affinity maturation

Antibodies produced in the secondary response have higher affinity for antigen than those produced in the primary response due to (a) more memory cells after antigenic challenge, of which those with the highest affinity antigen receptors compete successfully for limited amounts of antigen, and (b) point mutations in the DNA of the variable regions of the antibody L- and H-chains, which result in antibodies with increased affinity for antigen.

Class switching

IgM antibodies are produced first in an immune response followed by a switch to IgG, IgA or IgE. Class switch depends on (a) interaction of CD154 on T cells with CD40 on B cells and (b) the cytokines produced by the T helper cell: IL-4 induces switch to IgE; IL-5 to IgA; IFNγ to IgG1.

Related topics

Antibody classes (F2)
Generation of diversity (F3)
Cytokine families (G2)

T helper cells (K3)
Genes, T helper cells and cytokines (N3)

Affinity maturation
Antibodies produced in the secondary response usually have higher affinity for (tighter binding to) the antigen than those produced in the primary response. This is partly due to clonal selection and the presence of larger quantities of memory cells after antigenic challenge. In a secondary response there are more antigen binding B cells than during the primary response, and the quantity of antigen may be insufficient to stimulate all cells that could bind the antigen. Thus, when antigen is limited, the cells with the highest affinity antigen receptors will compete most successfully for the antigen. These cell populations are stimulated and give rise to plasma cells making their higher affinity antibody and thus the total pool of antibody will increase in affinity. In addition, affinity also increases after class switching because of increased point mutations in the DNA of the variable regions of the antibody L- and H-chains. Although some of these mutations result in loss of binding activity of the antibody, others will result in antibodies with increased affinity for their antigen. B cells with these antibodies as receptors will compete more effectively for antigen and be more likely to be stimulated to proliferate and differentiate. The resulting plasma cells make the higher affinity antibody and overall the affinity of the antibody population to that antigen increases. This process mainly takes place in germinal centers in lymphoid tissues (Topic D2).

Class switching   IgM antibodies are produced first in an immune response followed by a switch to
IgG or other antibody classes. This occurs on an individual cell basis, since each
cell initially expresses IgM antibodies and after activation undergoes switching to
a different class of antibody without changing its specificity for antigen (Topic F3).
This class switch is dependent on signaling by a T helper cell and in particular
requires binding of the CD40 ligand (CD154) on T cells to CD40 on B cells. In
addition, the cytokines produced by the T helper cell influence the constant region
gene to which class switching occurs. Th2 cells producing IL-4 (Topic G2) induce
B cells to class switch to IgE; IL-5, which is also produced by Th2 cells, induces B
cells to class switch to IgA; IFNγ produced by Th1 cells induces class switching to
IgG1 (*Fig. 1*).

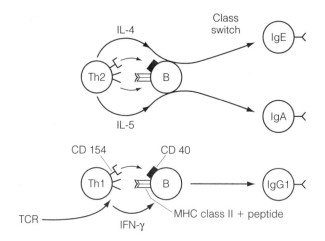

Fig. 1.   Class switching is mediated through Th/B cell interactions and specific cytokines.

J3 ANTIBODY RESPONSES IN DIFFERENT TISSUES

Key Notes

Blood	Antigens introduced into the blood are picked up by splenic macrophages, dendritic cells and B cells. These cells process and present the antigen on MHC class II molecules to T helper cells, which induce B cell differentiation and class switch to IgG.
Mucosa	Antigen introduced into mucosal areas contact B cells underlying these areas, which in turn interact with Th2 cells which induce class switch to IgA or IgE. Dimeric IgA binds to the poly-Ig receptors on epithelial cells and is transported to the lumen, where it mediates protection.
Lymphatics	Antigen introduced into tissues is channeled through the lymphatics to lymph nodes, where APCs process and present it to T cells which provide help to antigen specific B cells.
Related topics	Lymphoid organs and tissues (D2)
	Mucosa-associated lymphoid tissues (D3)
	Lymphocyte traffic and recirculation (D4)
	B cells are produced in the bone marrow (E3)

Blood

The localization and mechanism of elimination of antigen depend to a large extent on the route of its introduction. When introduced into the blood, antigens are eventually trapped in the spleen. The antigen is picked up by splenic macrophages and dendritic cells which process and present pieces of the antigen (antigenic determinants) on MHC class II molecules. T helper cells recognize these MHC-peptide complexes and provide help to B cells presenting the same antigen. These T helper cells also induce class switching to IgG.

Mucosa

When introduced into mucosal areas, the antigen comes into contact with lymphocytes underlying the mucosal areas, including those in the tonsils, the appendix and Peyer's patches. As in the spleen, B cells interact with antigen through cell-surface antibodies which function as their antigen-specific receptor. T cells interact with antigen that is processed and presented by B cells, and a humoral immune response is stimulated. In this case, the T helper cell population is a Th2 cell that usually induces B cell class switch to IgA, but sometimes to IgE. Dimeric IgA is released from plasma cells, binds to the poly-Ig receptor on epithelial cells and is transported through the cell to the lumen, where it has its primary protective role (*Fig. 1*).

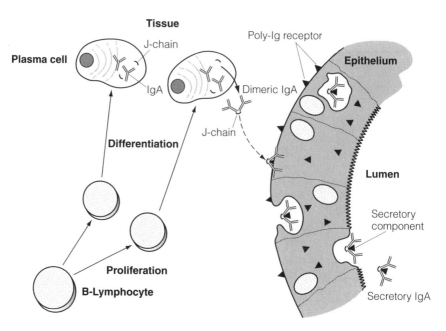

Fig.1.   Transport of IgA across the epithelium.

Lymphatics

Antigen introduced into tissues is channeled through the lymphatics to the lymph nodes, where again, B cells, macrophages or dendritic cells trap, process the antigen and present it to T cells for initiation of specific immune responses. Antigen is also picked up by dendritic cells (Langerhans cells) in the dermis, processed and carried via the lymphatics to the draining lymph nodes where it is presented to T helper cells. B and T cells are concentrated in different parts of the lymph nodes, the B cells in follicles and the T cells in the paracortical areas. The center of each follicle is the germinal center and is made up of rapidly dividing B cells (Topic D2).

J4 ANTIGEN/ANTIBODY COMPLEXES (IMMUNE COMPLEXES)

Key Notes

Immune complexes *in vitro*	Combination of antibody (Ab) with a multideterminant antigen (Ag) results in a lattice of alternating molecules of Ag and Ab, which grows until large precipitating aggregates are formed (equivalence). In Ab excess or in Ag excess, less lattice formation occurs and soluble complexes form.
Immune complexes *in vivo*	Introduction of Ag *in vivo* results in an immune response in which there is initially Ag excess. Within days, as Ab is produced, equivalence is reached and the resulting immune complexes are removed by phagocytic cells. After Ag removal, B cell stimulation stops, and the Ab concentration in the serum decreases as a result of normal catabolism.
Immune complexes and tissue damage	Persistence of Ag (microbial or self) may result in continual formation of immune complexes that with an 'overwhelmed' phagocytic system are deposited in tissues resulting in damage (type III hypersensitivity) mediated mainly by complement and neutrophils.
Related topics	Phagocytes (B1)
	Basic structure (F1)
	The acute inflammatory response (I)
	Immune-complex mediated (type III) hypersensitivity (T4)

Immune complexes *in vitro*

Immunogens have more than one antigenic determinant per molecule (are multideterminant). Immunization with antigen therefore results in many antibody populations, each directed toward different determinants on the protein. Since one molecule of Ab (IgG) can react with two molecules of Ag, and one molecule of Ag can react with many molecules of Ab, a lattice or framework consisting of alternating molecules of Ag and Ab is produced which precipitates. The extent to which a lattice forms depends on the relative amounts of Ag and Ab present (*Fig. 1*). As the amount of Ag added increases, the amount of precipitate and Ab in the precipitate increases, until a maximum is reached, and then decreases with further addition of Ag. When there is both sufficient Ag and sufficient Ab, the combination of Ag and Ab proceeds until large aggregates are formed, which are insoluble and precipitate (**equivalence**). However, in **Ab excess** or in **Ag excess**, less lattice formation occurs and more soluble complexes are formed.

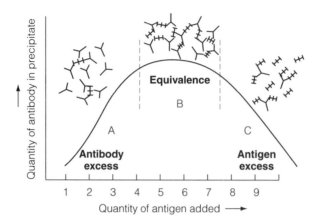

Fig.1. Immune complex formation and precipitation. The same amount of Ab to a protein was added to each of a series of tubes (1–9), followed by the addition of increasing amounts of the protein Ag to each successive tube. (A) The zone of Ab excess; (B) Zone of equivalence in which all of the Ag and Ab are incorporated into a precipitate; and (C) The zone of Ag excess.

Immune complexes *in vivo*

These reactions occur *in vivo* during an immune response. Initially, there is Ag excess as no Ab to the Ag is present at the time of first contact with the Ag. Within days however, plasma cells develop, producing Ab to the Ag which complex with it (Ag excess). As more Ab is produced, equivalence is reached resulting in large Ag–Ab complexes which are removed by phagocytic cells through interaction with their Fc and complement receptors. Plasma cells continue to produce Ab during their short life, increasing the Ab concentration in the serum (Ab excess). However, as Ag has been removed, no further restimulation of B cells occurs and no more plasma cells develop. Thus, the Ab concentration in the serum begins to decrease as a result of normal catabolism.

Immune complexes and tissue damage

If the Ag persists (e.g. with some infectious organisms such as *Streptococcus*) or is self Ag, immune complexes are continually formed and may not readily be removed due to an 'overwhelmed' phagocytic system. This can lead to the deposition of immune complexes in tissues resulting in damaging reactions (type III hypersensitivity, Topic T4). The complexes activate complement and induce an acute inflammatory response (Topic I1). Direct interaction of the immune complexes with Fc and complement receptors on the neutrophils causes the release of proteolytic enzymes which damage surrounding tissues.

K1 CELL MEDIATED IMMUNITY

Key Notes

T cell-mediated immunity	Cell mediated immunity (or T cell-mediated immunity) is due to the direct action of T cells, and can be transferred by cells, which distinguishes it from humoral immunity, which is mediated by, and can be transferred by, antibodies.
Functionally distinct T cell subpopulations	T cells have two major roles which are carried out by two distinct subpopulations. T helper (Th) cells help other cells carry out their functions, whilst T cytotoxic (Tc) cells directly kill cells infected with intracellular microbes. Both Tc and Th cells need to interact directly with the cells they are going to kill/help and they do this through specific recognition mechanisms. This is mediated through interaction with MHC molecules on the surface of the cells being targeted for help or cytotoxicity.
Cell-mediated immunity in context	Antigen presenting cells (APCs) initially process and present microbial peptides via the exogenous pathway in association with MHC class II molecules. Th cells recognize and are activated by interaction with these cells, and in turn influence APC function by direct interaction and cytokines. These APCs may then present antigen more efficiently in association with MHC class I to CTLs and class II to Th cells. Specific Th cells activate macrophages (by release of IFNγ); specific CTLs kill infected cells expressing viral antigens in association with MHC class I.
Related topics	The major histocompatibility complex and antigen processing and presentation (H4)
	Immunity to different organisms (O2)

T cell-mediated immunity

Cell mediated immunity is due to the direct action of T cells, which distinguishes it from immunity mediated by antibodies (humoral immunity). These terms evolved from the finding that immunity to certain antigens could be transferred to other animals by either cells, if they were of the same inbred strain, or antibodies. T cell immunity provides protection against intracellular microbes (viruses and some bacteria) but is also important in providing help for the development of humoral immunity, needed to combat extracellular microbes and those in transport to sites of intracellular habitat (e.g. some viruses: Topics O1 and O2).

Functionally distinct T cell subpopulations

Cell mediated immunity is a function of two distinct T cell subpopulations. In particular, T helper (Th) cells are required for activation and differentiation of certain other cells (e.g. B cells) of the immune system, whilst cytotoxic T cells (Tc) directly kill cells infected with intracellular microbes. Both Tc (also referred to as cytotoxic T lymphocytes, CTLs) and Th cells need to interact directly with the cells they are going to kill/help, and do this through specific recognition mechanisms. In addition to specifically binding appropriately presented antigen, Th cells also have receptors which bind to the nonpolymorphic region of MHC class II, restricting these cells to recognize only peptides presented on MHC class II molecules. This interaction activates Th cells to produce cytokines and to proliferate and differentiate into memory T cells. In turn, the Th cell provides essential help for activation, proliferation and differentiation of the antigen presenting cell (e.g. dendritic cells, macrophages and B cells). Th cells are also subdivided into Th1 and Th2 cells based on their cytokine profiles and functional activity. Like Th cells, Tc cells also specifically bind appropriately presented antigen, but these cells have receptors which bind to the nonpolymorphic region of MHC class I, restricting them to recognize only peptides presented on MHC class I molecules. Tc cells kill virus infected cells by induction of apoptosis (programed cell death).

Cell-mediated immunity in context

To understand and appreciate the various functional activities of the different T cell subpopulations, it is important to first put these cells and their properties into a relevant context, e.g. to consider the role of these cells in immunity to an infectious organism. Microbes first entering the body are taken up into dendritic cells or macrophages (antigen presenting cells) through interaction with innate immune system receptors (*Fig. 1*; Topic H1). If the microbe has been previously encountered, this uptake may be enhanced by opsonization of the microbe with antibody and/or complement and subsequent interaction with Fc and complement receptors, respectively. These antigen presenting cells process microbial proteins via the exogenous pathway displaying peptides from these proteins on their surface in association with MHC class II molecules. Th cells recognizing antigen on these APCs are activated (Topic L2) to produce cytokines, including IFNγ or IL-4. In addition, the interaction of the Th cell with the antigen presenting cell along with the cytokines produced, 'conditions' the antigen presenting cell such that it can interact with and prime CTLs. Dendritic cells, in particular, when primed are able to pick up exogenous antigen and present it on MHC class I molecules to CTL, as well as on MHC class II molecules to Th cells. That is, there is some crossing of exogenous antigen into the endogenous pathway with the consequence that some peptides become associated with MHC class I molecules. Thus, in the presence of antigen and cytokines, specific Th *and* CTLs are generated. The 'primed' Th and CTLs are 'effector cells' which can then deal with infected cells. Specific Th1 cells will attach to macrophages presenting antigen in association with MHC class II molecules and produce IFNγ, resulting in activation of killing mechanisms in the macrophage. Other Th cells will interact with antigen presented by B cells and help them to produce antibodies to deal with those microbes accessible to antibody and complement (Topic F5). Conversely, specific CTLs attaching to virus infected cells via antigen presented in MHC class I molecules will be activated to release perforins and granzymes and kill the infected cell.

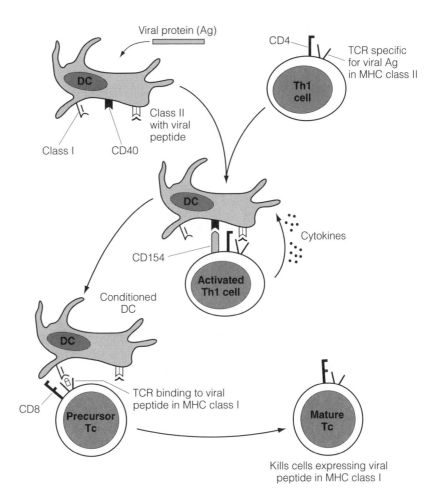

Fig. 1. Dendritic cells (DC) conditioned (licensed) by Th1 cells present antigen to Tc via MHC class I. Interaction of specific Th1 cells with peptide (e.g. from a virus or tumor cell protein) presented in MHC class II on the DC involves adhesion molecules as well as binding of B7 to CD28. This series of interactions induces expression on the Th1 cells of CD154 which then binds CD40 on the DC. This triggering through CD40, in the presence of cytokines also released by Th1 cells, conditions the DC to present antigen in MHC class I to peptide specific Tc precursor cells, inducing their maturation into Tc cells.

K2 T CYTOTOXIC CELLS

Key Notes

Peptide recognition and activation of cytotoxic T cells	CTLs express CD8 on their surface to interact with MHC class I molecules presenting peptides derived from an intracellular microbe (usually virus). CD8 binding to the nonpolymorphic MHC class I molecules on infected cells stabilizes the Tc:target cell interaction, and thus facilitates TcR binding to specific peptides in the polymorphic part of MHC class I. Activation of CTLs by interaction with virus infected cells induces expression of Fas ligand (FasL) which is important in killing virus infected cells expressing Fas.
Mechanisms of cytotoxicity	Cytotoxicity by Tc can be mediated through (a) lytic granule release of perforin and granzymes onto the surface of the target cell, and (b) interaction of FasL on the CTL with Fas on infected cells. Both mechanisms result in programed cell death (apoptosis) of the infected cell.
Related topics	The major histocompatibility complex and antigen processing and presentation (H4) T cell activation (L2) Immunity to different organisms (O2)

Peptide recognition and activation of cytotoxic T cells

Peptides derived from proteins of intracellular microbes are processed via the endogenous route and are presented on the cell surface in MHC class I molecules, marking this cell as infected and as a target for CTL killing. CTLs express cell surface CD8 which binds to the nonpolymorphic region of MHC class I (expressed on all nucleated cells), restricting these killer T cells to recognizing only cells presenting peptide in MHC class I molecules (Topic H3). This interaction also serves to stabilize the interaction of the T cell receptor with specific peptides bound to the polymorphic part of the MHC class I molecule (*Fig. 1*). Other surface co-stimulatory and adhesion molecules are important for close interaction of the CTL with the infected cell and for activating its cytotoxic machinery (Topic L2). This activation step also induces the expression of FasL on the Tc and this can interact with the Fas expressed on the surface of the virus-infected cell.

Mechanisms of cytotoxicity

CTL induction of programed cell death (apoptosis) of virus infected cells is mediated through two distinct pathways: (a) Release of lytic granules containing perforin and granzymes which enter the target cell; (b) Interaction of FasL with Fas on the CTL and target cell, respectively.

CTL contain large cytolytic granules and are difficult to distinguish morphologically from NK cells (also called large granular lymphocytes;Topic B2). These intra-cytoplasmic granules contain proteases, granzyme a and granzyme b, and perforin, a molecule similar to C9 of the complement pathway. On interaction of the CTL with a virus infected cell, the granules move toward the portion of the membrane close to the point of contact with the target cell. On fusion with the

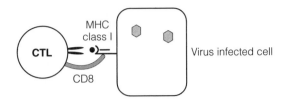

Fig. 1. CTL recognise peptides associated with MHC class I molecules. CD8 binds to non-polymorphic MHC class I stabilizing this interaction and enhancing killing.

membrane, the granules release perforins which polymerize in the membrane of the infected cell creating pores that allow entry of the proteases (*Fig. 2*). These enzymes cleave cellular proteins, the products of which initiate induction of programed cell death (apoptosis). CTL then re-synthesize their granular contents in preparation for specific killing of another infected cell. Nucleated cells of the body infected with some viruses upregulate expression of Fas (CD95). CTL activated to release their granules by their first encounter with antigen, presented in MHC class I molecules, are induced to upregulate FasL which then also allows them to kill specific virus infected cells by an additional mechanism through interaction with surface CD95 (*Fig. 3*). The importance of apoptosis as a killing mechanism used by the immune system is that targeted cells can be removed rapidly by phagocytes without any inflammatory response. Another mechanism of cell death – necrosis – follows tissue trauma or certain kinds of infection and leads to acute inflammation through the production of inflammatory cellular products. This then leads to tissue repair mechanisms (Topic I1).

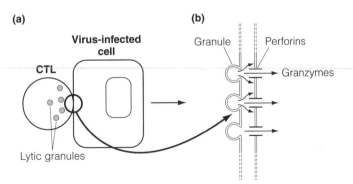

Fig. 2. Apoptosis induced by release of lytic granules. Perforins polymerize in the membrane leading to passage of granzymes into the cell. (a) Lytic granules containing perforin and granzymes accumulate at the point of contact of CTL (via TCR/MHC and other molecules) with virus infected cell. (b) The granule contents are released, the perforin polymerizes and inserts itself into the infected cell membrane allowing entry of granzymes which induce apoptosis.

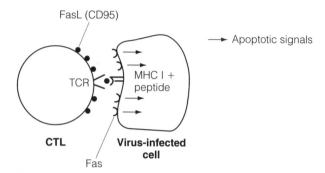

Fig. 3.   Apoptosis induced by Fas/FasL interactions. CTL have preformed FasL in their granules which is rapidly expressed on their surface when they attach via their TCR to the target cell. Ligation of Fas on the target is an additional mechanism for induction of apoptosis of the infected cell.

K3 T HELPER CELLS

Key Notes

T helper cells

Th cells express CD4 on their cell surface which interacts with MHC class II molecules on cells requiring help. They function in two complementary ways: (a) through molecular interactions during contact of the Th cell with the antigen presenting cell; (b) through production of cytokines.

Two types of T helper cells – Th1 and Th2

T helper cells are divided into two main types dependent on their cytokine profiles. Th1 cells or inflammatory T cells produce high levels of IFNγ and TNFα which primarily act on macrophages to cause their activation and Th2 cells which are characterized by production of IL-4, IL-5 and IL-6 and are involved mainly in B cell differentiation and maturation.

Related topics

Cytokine familes (G2)
Affinity maturation and class
  switching (J2)

Genes, T helper cells and
  cytokines (N3)
The microbial cosmos (O1)

T helper cells

T helper cells express CD4, a ligand for MHC class II, which restricts the interaction of Th cells to those cells in the body which express MHC class II molecules (Section H). This binding of CD4 on the Th to MHC class II on cells requiring help permits more productive interaction of the T cell receptor with specific peptides bound in the MHC class II groove.

Th cells carry out their function in two complementary ways: (a) through molecular interactions during contact of the Th cell with the antigen presenting cell; (b) through production of cytokines. The resulting signals and cytokines activate and/or modulate functions of the antigen presenting cell, e.g. B cells are induced to undergo class switching and proliferation (Topics F2, G2, J2, L3).

Two types of T helper cells – Th1 and Th2

CD4 T cells can differentiate down at least two pathways to become inflammatory T cells (Th1), or Th2 cells which help B cells. Th1 cells are predominately involved in mediating inflammatory immune responses (through the activation of macrophages), while Th2 cells are primarily involved in the induction of humoral immunity (via the activation of B cells). Th1 cells produce cytokines that primarily act on macrophages (IFNγ and TNFα) whilst Th2 cells are involved mainly in B cell differentiation and maturation (via IL-4, IL-5 and IL-6). It is important to remember, that in most cases, an immune response elicits both Th1 and Th2 activities, although there are some instances where one or the other is more effective in mediating protection.

Th2 cells (humoral immunity)
Participation of T cells is required for B cell responses to most antigens (Topic L3). T cells most effective in inducing the production of antibody from B cells,

especially of the IgA and IgE isotype, are the helper CD4 T cells. Th2 cells are able to induce B cells to produce Ig, switch the isotype of Ig being produced, and induce affinity maturation of the Ig. This involves not only cytokines but direct engagement of surface molecules on the T and B cells (cognate interactions) which trigger their activation.

Th2 cells recognize antigenic peptides on the surface of antigen-specific B cells and through interaction with other surface molecules are activated (Topics H4 and L2). Cell–cell interactions involving especially Th cell CD40L binding to CD40 on B cells, as well as cytokines produced by the Th2 cells, are important in inducing B cell proliferation and further differentiation into plasma cells and class switching into IgE and IgA producing cells (Topic J2, *Fig. 1*).

Th1 cells (inflammatory immune responses)

The response to a variety of intracellular parasites is dependent upon functionally intact inflammatory T cells. For example, the immune responses to *Leishmania* and mycobacteria are severely diminished if the host cannot produce IFNγ and TNF. This is because, in the absence of these mediators, infected macrophages cannot become activated to kill the pathogen. Although other cytokines can augment macrophage activities, both IFNγ and TNF are critical for effective macrophage activation.

Th1 cells when activated also produce cytokines that assist in the recruitment of macrophages to the site of infection. These include two hematopoeitic growth factors; granulocyte-macrophage stimulatory factor (GM-CSF) and IL-3, which heighten the production and release of macrophages from the bone marrow. Secondly, TNF from Th1 cells alters the surface properties of endothelial cells to promote the adhesion of macrophages at the site of infection. The coordinated production of these mediators allows the infiltration of T cells and macrophages to the site of inflammation where their interaction leads to macrophage activation and the elimination of the pathogen (*Fig. 1*).

Th1 cells may also be involved in inducing B cells to produce Ig, switch the isotype of Ig produced, and to undergo affinity maturation of the Ig (Topic J2, *Fig. 1*). As with Th2 cells, this involves both cytokines and the expression of cell surface molecules that directly engage the cognate B cell and trigger its activation. However, a different set of cytokines (IFNγ and TNFα) are involved than those associated with Th2 cells, resulting in signals and help for the development of B cells that produce primarily IgG antibodies.

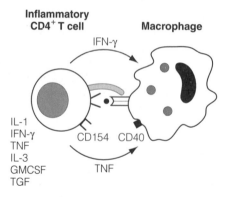

Inflammatory CD4+ T cell

Macrophage

IFN-γ

IL-1
IFN-γ
TNF
IL-3
GMCSF
TGF

CD154   CD40

TNF

Fig. 1.   Macrophage activation by CD4+ inflammatory T cells. Cytokines released by Th1 cells, as well as signaling through direct contact of cell surface receptors, increase: (a) fusion of lysozomes and phagosomes; (b) production of nitric oxide and oxygen radicals for killing pathogens; and (c) expression of MHC class II molecules and TNF receptors. Note that CD154/CD40 interactions are also important in activation of the macrophage.

L1 RECEPTORS, CO-RECEPTORS AND SIGNALING

Key Notes

Receptor–ligand interactions	Lymphocytes need to be activated in order to carry out their function. Binding of the lymphocyte to an antigen via its antigen receptor, *signal 1*, is necessary, but not sufficient to stimulate it and leads to anergy. Accessory and co-stimulatory molecules on the surface of T and B cells and APCs are required for cell–cell interaction and the signal transduction events leading to activation (*signal 2*).
Signaling by co-receptors	T cell signaling is initiated through CD3, which is associated with the TcR. B cell signaling is initiated through the CD79a/b complex associated with the BcR. Both initiate phosphorylation of tyrosine motifs (ITAMs), which is followed by an ordered series of biochemical events involving kinases and phosphatases. These events are modulated by signals from co-receptors. Second messengers lead to activation of transcription factors and thus to activation of lymphocyte function.
Related topics	Dendritic cells (B4) Lymphocytes (D1) B cell recognition of antigen, the B cell receptor complex and co-receptors (H2) T cell recognition of antigen, the T cell receptor complex (H3) The major histocompatibility complex and antigen processing and presentation (H4)

Receptor–ligand interactions

Lymphocytes need to be activated in order to carry out their function. At the molecular level this means receiving a message from outside the cell via interaction with a cell surface receptor. This signal is then passed through the cytoplasm to the nucleus (signal transduction) to induce the gene transcription required for cell proliferation and synthesis and release of effector molecules e.g. cytokines and antibodies. Although binding of the lymphocyte to an antigen via its antigen receptor (*signal 1*) is necessary to stimulate the cell, it is not sufficient and usually results in anergy. Certainly, the binding of accessory cell surface molecules (e.g. CD4 or CD8, LFA-1, CD2 and CD28 on T cells) with their counter receptors on other cells is important, as these interactions increase the avidity of cell–cell interaction. In addition, co-stimulatory molecules (some of which are also accessory molecules) modulate the signal transduction events leading to activation by providing the critical second signal (*signal 2*). T cells are stimulated via their TcR by peptide antigen bound to MHC molecules (Topic H3). B cells are activated with and without the requirement of T cells. Multimeric antigens can stimulate B cells directly whilst responses to protein antigens require T cell help.

Signaling by co-receptors   Neither of the antigen receptors on T or B cells have intracytoplasmic tails of sufficient length and amino acid composition to act as signaling molecules. Thus, T cell signaling is initiated through CD3, which is associated with the TcR, and B cell signaling through CD79a/b, which is associated with the BcR (Topic H2). These molecules have tyrosine motifs (ITAMs) that are phosphorylated by kinases to initiate the activation process. An ordered series of biochemical events then occurs via kinases and phosphatases, which is modulated by signals from other co-receptor cell surface molecules. Second messengers are produced which are eventually responsible for activation of transcription factors inside the nucleus and for production of cell cycle proteins and molecules required for lymphocyte effector functions. Cytokines induce proliferation and further differentiation of activated B and T cells.

L2 T CELL ACTIVATION

Key Notes

Accessory molecules	Initial recognition of processed antigen by T cells is via the T cell antigen receptor. Accessory molecules further link the APC and the T cell leading to a stronger cell interaction. For example CD4 binds to the constant region domain of class II MHC molecules whilst CD8 binds to class I MHC molecules. Other ligand–receptor pairs such as LFA-1 and ICAMS are also important.
Co-stimulatory molecules: two signals are required for Th cell activation	Full activation of antigen-specific T cells requires **two signals** – one signal coming via the TcR and the other signal through engagement of co-stimulatory molecules. T cells receiving one signal via their TcR are turned off (become anergic), whilst those receiving two signals e.g. via T cell CD28 binding to B7 on the APC induce T cell lymphokine production and T cell proliferation.
Super-antigens and Th cell activation	Some protein products of bacteria and viruses can initiate T cell activation by linking the TcR on T cells to the MHC class II–peptide complex on APCs without the need for antigen processing. These super-antigens include *Staphylococcal enterotoxins (SE)* that cause common food poisoning and the toxic shock syndrome toxin (TSST).
Activation of cytotoxic T cells	CD8$^+$ Tc cells also require activation to produce functional CTLs containing granules and perforin. This is mediated through attachment of their TcR to MHC class I–peptide complexes on APCs (Signal 1). In this case, however, it appears that, the second signal can only be supplied by APCs that have been conditioned by Th cells. As with Th activation, cytokines produced by Th cells and APCs are important for Tc activation.
Biochemical events leading to T lymphocyte activation	In order for a T cell to function it must convey a signal from the cell surface to the nucleus. This *signal transduction* is brought about by phosphorylation and dephosphorylation of particular amino acids thus activating them in a sequential fashion leading eventually to activation of specific transcription factors in the nucleus and production of functional proteins. Initiation of the process is through activation of a CD4 associated kinase (lymphocyte kinase; lck) by CD45 (a phosphatase) on the APC, which then phosphorylates ITAM tyrosines on the zeta chain of CD3.
Related topics	T cell recognition of antigen, the T cell receptor complex (H3) The major histocompatibility complex and antigen processing and presentation (H4)
	T cytotoxic cells (K2) Peripheral tolerance (M3) Genes, T helper cells and cytokines (N3)

Accessory molecules

Pathogens or antigens infecting peripheral sites are typically trapped in the lymph nodes directly downstream of the site of infection. Blood borne pathogens are trapped in the spleen. These secondary lymphoid organs contain APC (dendritic cells and macrophages) that efficiently trap antigen for processing and presentation. Naive T cells recirculate through these sites looking for appropriate processed antigen (Topic H3).

Initial recognition of processed antigen by T cells is via the T cell antigen receptor. To strengthen the cellular associations between the antigen-specific T cells and the APC and accessory molecules provide additional linkages between the APC and the T cell (*Fig. 1*). CD4 binds to the constant region domain of class II MHC molecules thereby strengthening the association of the TCR with peptide-class II MHC molecules. Likewise, CD8 binds to class I MHC molecules to strengthen the association of the TCR with class I MHC molecules. In addition to engagement of these ligand–receptor pairs (*Fig. 1*), additional adhesion molecules, integrins, become engaged. These include the intercellular adhesion molecules (ICAMs) and lymphocyte function-associated antigens (LFA). Some of these accessory molecules are also important in regulating early activation events through signaling, e.g. CD4 and CD8, and are sometimes termed co-receptors, as they are part of the T cell receptor complex (Topic H3).

Co-stimulatory molecules: two signals are required for Th cell activation

Ligation of the TCR on its own does not stimulate T cell clonal expansion or lymphokine production. The full activation of antigen-specific T cells requires **two signals**. Signal **one** is provided by the engagement of the T cell antigen receptor and signal **two** is provided by engagement of a co-stimulatory molecule. The best characterized co-stimulatory molecule is B7, which is on many APC and binds to CD28 on the T cell. Signals emanating from this TCR and CD28 synergize to induce T cell lymphokine production and T cell proliferation. If the T cell receives signal 1 (TCR binding) and not signal 2 (co-stimulation) the T cell is turned off (*Fig. 2*; Topics M3 and U3).

Superantigens and Th cell activation

Some protein products of bacteria and viruses produce proteins known as super-antigens that bind to lateral surfaces of the MHC class II molecules (not in the peptide binding groove) and the V region of the β subunit of the TCR. These antigens are not processed into peptides as conventional antigens, but are able to bind to a specific family of TCR. In a sense they 'glue' T cells to APC (*Fig. 3*) and cause stimulation of the T cell. However, these T cells are not specific for the

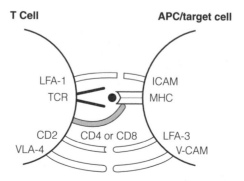

Fig. 1.   Pairs of molecules which strengthen the association of T cells with antigen presenting and target cells.

pathogen, since all members of a particular family of TCR are activated. The consequence of binding to a large percentage of the T cells is the massive production of cytokines leading, in some cases, to lymphokine-induced vascular leakage and shock. Among the bacterial superantigens are the *staphylococcal enterotoxins* (SE) that cause common food poisoning and the toxic shock syndrome toxin (TSST).

Activation of cytotoxic T cells

CD8 cytotoxic T cells also need to be activated to produce functional CTLs containing granules and perforin. This requires attachment of their TcR to MHC class I–peptide complexes on APCs (Signal 1). In addition, a second signal is provided, the nature of which is unclear but can only be supplied by APCs that have been conditioned by Th cells (see Topic K1, *Fig. 1*). As with Th activation, cytokines produced by Th cells and APCs are important for Tc activation. Of note, although other Th conditioned APCs may be able to provide the necessary signals for Tc activation, dendritic cells are the only cells which have a significant cross-over of processed antigen into exogenous and endogenous pathways (Topics H4 and K1). Moreover, they are, in general, the most efficient of the antigen presenting cells.

Biochemical events leading to T lymphocyte activation

In order for a T cell to fulfill its function it has to convey a signal from the cell surface via the cytosol into the nucleus to give rise to specific gene transcription. This *signal transduction* is brought about by several molecules at the cell surface (*Fig. 4*). The key players in this amplification process are enzymes which phosphorylate (kinases) and dephosphorylate (phosphatases) particular amino

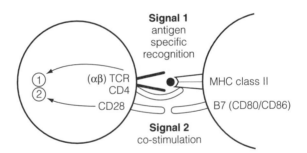

Fig. 2.   The role of co-stimulation in T cell activation.

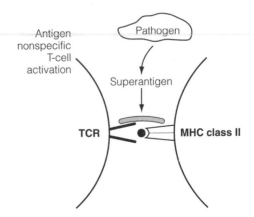

Fig. 3.   Superantigen activation of T cells by bridging TCR and MHC class II.

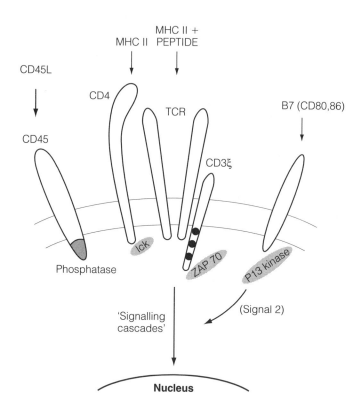

Fig. 4. CD45 and B7 (CD80/86) are important cell surface molecules involved in T cell activation. Ligation of surface receptors leads to activation of CD45 (a phosphatase) and several kinases (e.g. lck, ZAP 70, PI3 kinase). Activity of these enzymes results in 'signaling cascades' leading ultimately to transcription of specific genes. Co-stimulation via CD28 (signal 2) is necessary for cell activation and proliferation.

acids thus activating them sequentially leading eventually to activation of specific transcription factors in the nucleus and production of functional proteins. Initiation of the process is through activation of a CD4 associated kinase (lymphocyte kinase – lck) by CD45 (a phosphatase), one of its functions being to phosphorylate tyrosines of the immunostimulatory tyrosine-based activation motifs (ITAMS) on the zeta chain of CD3 (*Fig. 5*). This, in turn, activates another protein tyrosine kinase ZAP 70 which activates an enzyme responsible for activating the phosphatidyl inositol pathway and further downstream events leading to the activation of transcription factors regulating production of IL-2 and other important proteins.

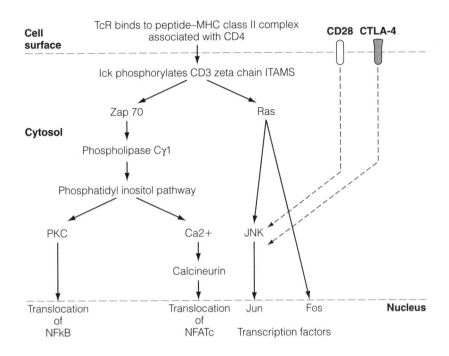

Fig. 5.   Signaling pathways leading to Th cell activation. Ligation of CD28 on the T cell (signal 2) modulates the JNK biochemical pathway in a positive way and ligation of CTLA-4 is thought to negatively influence the activation pathway thus resulting in damping down of the Th cell response. The important outcome of these processes is the production of receptors e.g. IL2R and cytokines by the cell. PKC, protein kinase C; JNK, June kinase.)

L3 B CELL ACTIVATION

Key Notes

Thymus independent (T-I) antigens

Although B cell responses to most antigens require T cell help, activation of B cells by certain antigens does not. These T independent antigens (T-I) are of two types, both of which generate primarily IgM antibodies of low affinity. Type 1 antigens are bacterial polysaccharide mitogens that activate B cells independent of their antigen receptors. Type 2 antigens are linear, poorly degradable antigens, e.g. pneumococcus polysaccharide. These antigens persist on the surface of macrophages and directly stimulate B cells through cross-linking of their surface receptors.

Thymus dependent (T-D) antigens

Th cells induce B cells to produce antibodies, to switch the isotype of antibody being produced and to undergo affinity maturation. Binding of most antigens to antigen receptors on B cells provides one signal whilst the cytokines produced by the Th cells, and the engagement of complementary surface molecules on the *cognate* B cell provides the second signal resulting in B cell activation. Th cells recognize antigenic peptides on the surface of antigen-specific B cells because the B cells can capture antigen specifically via membrane Ig and associate it with class II MHC molecules. Once triggered via the TCR, Th cells express CD40L which triggers B cell activation via its CD40 surface receptor. Activated B cells reciprocally co-stimulate T cells via CD28, which produce IL-2, IL-4 and IL-5. As a result, both the T cells and B cells clonally expand and differentiate.

Biochemical events leading to B lymphocyte activation

CD79a/b molecules transmit the first signals following B cell interaction with antigen through ITAMs of their intracytoplasmic tails. Co-receptors of the B cell receptor complex (CD21, CD19 and CD81) modulate these initial signals. CD21 binds to C3d if it is bound to the specific antigen and provides an additional positive signal in B cell activation. Cross-linking of membrane receptor antibodies on B cells by T-I antigens induces clustering of co-receptors leading to multiple signals enhancing activation of kinase networks and of IgM producing B cells. B cells primed by a T-D antigen receive a second signal when the Th cell CD40L binds to CD40 on the B cell. Together with cytokines such as IL-2, IL-4, etc., this signaling induces proliferation and differentiation of the B cells into plasma cells or memory cells.

Related topics

B cells are produced in the bone marrow (E3)

B cell recognition of antigen, the B cell receptor complex and co-receptors (H2)

The major histocompatibility complex and antigen processing

and presentation (H4)

Genes, T helper cells and cytokines (N3)

The role of antibody (N4)

Primary/congenital (inherited) immunodeficiency (S2)

Thymus independent (T-I) antigens

Although B cell responses to most antigens require T cell help, activation of B cells by certain antigens does not. For the most part, these T-independent (T-I) antigens generate primarily IgM antibodies of low affinity, whereas T-dependent (T-D) antigens generate much higher affinity antibodies of the other classes. T-I antigens are of two types.

Type 1 antigens
Bacterial polysaccharides have the ability, at high enough concentration, to activate the majority of B cells independently of their specific antigen receptors. They do this through a mitogenic component which bypasses the early biochemical pathways initiated through the antibody receptor. The B cell focuses the polysaccharide antigen and at sufficiently high concentrations drives its activation (*Fig. 1*).

Type 2 antigens
Some linear antigens that are not easily degraded and have epitopes spaced appropriately on the molecule, e.g. pneumococcus polysaccharide, can directly stimulate B cells in a T cell independent fashion. These antigens persist on the surface of splenic marginal zone and lymph node subcapsular macrophages and directly stimulate B cells through cross-linking of their surface receptors (*Fig. 2*). Although activation is independent of T cells, cytokines produced by T cells can amplify these responses.

Thymus dependent (T-D) antigens

The production of antibody to most antigens requires the participation of T cells. In particular, Th cells induce B cells to proliferate, differentiate and produce antibodies. In addition, Th cells induce switching of the class of antibody being produced and affinity maturation. To accomplish this, Th cells produce critical cytokines and directly engage the *cognate* B cell and trigger its activation through cell surface receptors. This T cell *collaboration* with B cells is necessary since binding of most (non multimeric) antigens to antigen receptors on most B cells provides one signal that, in the absence of a second signal, is an anergic signal, i.e.

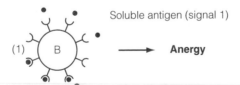

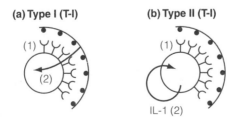

Fig. 1.   Activation of B cells through T cell independent antigens. Soluble antigen interaction with the B cell antigen receptor (antibody) results in anergy (signal 1 only). Signal 2 is provided by a mitogenic component of the type 1 antigen (a) and via autocrine activity of IL-1 for type II antigen (b).

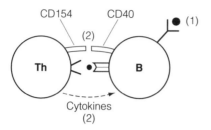

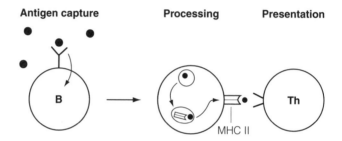

Fig. 2.   T cell activation of B cells. T cells provide the 2nd signal to B cells via ligation of CD40 by CD154 (CD40 ligand) but also via cytokines.

Fig. 3.   Activation of B cells through T cell help. Captured soluble antigens are processed and presented to Th cells which provide the 2nd signal required for B cell activation (see L3 Figure 2).

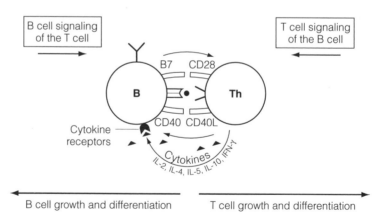

Fig. 4.   Reciprocal activation of T and B cells.

turns off the B cell. The cytokines produced by the Th cells and the engagement of complementary surface molecules provide the essential second signals to the B cell resulting in its activation (see above for T cells: *Fig. 3*).

More specifically, Th cells recognize antigenic peptides on the surface of antigen-specific B cells because the B cells are able to capture antigen specifically via membrane (m) IgM and mIgD. This feature of B cells, to capture, process and present specific antigen, makes them unique amongst the antigen-presenting cells which normally take up antigen via scavenger and other receptors (Section H). The antigen is then endocytosed, degraded via the exogenous processing pathway and peptides are associated with class II MHC molecules (*Fig. 4*; Topic H4).

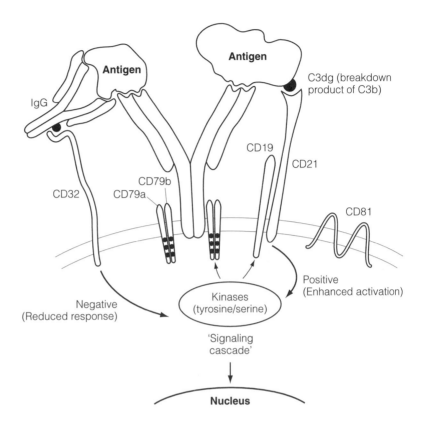

Fig. 5. Activation of B cells via the BCR and co-receptor complex. Attachment of antigen results in activation of several kinases and CD79a/b are phosphorylated on their ITAMs. Binding of CD21 to antigen bound to complement (C3dg) regulates signaling via CD19 in a positive way, whilst interaction of CD32 with IgG antibody bound to antigen and the antigen receptor, provides a negative signal (see Topic N6).

Th cells whose TCR are specific for that peptide–MHC complex, recognize and bind to B cells via TCR-MHC interactions and through engagement of adhesion molecules.

Once triggered via the TCR, the Th cells express CD40 ligand (CD40L), the ligand for the B cell surface molecule CD40. This Th cell now triggers the activation of the B cell via the CD40 surface receptor (*Fig. 5*). As a result, the activated B cell reciprocally co-stimulates the Th cell via CD28. At this time, both the T cell and B cell are stimulated. T cells then produce cytokines including IL-2 (autocrine growth factor for the Th cells) and IL-4 and IL-5 (growth and differentiation factors for the activated B cells). As a result, both the T cells and B cells clonally expand and differentiate. Ligation of B cell CD40 by CD40L on T cells is also important in that it rescues B cells with mutated antibody receptors from death in germinal centers (Topic E3).

Biochemical events leading to B cell activation

The transmembrane surface immunoglobulin antigen receptors on B cells, like the TcR on T cells have short intracytoplasmic tails unable to transduce signals themselves. Therefore, on engagement of the B cell antigen receptor, other molecules associated with these receptors mediate signaling. In particular, CD79a and b of the B cell receptor complex (Topic H2) contain ITAMs which are phosphorylated

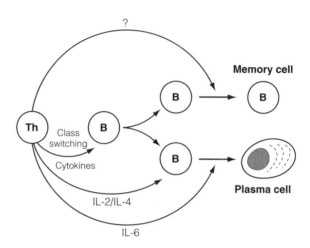

Fig. 6.   The roles of cytokines in maturation of B cells into memory and plasma cells.

during the early stages of activation and initiate the B cell signaling cascade. Other members of the B cell receptor complex (*Fig. 5*) modulate the initial signals mediated through antigen binding and enhance the strength of cell–cell interaction. For example, CD21, a complement receptor which binds C3d, may provide an additional positive signal in B cell activation as a result of binding to C3d associated with antigen. As with T cell activation, these processes in B cells are mediated through phosphatases and kinases. The importance of one kinase, btk, is indicated by the observation that mutation of the gene encoding it results in the absence of B cells (Bruton's agammaglobulinemia: Topic S2).

B cells like T cells require two signals for their activation. Binding of soluble antigen to the antibody receptor alone (signal 1) results in apoptosis. This is seen experimentally using antibodies to the sIgM on B cells. Proliferation is induced in the presence of another second signal such as that provided by IL-2. The physiological second signal for B cell activation is provided by interaction of Th cell CD40L with CD40 on the B cell surface. This is also an absolute requirement for class switching. Other cytokines produced by Th cells induce appropriate signals important to differentiation of the B cells into plasma or memory cells (*Fig. 6*). After initial B cell activation and following class switching to IgG, B cells are susceptible to regulation by concomitant binding of FcγRII (CD32) and the B cell antigen receptor. In particular, further activation of these cells can be inhibited by their binding of specific antigen attached to IgG. As a result, CD32 transmits a negative signal to the B cell and prevent its activation ('negative feedback': Topic N4).

TI antigens, which do not induce IgG responses (since their CD40 molecules are not ligated), receive their second signal via the 'mitogenic' component of T-I 1 antigens and probably via antibodies on B cells by T-I antigens with repeating antigenic units allows clustering of co-receptors which is also likely to enhance signaling. In these cases, the signals transduced are quite different from those resulting in activation of T-D B cells.

M1 CELL RECOGNITION OF SELF AND NON SELF

Key Notes

Cell recognition	It is of utmost importance that the cells of the immune system are able to recognize and kill invading microbes, and thus to be able to distinguish what is 'foreign' (i.e. non self) from self.
The innate immune system	In the innate immune system, phagocytes only recognize self cells if they are damaged or dying; natural killer cells are normally inhibited from killing self cells through inhibitory receptors; complement cannot be activated on the surfaces of normal cells due to inhibitory molecules.
The adaptive immune system	In the adaptive immune system, some lymphocytes develop which have anti-self reactivity, others develop with receptors specific for foreign antigens. Self tolerance is the state of immunological unresponsiveness to self antigens maintained through a number of different mechanisms in central and peripheral lymphoid organs. These include deletion and inactivation (anergy) mechanisms.
Related topics	Phagocytes (B1) Natural killer cells (B2) Complement (C2) Nonself recognition by the innate immune system (H1)

Cell recognition

All cells of the body recognize each other when they come into contact. Thus, in a developing embryo, cells produced from one germ layer attach to each other and not to the cells produced by other germ layers. This is maintained by cell surface molecules/receptors which interact with each other. Cells of the immune system must be able to recognize and eliminate microbes and thus to distinguish what is 'foreign' (i.e. non self) from what is self.

The innate immune system

In the case of the cells and molecules of the innate immune system which have evolved to be aggressive towards microbes there are two ways in which self reactivity is prevented: lack of recognition (ignorance) of self cells unless they change their surface structure; and the presence of inhibitory structures/receptors on the nonimmune cells.

Phagocytes
Self cells are not normally phagocytosed unless they are aging (erythrocytes), dying or dead. Phagocytes recognize microbes through receptors for sugars, e.g.

mannose. These are either absent or concealed by other structures e.g. sialic acids on the surface of mammalian cells. When an erythrocyte ages, it loses sialic acid exposing N-acetyl glucosamine which the phagocyte now recognizes as non self and phagocytoses it (*Fig. 1*). When cells die, a large number of surface molecules are exposed which are recognized by phagocytes.

Natural killer cells

These cells play an important role in killing virus infected cells. They are prevented from killing the non-infected nucleated cells of the body through a balance in signaling through killer activation receptors (KAR) and killer inhibitory receptors (KIR) recognizing molecules on self cells. However, when certain viruses infect cells they down regulate expression of molecules recognized by KIR giving rise to an overriding activation through KAR leading to death of the infected cells (*Fig. 2*).

The complement system

C3 is activated through the alternative pathway by stabilization of appropriate enzymes on the surface of some microorganisms. This cannot occur on the body's cells since they all have inhibitory molecules on their surface membranes (*Fig. 3*).

The adaptive immune system

A fundamental requirement of the immune system is that it destroy, eliminate or inactivate all foreign viruses, bacteria and parasites without destroying self cells or molecules. **Self tolerance** is the 'State of immunological unresponsiveness to self antigens'. It is maintained through a number of different mechanisms in central and peripheral lymphoid organs. The fundamental basis for self tolerance is that interaction of antigen with immature clones of lymphocytes already expressing antigen receptors, would result in an unresponsive state. This theory, for which Burnet and Medawar received the Nobel Prize in 1960, is now recognized to involve a mechanism that causes self-reactive lymphocytes to be eliminated (**clonal deletion**) on contact with self antigens. Immature cells derived from bone marrow stem cells migrate to the thymus to mature into immunocompetent T cells or mature in the bone marrow to become B cells. In the thymus, self-reactive T cells are clonally eliminated by negative selection as part

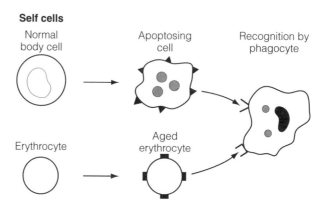

Fig. 1.   Recognition of aged/damaged self cells by phagocytes.

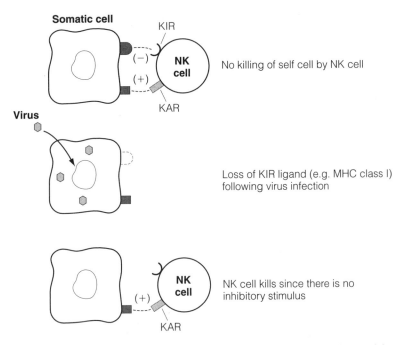

Fig. 2. *Inhibition of NK cell activity. NK cells recognize self-antigens and travel around the body in search of aberrant self-cells. When they come into contact with a healthy cell they receive two signals – a positive signal to kill via their KAR (killer activation receptors) and a negative signal via their KIR (killer inhibitory receptors). These two signals cancel each other out and the NK cell goes on its way. Some viruses inhibit expression of the self-molecules recognized by the KIR (e.g. MHC class I, HLA-A, B, C in man) which means that the negative signal is absent and the NK cell carries out its lethal duty.*

of maturation of the functional T cell repertoire. This is also termed **central tolerance** (Topics E2 and M2). In the bone marrow, self reactive B cells are also eliminated. Lymphocytes escaping tolerance in the primary lymphoid organs are eliminated or anergized in the peripheral lymphoid organs through **peripheral tolerance** mechanisms.

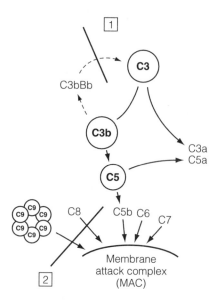

Fig. 3. Inhibition of complement activation on self-cell surfaces by regulatory proteins. ① Inhibition of C3 convertase by membrane cofactor proteins (CD46) and decay accelerating factor (CD55). ② Blocking of attachment of C8 and C9 of MAC to membrane, inhibiting active lysis (MIRL; CD59).

M2 CENTRAL TOLERANCE

Key Note

Central tolerance	Central tolerance is the process whereby immature T and B cells acquire tolerance to self antigens during maturation within the primary lymphoid organs/tissues (thymus and bone marrow, respectively). It involves the elimination of cells with receptors for self antigens.
Related topics	T cells are produced in the thymus (E2) Receptors, co-receptors and signaling (L1)
	B cells are produced in the bone marrow (E3)

Central tolerance T cells with specificity for self appear during normal development in the thymus as the result of the expression of combinations of germ line minigenes (Topics E2, E3 and F3). These self-reactive T cells must be eliminated to prevent autoimmunity. T cells with receptors with weak binding to MHC class I and II antigens are permitted to survive, **positively selected** (*Fig. 1*). T cells which bind MHC class I and II, alone or carrying self peptides (Topics E2 and H2), with high affinity are induced to die through the process of apoptosis. This **negative selection** leads to elimination of some but not all self-reactive T cells. Cortical epithelial cells expressing class I MHC antigens are the main players in the positive selection process whereas macrophages and interdigitating dendritic cells expressing both class I and class II MHC antigens play a leading role in negative selection. This 'education' process within the thymus leads to suicide of greater than 90% of the T cells. Thus, only a small percentage of the T cells generated survive to emigrate to the peripheral tissues. These T cells are the ones capable of recognizing foreign non self peptide antigens in the context of self MHC molecules.

A similar process of negative selection occurs during B cell development in the adult bone-marrow. As in the thymus, receptor diversity for antigen is created from germ-line mini genes resulting in B cells having membrane antibodies with self reactivity. **B cell tolerance** occurs as a result of clonal deletion, through apoptosis, of immature B cells reactive to self antigens (*Fig. 2*). Immature B cells expressing surface IgM that react with self antigens are rendered unresponsive or anergic. Thus, only those B cells that do not react with self antigens are allowed to migrate to the periphery and mature.

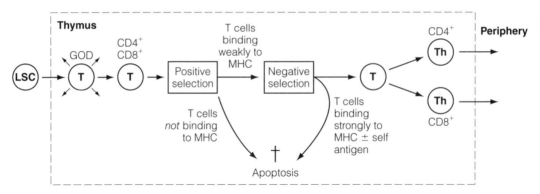

Fig. 1.   Central tolerance: T cells. T cell precursors derived from lymphoid stem cells (LSC) enter the thymus where they develop T cell antigen receptors through generation of diversity (GOD). They also acquire CD4 and CD8 molecules and undergo positive and negative selection. They leave the thymus as CD4+ helper or CD8+ cytotoxic T cells and migrate to the secondary lymphoid organs/tissues.

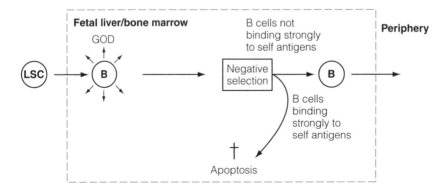

Fig. 2.   Central tolerance: B cells. B cell precursors develop diverse antigen receptors (GOD). They undergo negative selection and the surviving cells leave for the peripheral (secondary) lymphoid organs/tissues.

M3 PERIPHERAL TOLERANCE

Key Notes

Introduction	Peripheral tolerance is the process whereby mature lymphocytes acquire tolerance to self antigens in the peripheral tissues through elimination, lack of costimulatory signals, activation induced cell death or regulation through the idiotypic network.
The importance of peripheral tolerance	Self-reactive lymphocytes cannot all be eliminated by central tolerance mechanisms due to the absence of most self antigens in the primary lymphoid organs, and to the generation of new specificities, including to self, in germinal centers.
T cell anergy	This is the main mechanism by which peripheral T cells are made tolerant. It is due to the absence of a second signal given by costimulatory molecules (i.e. B7) on antigen-presenting cells (APCs) which, in addition to the signal via the TCR, is necessary for T cell activation.
B cell anergy	Most B cells require help from T cells to develop into plasma cells. This occurs through costimulatory signals which include costimulatory molecules and cytokines. In the absence of these signals they may undergo a state of unresponsiveness (anergy).
Activation induced cell death	Activated lymphocytes may express the receptor protein Fas and its ligand FasL. Fas/FasL interactions may be of primary benefit in maintaining immunological and physiological homeostasis by eliminating unnecessary cells.
Other mechanisms	Anti-idiotypic immune responses, produced as part of a natural network, may anergize T and B cells.

Related topics	Antibody responses in different tissues (J3)	Other control mechanisms (N5)
	Cell mediated immunity (K1)	Mechanisms leading to the development of autoimmune
	T cell activation (L2)	disease (U3)
	B cell activation (L3)	

Introduction

A variety of different mechanisms have been suggested to explain tolerance to self antigens that occurs in the periphery (peripheral tolerance). These include clonal deletion, anergy and activation induced cell death (AICD). As distinct from central tolerance, peripheral tolerance is associated with anergy as well as deletion of lymphocytes and in some instances peripheral tolerance may be transferred from host to host.

The importance of peripheral tolerance

Most self-reactive lymphocytes cannot all be eliminated in the primary lymphoid organs for two reasons. Firstly, many self antigens are neither present in the primary lymphoid organs nor supplied to them via the blood stream. Moreover, with the exception of self antigens that do not normally come in contact with the immune system, 'sequestered antigens' such as lens proteins in the eye, most self antigens expressed as the result of differentiation of cells and tissues in the major organs of the body do not 'pass through' the primary lymphoid organs. Certainly, lymphocytes in the periphery do come into contact with these antigens. Secondly, different receptor specificities may be generated as the consequence of somatic mutation of the antibody genes in B cells in the germinal centers in secondary lymphoid organs/tissues (Topics D2, E3 and J2). Unlike B cell antigen receptors, it is believed that TCRs do not normally mutate.

T cell anergy

Peripheral self-reactive T cells can be deleted as described above or anergized. The main mechanism preventing autoreactivity in the periphery involves development of anergy. Naive T cells require two main signals to respond to an antigen. One comes via the TCR, the other comes from costimulatory molecules. The glycoproteins B7.1 (CD80) and B7.2 (CD86) are essential costimulatory molecules, found almost exclusively on professional antigen-presenting cells (APCs). Interaction of these B7 molecules on APCs with CD28 on T cells is required for T cell activation (*Fig. 1*). Thus, in the absence of professional presentation of self antigens and engagement of costimulatory molecules (signal 2), the binding of self antigens presented in MHC molecules to the TCR on naive T cells, as they migrate through the peripheral tissues, results in anergy. Moreover, if naive T cells do become activated they express an additional receptor called CTLA-4 which has a greater binding affinity for the B7 molecules than CD28. Binding of CTLA-4 to B7 results in a negative signal to the T cells resulting in inhibition of T cell activity.

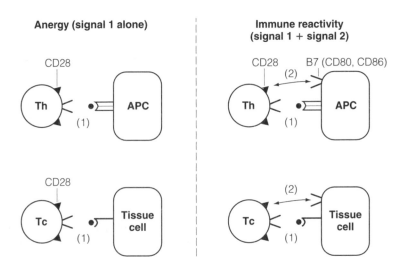

Fig. 1. T cell anergy. Th and Tc (including those that are self reactive) cannot be activated by one signal. Binding of B7 (CD80, CD86) on the APC/tissue cell to CD28 provides a second signal to the T cells leading to their activation.

B cell anergy   Self reactive B cells require T cell help in order to respond to T dependent antigens. Since most self-reactive T cells have been deleted during thymic maturation, self reactive B cells on contact with self antigens do not receive the required costimulatory signals (signal 2) from T helper cells and consequently become anergic (*Fig. 2*). Engagement of the B cell costimulatory molecules CD40 and B7 by CD154 and CD28 on T cells, as well as certain cytokines (IL-2, IL-4, IL-5, IL-6), are required for activation.

Activation
induced cell death   Fas/FasL (CD95/CD95L) interaction is directly responsible for AICD. This may be of primary benefit in maintaining immunological as well as physiological homeostasis by eliminating unnecessary cells through apoptosis. Activated T lymphocytes can express both the receptor protein Fas and its ligand (FasL), whereas B cells mainly express Fas. Peripheral tolerance may be facilitated by interaction between activated T cells and B cells (and, perhaps under certain conditions, other T cells) resulting in apoptosis (*Fig. 3*). In addition, T cells activated to kill self cells may be prevented from doing so by interaction with FasL expressed by certain somatic cells e.g. eye and testis (Topic U3). This may also be a strategy used by tumor cells to prevent their demise by cytotoxic T cells.

Other mechanisms   In 1955, Neils Jerne introduced the theory that lymphocytes were produced to not only recognize foreign antigens but also to recognize self antigen receptors (in particular the binding regions of T and B cell antigen receptors). He proposed that this helped maintain homeostasis resulting in lymphocyte anergy to self antigens (idiotype network). A breakdown in regulation of this network might give rise to autoreactivity (Topic N5).

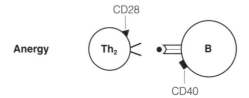

No help from T cells (no signal 2)

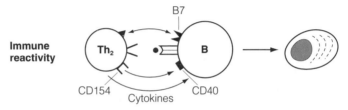

Help from T cells (signal 1 + signal 2)

Fig. 2.   B cell anergy. B cells require triggering through their CD40 molecules to progress through activation and maturation. Interaction of CD28 on T cells with B7 on B cells is necessary to induce expression of CD154 (CD40 ligand). This binds to CD40 on the B cell, acting as the second signal for activation.

Self reactive T and B cells

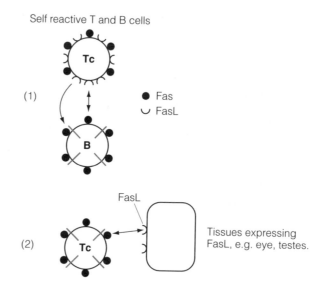

Fig. 3. Activation induced cell death (AICD) in peripheral tolerance. Tc cells may kill self-B cells expressing Fas (1) and may themselves be killed by tissue cells expressing FasL (2).

M4 ACQUIRED TOLERANCE

Key Notes

Introduction

That tolerance can be induced to certain antigens under appropriate conditions has considerable importance to immune defense as well as to modulating immunity to self antigens. Acquired tolerance is primarily associated with tolerance to non self antigen and may involve anergy, deletion and active suppression by Th2 cells. These mechanisms are influenced by the nature of antigen, its route of administration and concentration and the maturity of the immune system.

Nature of antigen

The chemical makeup and complexity of the antigen, as well as how similar it is to the species into which it is being introduced determines its ability to induce tolerance or immunity. The closer the similarity with self the easier it is to induce tolerance.

Maturity of the immune system

Tolerance is easier to achieve before birth or in early neonatal life, perhaps related to immaturity of T, B and/or antigen-presenting cells. It is more easy to tolerate T cells than B cells.

Route of administration

The route of administration may determine whether tolerance is induced or not. Antigens introduced intraperitonealy or intravenously are often more tolerogenic than when the same antigens are given subcutaneously or intramuscularly. Exposure to antigens via the oral route can result in both immunity or peripheral tolerance. Immunity to an antigen may, in some instances, be prevented by feeding these antigens orally.

Dose of antigen

Low or high doses of antigen may induce systemic tolerance, whereas intermediate doses may elicit an immune response. Larger doses are needed for tolerance in adults compared to neonates.

Related topics

Introduction

Under appropriate conditions tolerance can be induced to certain antigens. This has considerable importance to immune defense as acquired tolerance to critical epitopes on microbes may compromise protective immune responses to the organism. Acquired tolerance also has the potential for modulating immunity to self antigens (e.g. MHC molecules, permitting grafting of MHC incompatible organs) or allergens. The mechanisms that lead to the induction of acquired tolerance to foreign antigens are not clearly understood. Three basic mechanisms have been suggested based on experimental data. These include active suppression by Th2 cells, anergy and deletion.

● Active suppression requires the production of inhibitory cytokines such as TGFβ and IL-10 and can be adoptively transferred by lymphocytes from one animal to another (using inbred strains of mice).
● Anergy results when the antigen sensitive cell becomes unresponsive and goes into a resting state.
● Deletion involves the removal of the reactive cell by apoptosis.

There are many factors that may influence the induction of tolerance systemically:

● Nature of the antigen;
● Maturity of the immune system (age of host);
● Route of immunization of the antigen;
● Dose of antigen.

Moreover, T and B cell tolerance may differ. The genetic background of the host may also influence the development of tolerance as the immune response is under the control of immune response genes (IR genes, Topic N3).

Nature of antigen   The more dissimilar and complex the foreign antigen is in composition and structure to the host, the more difficult it is to induce tolerance. The closer the composition and structure of the antigen is to self antigens, the easier it is to induce tolerance. Aggregated antigens or antigens with multiple different epitopes are usually good 'immunogens' (i.e. able to induce immunity) but poor tolerogens, whereas soluble antigens are poor immunogens but good tolerogens.

Maturity of the   Tolerance is easier to achieve before birth or in early neonatal life. This may be
immune system   related to the immaturity of both T and B cells and/or APCs. It is also easier to induce tolerance in immune compromised individuals e.g. immunodeficient individuals or animals that are recovering from irradiation (Topic S3). Moreover, it is easier to induce tolerance in T cells than in B cells and, once attained, this tolerance lasts longer. Relative to B cell tolerance, T cell tolerance is achieved with lower doses of antigen and occurs more quickly after exposure.

Route of   The route of administration of antigen may influence the nature of the immune
administration   response. Antigens given subcutaneously or intramuscularly may be more immunogenic than when given intravenously or intraperitoneally.

Antigens introduced into an individual by the oral route (feeding) can induce oral tolerance. At least three mechanisms are involved, including active suppression, clonal anergy and deletion. Active suppression probably involves the release of inhibitory cytokines such as TGFβ and IL-10 and can be adoptively transferred. In animal models of oral tolerance, active suppression can be adoptively transferred by both CD4 and CD8 cells. Clonal anergy is usually induced by exposure to low or high doses of antigen. Thus, in the absence of costimulatory accessory signals, T or B cells may undergo anergy. Deletion results when high doses of antigen are fed, and has been shown to induce lymphocytes to undergo apoptosis in the Peyers patches. The requirements for tolerance induction may be different for different antigens and may also depend on the context of the stimulus. Antigens seen in the context of microbial infection may induce immune reactivity instead of tolerance.

Dose of antigen   Tolerance, rather than immunity is induced by extremes in antigen dose. The tolerance induced by the administration of high doses of antigen is called 'high zone tolerance'. In mature animals, a much larger dose is required than may be necessary in neonates. Tolerance can also be induced by extremely low doses of antigen, so called 'low zone tolerance'.

N1 COMPONENTS INVOLVED IN IMMUNE REGULATION

Key Note

Components involved in immune regulation	The regulation of the immune system is maintained through positive and negative events. Antigen is required to drive the immune response, the magnitude of which is under genetic control (e.g. MHC locus genes). Th cells regulate the type and extent of the immune response through cytokines and by signaling during direct cell–cell contact, and can be negative as well as positive. Specific antibody may enhance or inhibit further antibody production, with the idiotype network potentially involved in regulating the immune response, and overall control maintained by the neuroendocrine system.

Related topics	Peripheral tolerance (M3)	The role of antibody (N4)
	The role of antigen (N2)	Other control mechanisms (N5)

Components involved in immune regulation

The regulation of the immune response requires a fine balance between positive and negative events. Antigen is required to drive the immune response, the magnitude of which is under genetic control (e.g. MHC locus genes). The nature of the antigen is also important, since its size, state of aggregation, composition (e.g. protein vs carbohydrate), etc., significantly influence the type of response and its strength. Removal of the antigen and therefore the stimulus results in the response subsiding. Helper T cells are involved in regulating this response and in modulating the functions of other cells, including dendritic cells, NK cells, macrophages, and cytotoxic T cells. Although this modulation is often mediated through cytokines, it may also involve direct cell–cell interactions. The influence of Th cells can significantly effect the type of response depending at least partly on the kinds of cytokines produced and the particular cell participating in the response. Antibody itself can, in some instances, either enhance (IgM) or inhibit (IgG: negative feedback) further antibody production. The idiotype network, first described by Neils Jerne, may also play a role in regulation of the immune response. Finally, it is important to note that the immune system does not function in isolation, but rather is influenced by other body systems. In particular, the neuroendocrine system plays an important role in modulating immune responses. Defective regulation of the immune system leads to breakdown of tolerance (Topic U3) and overreactivity (Topic T1).

N2 THE ROLE OF ANTIGEN

Key Notes

Stimulation of the response	Antigen initiates the immune response via presentation of its peptides by antigen presenting cells (dendritic cells and macrophages) to antigen specific Th cells. Th cells then help B cells produce antibody, or CTLs develop. The physical state (e.g. aggregation) and composition (e.g. protein) of the antigen are also important.
Removal of antigen	Removal of antigen by antibody, and ultimately through phagocytic cells, is the most effective means of regulating an immune response, since in its absence, the restimulation of antigen specific T and B cells stops. This appears to be the mechanism by which anti-RhD+ antibodies given to RhD− mothers inhibits their production of anti-RhD+ antibodies in future pregnancies. Moreover, maternal IgG in the newborn may bind antigen and remove it, thereby interfering with development of active immunity. Persistent antigen, as found with some viruses and bacteria, maintains production of specific immune responses.
Related topics	Antigens (A4) Immunization (R2)
	Immunity in the newborn (E4) IgG and IgM-mediated type II
	The cellular basis of the antibody hypersensitivity (T3)
	response (J1)

Stimulation of the response

Antigen is an absolute requirement for the initiation of an immune response. Recognition of microbes as foreign or nonself is initially mediated through microbe pattern recognition by receptors of the innate immune system or antigen specific receptors on lymphocytes (Topics H1, H2 and H3). The nature of the antigen is also important in that particulate antigens produce stronger immune responses than soluble forms of the same antigen. This may in part be due to the ability of soluble antigens to produce a tolerogenic response rather than an immune response. Aggregated antigens are also more likely to be taken up and processed by antigen presenting cells.

Removal of antigen

The successful generation of an antigen driven cell-mediated and/or antibody response, leads in most cases to removal of the invading microbes. Microbial remains and dead virus infected cells are cleared by the phagocytic system, thus removing the antigenic source and therefore the stimulus. In particular, as a result of elimination of antigen by antibody, restimulation of antigen specific T and B cells stops, preventing more specific antibodies from being made at a time when antigen is being effectively cleared from the system. The ability of preformed antibodies to inhibit specific unwanted host responses to antigens has been shown clinically by passive immunization. Injection of RhD+ antibodies into RhD− mothers immediately after birth of an RhD+ infant removes RhD+ erythrocytes that may have passed into the maternal circulation. This prevents the development of hemolytic disease of the newborn from occurring as a result of future pregnancies (Topic T3). This results from the simple removal of antigen (RhD+ erythrocytes), such that the mother never develops a memory response to RhD antigen.

In addition, unresponsiveness of the newborn to certain antigens may be related to the passive immunity acquired from the mother (Topic E4). Due to transfer of maternal IgG across the placenta during fetal life, the infant at birth has all of the IgG antibody mediated humoral immunity of the mother. Furthermore, maternal IgA obtained by the infant from colostrum and milk during nursing coats the infant's gastrointestinal tract and supplies passive mucosal immunity. Thus, until these passively supplied antibodies are degraded or used up, they may bind antigen and remove it, thereby interfering with development of active immunity.

Of note, some microbes persist and continuously stimulate specific T and B cells. For example, Epstein–Barr virus, which causes glandular fever, persists for life at low levels in the pharyngeal tissues and B cells, continually restimulating immunity to the virus.

N3 GENES, T HELPER CELLS AND CYTOKINES

Key Notes

Genetic control of immune responses	Although many genes are involved in control of immune responses, the major gene locus which regulates the T cell response to a variety of antigens is the major histocompatibility complex (MHC). Polymorphism of the locus provides the human population as a whole with the chance of binding new peptides and of thus producing protective responses to new pathogenic microbes which might arise through mutation.
T helper cells	The type of immune response is determined by the nature of the antigen and by regulatory T cells and their cytokine products. Th1 cells produce pro-inflammatory cytokines important for killing of intracellular microbes and the generation of T cytotoxic cells, whereas the anti-inflammatory cytokines, IL-4, IL-10 and IL-13, produced by Th2 cells are important for B cell proliferation and differentiation and immunoglobulin class switch to IgA or IgE, antibody isotypes important for immune defense of mucosal surfaces. Th1 and Th2 cytokines are self regulating and inhibit each others functions.
Stimulatory and inhibitory cytokines	Cytokines promote cell growth, attract specific immune cells (chemokines) or contribute to cell activation. Other cytokines suppress cell proliferation (e.g. TGFβ and IFNα) or inhibit activation of macrophages (e.g. TGFβ).
Related topics	Cytokine families (G2) The major histocompatibility antigens and antigen processing and presentation (H4)	Genes, T helper cells and cytokines (N3) Transplantation antigens (Q2)

Genetic control of immune responses

It has been well established that many genes are involved in regulation of immune responses. Many of these undoubtedly code for the large number of receptors, signaling proteins, etc., which are critical to the specific immune response. However, the major gene locus which regulates the T cell response to most antigens is the major histocompatibility complex (MHC). This complex, which is composed of six major loci (Topics H4 and Q2) is polymorphic with allelic forms which encode different amino acids within the peptide binding region of the MHC class I and class II molecules. This polymorphism is believed to provide the human population as a whole with the chance of binding any new peptides which might arise through mutations of microbes. Those individuals who have an MHC able to bind a rare new peptide would be selected in a Darwinian way.

T helper cells

Th cells are an absolute requirement for immune responses to protein antigens in general, and for helping B cells to make the different classes of antibodies. The type of response is, in some instances, determined by the nature of the antigen and its mode of entry as well as the effect of regulatory $CD4^+$ T helper subsets, Th1 and Th2, and their cytokine products. The pro-inflammatory cytokines, IL-2, TNFα and IFNγ, produced by Th1 cells are important for killing of intracellular microbes and the generation of T cytotoxic cells, whereas the anti-inflammatory Th2 cytokines, IL-4, IL-10 and IL-13, are important for B cell proliferation and differentiation and immunoglobulin class switch to IgA and IgE as well as the IgG2 response to the polysaccharide antigens associated with encapsulated bacteria such as *Pneumococcus*. Th2 cytokines are also important in helping to eradicate parasitic infections as they lead to the production of IgE and the recruitment of eosinophils which have powerful anti-parasitic functions. Th1 and Th2 cytokines are self regulating as well as inhibiting each other's functions (*Fig. 1* and Topic G1). For example, IL-4 and IL-10 down regulate Th1 responses whereas IFNγ has an antagonistic effect on Th2 cells. Down regulatory mechanisms are necessary to prevent collateral damage as well as being energy conserving. Patients with atopy, i.e. with a genetic predisposition to having high levels of IgE, are believed to poorly regulate their Th2 cells (Section T). In addition, in AIDS there is some suggestion that the response is biased in favour of a Th2 rather than Th1 response.

Stimulatory and inhibitory cytokines

Most cytokines promote growth of particular cell lineages, attract specific immune cells (chemokines) or contribute to cell activation. Other cytokines can be suppressive. TGFβ inhibits activation of macrophages and the proliferation of B and T cells. IFNα also has cell growth inhibitory properties. The action of these suppressive cytokines is a primary way that T cells and macrophages regulate immune responses. In addition, the stimulatory and inhibitory action of cytokines produced by Th1 and Th2 cells on each other also plays a major role in determining the type and extent of an immune response (Topic G1).

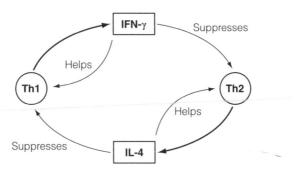

Fig. 1. *Reciprocal regulation of Th1 and Th2 cells. Th1 cells release IFNγ which suppresses proliferation of TH2 cells and their IL-4 production. Th2 cells release IL-4 (and IL-10) which suppresses IFN-γ production by Th1 cells and their proliferation.*

N4 THE ROLE OF ANTIBODY

Key Notes

Positive effects of antibodies	Antibodies of the IgM class may regulate the immune response through complement activation. Thus, interaction of antigen-IgM-complement complexes with antigen-specific B cells may enhance the response.
Negative feedback by IgG	IgG-antigen complexes may specifically inhibit further responses by antigen-specific B cells as a result of a negative signal transduced by FcγRII (CD32) on binding of the IgG component of the complex.
Related topics	Complement (C2) cell receptor complex and B cell recognition of antigen, the B co-receptors (H2)

Positive effects of antibodies

Antibodies of the IgM class appear to be important in enhancing humoral immunity. In particular, antigen-IgM-complement complexes which bind to specific antibody of the B cell antigen receptor stimulate the cell more efficiently than antigen alone (*Fig. 1*). This is probably the result of interaction of the C3b component of complement with the CD21 molecule of the antigen receptor complex which then transduces a positive signal to the B cell.

Negative feedback by IgG

The interaction of IgG-antigen complexes with antigen-specific B cells through the simultaneous binding of both the B cell antigen receptor and the FcγRII molecule

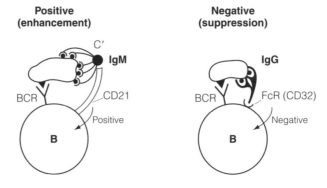

Fig. 1. Regulation of B cell activity by antibody. IgM bound to antigen recognized by the BCR fixes complement which then interacts with CD21 giving a positive signal to the B cell. However, IgG bound to antigen attached to the BCR binds to FcγR (CD32) and delivers a negative signal to the B cell.

of the B cell receptor complex can deliver a negative signal to the B cell (*Fig. 1*). Thus, IgG, which is produced later in the antibody response, could interact with antigen (if present) forming a complex that, on binding to antigen specific B cells, may provide feedback inhibition mediated via FcγRII, decreasing the amount of antigen-specific antibody being produced.

N5 OTHER CONTROL MECHANISMS

Key Notes

The idiotype network
The ability of the immune system to produce anti-idiotypic responses (immune responses to the variable region of immunoglobulin molecules) has been proposed as a mechanism by which immune responses can be regulated.

Neuroendocrine system: the HPA axis
The hypothalamus/pituitary/adrenal (HPA) axis exercises control over the immune response through the release of mediators such as corticotrophin-releasing hormone (CRH), opioids, catecholamines and glucocorticoids. Glucocorticoids have wide-ranging regulatory effects on the immune system and are powerful down regulators of the pro-inflammatory response. In turn, the immune system, through cytokines such as IL-1, directly affects the HPA axis by, for example, inducing the production of glucocorticoids. Thus, immune effector mechanisms are tightly integrated into a network that includes the nervous and endocrine systems.

Related topics
Allotypes and idiotypes (F4)

Diagnosis and treatment of autoimmune disease (U5)

The idiotype network

The hypervariable region, the idiotype, of the immunoglobulin molecule (Topic F4) is immunogenic, and thus antibody and T cell responses can be produced to this region. It has been suggested that these immune responses to idiotypes have an immunoregulatory role. That is, antibodies or T cells directed to the idiotype of an antigen-induced antibody may, by interacting directly with the B or T cell, regulate with its further proliferation and differentiation. Anti-idiotypic antibodies or T cells may thus form networks of connectivity and act as inducers and regulators of their own responses. In the absence of antigen, B cells or T cells with idiotypic and anti-idiotypic antigen receptors may directly anergize other B and T cells through direct contact of the antigen receptors.

In addition, it has become clear that two different sets of antibodies can be produced against the idiotype of an antibody molecule. One set of antibodies may express anti-idiotype binding sites that resemble the antigenic determinant on the original antigen. Thus, an antibody directed against an antigenic determinant on a microbe, for example, may produce an anti-idiotypic response with antibodies with variable regions that resemble the antigenic determinant on the microbe molecule (*Fig. 1*). Antibodies so produced can potentially mediate protection against the microbe.

Moreover, anti-idiotypes can behave as surrogate antigens. For example, antibodies to hepatitis B antibodies have been used as vaccines for hepatitis B.

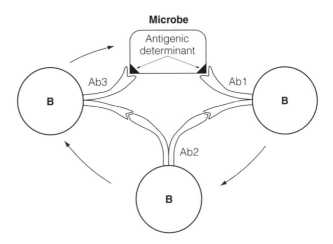

Fig. 1. Idiotype-mediated regulation of the immune response. A microbe stimulates development of Ab1 antibodies, which, acting as neoantigens, stimulate production of Ab2, which in turn can stimulate further anti-idiotype responses, giving rise to Ab3. Note that Ab2 looks like the original antigenic determinant on the microbe and may behave as a surrogate antigen to stimulate a cross reactive immune response. Other idiotype interactions could lead to negative regulation of B cell responses. It is thought that T cells interact with idiotypic determinants on B cells and in this way amplify and suppress their responses.

Anti-idiotype antibodies behaving as surrogate antigens may permit the immune system to boost its own response during infection. In this way, during an immune response to a microbe, antibodies mimicking microbial antigens or idiotypic antigen receptors on lymphocytes may amplify the immune response without the destructive effects of the real microbes.

Neuroendocrine system: the HPA axis

The activity of the immune system is influenced by other systems and perhaps most importantly by the neuroendocrine axis. Thus, lymphocytes are not only susceptible to regulation by cytokines of the immune system but also by hormones and neurotransmitters. The hypothalamus/pituitary/adrenal (HPA) axis exercises powerful control over the immune response through the release of mediators such as corticotrophin-releasing hormone (CRH), opioids, catecholamines and glucocorticoids (*Fig. 2*). While the effector mechanisms for some of these mediators are not fully understood, it is known that they act on both the sensory (mast cells) and cognitive (lymphocytes) cells of the immune system.

Glucocorticoids have wide-ranging regulatory effects on the immune system, including: reducing the number of circulating lymphocytes, monocytes and eosinophils; quenching cell mediated immunity by inhibiting the release of the pro-inflammatory cytokines IL-1, IL-2, IL-6, IFNγ and TNFα; decreasing antigen presentation; and inhibiting mast cell function. Growth hormone and prolactin, which are produced by the pituitary, are apparently also able to modulate the activity of the immune system. It has been shown that rats who undergo hypophysectomy (destruction of the pituitary) have prolonged allograft survival that is reduced on the reintroduction of prolactin or growth hormone.

Neurotransmitters including adrenaline (epinephrine), noradrenaline, substance P, vasoactive intestinal peptide (VIP) and 5'hydroxytryptamine (5HT) can also have both wide-ranging and specific effects on immune function.

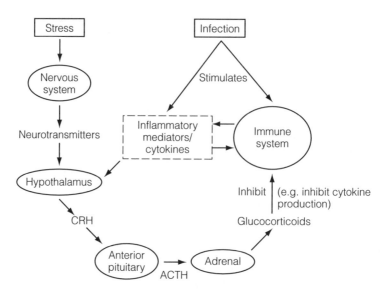

Fig. 2. The interconnectivity between the immune and neuroendocrine systems. Infection or stress can affect, either directly or indirectly, both the immune and the nervous systems. Inflammatory mediators/cytokines released in response to infection not only are involved in the development and regulation of immune responses, but also stimulate the release of immune modulators such as glucocorticoids, which downregulate immune responses. Stress and inflammatory mediators cause the release of corticotrophin releasing hormone (CRH) by the hypothalamus, which stimulates the pituitary to release ACTH. ACTH causes the adrenal gland to release glucocorticoids, which in turn downregulate the immune system.

Interestingly, the HPA axis is also directly influenced by the immune system as evidenced by the fact that the cytokines IL-1, TNFα and IL-6, which are released during the inflammatory response, directly effect the hypothalamus, anterior pituitary and adrenal cortex. Thus, immune effector mechanisms are tightly integrated into a network that includes the nervous and endocrine systems.

01 THE MICROBIAL COSMOS

Key Notes

Infection and its consequences	In the past, epidemics caused by plague and influenza have caused the deaths of large numbers of people as well as causing changes in social structures and behavior. Today, new and old diseases such as those caused by the human immunodeficiency virus (HIV), *Legionella*, *Helicobacter pylori* as well as the emergence of multi-drug resistant tuberculosis (TB), present new challenges to the immune system and man's inventiveness.
The microbial habitat and immune defense	Microbes (e.g. many bacteria and fungi) that live outside the cells of the body are usually dealt with by phagocytes, complement and specific antibodies. However, those having an intracellular habitat (e.g. viruses, some bacteria and protozoa) require the presence of neutralizing antibodies, cytotoxic T cells or NK cells to control them.
Pathogens have their own protective mechanisms	To avoid the multiple defenses of the immune system, microbes have evolved ways and means of evading the body's defense mechanisms and of causing infection. They can avoid recognition by having an intracellular habitat, by molecular mimicry (where antigens of the infectious agent are antigenically indistinguishable from host antigens) and by antigenic variation. They can also down modulate the effector arm of the immune response.
Damage caused by pathogens	Pathogens can cause tissue damage directly by production of toxins but also through an overzealous immune response. Mechanisms of immune mediated damage to the host include anaphylaxis, immune complex disease, necrosis and apoptosis.
Related topics	Phagocytes (B1) T helper cells (K3) Complement (C2) Hypersensitivity – when the Cytokine families (G2) immune system overreacts (T) T cytotoxic cells (K2)

Infection and its consequences

As well as being useful, microbes (and larger parasites) are still one of man's greatest threats to survival. In the past, diseases such as tuberculosis (TB) and epidemics caused by plague and influenza have caused the deaths of large numbers of people as well as causing changes in social structures and behavior. It is estimated that the 1918 flu epidemic killed between 40 and 100 million people and it is suggested that more people died from TB as a result of the Second World War than from the war alone. Today, new and old diseases such as those caused by the human immunodeficiency virus (HIV), *Legionella*, *Helicobacter pylori* as well as the emergence of multi-drug resistant TB, present new challenges to the immune system and man's inventiveness.

The microbial habitat and immune defense

The immune response to bacteria, viruses, fungi, protozoa and worms differ in the variety of defensive mechanisms used. In general, microbes (e.g. many bacteria and fungi) living outside the cells of the body are more likely to be opsonized by specific antibodies and engulfed by phagocytes or destroyed by the alternative or classical complement pathway, whereas those having an intracellular habitat (e.g. viruses, some bacteria and protozoa) may require the presence of antibodies (neutralization) as well as cytotoxic T cells or NK cells to provide effective protection. The immune response to fungi is poorly understood, and while antibodies may play a role in their elimination, the major mechanism of protection against these microorganisms appears to be through a cell mediated response (T cells and macrophages). Both humoral and cellular responses are required for protection against protozoa, which are difficult to immunize against. Immune protection against helminths (worms) is difficult to achieve because of size and complexity. The major response mechanisms include the production of antibodies, especially immunoglobulin (Ig)E, and a cellular response including eosinophils, mast cells, macrophages and CD4 T cells. Both mast cells and eosinophils degranulate in the presence of IgE antigen complexes, IgA complexes also cause eosinophils to degranulate. Mast cells release histamine, which causes gut spasms whereas eosinophils release cationic protein and neurotoxins. Helminth antigens direct the immune response towards a Th2 response that results in the preferential production of IgE.

Pathogens have their own protective mechanisms

Many microbes have evolved ways and means of evading the multiple and overlapping human immune defense mechanisms and of causing infection. Microbial strategies of escape from immune surveillance are essentially of two kinds. They can avoid recognition by having an intracellular habitat, by molecular mimicry (where critical antigens of the infectious agent are antigenically indistinguishable from host antigens) and by antigenic variation. They can also modulate the effector arm of the immune response by interference with complement activation, inhibiting phagocytosis, neutralization of antibody responses and modulation of Th1/Th2 responses. Microbes can invade the host through mucosal surfaces, skin, bites and wounds. Such invasion is usually countered by innate defense mechanisms, which act rapidly. In the event that the infectious agent still survives these first lines of defense, the adaptive immune system responds more specifically, but more slowly in an effort to eliminate the pathogen. In this way the adaptive and nonadaptive immune systems can be considered as brain versus brawn, respectively. The final pathway of defense usually results in immunological memory so that repeated infection with the causative microbe or parasite is minimized or, as is the case with infectious agents such as smallpox and measles, prevented.

Table 1.   Pathogens and hypersensitivity

Type I	Echinococcus – hydatid cyst, when it bursts it produces an anaphylactic response
Type II	Cross-reactions of antibodies to shared antigens, e.g. streptococci and heart tissues in rheumatic fever
Type III	Immune complex deposition in kidney, lung, blood vessel or joint causing glomerulonephritis (e.g. streptoccocal infection), bronchiectasis, vasculitis or arthritis, respectively
Type IV	Granuloma formation, e.g. TB and leprosy

**Damage caused
by pathogens**

Pathogenic organisms can cause tissue damage and disease directly through the production of toxins. For example, bacteria and protozoa produce exotoxins and endotoxins. In addition, most viruses have a lytic stage resulting in tissue damage. On the other hand, the immune system itself, in certain infectious disease, may be more destructive than the offending pathogen itself, especially in persistent states. Some examples (Section T) are listed in *Table 1*. Mechanisms of immune mediated damage to the host include anaphylaxis, immune complex disease, necrosis and apoptosis.

02 IMMUNITY TO DIFFERENT ORGANISMS

Key Notes

Immunity to bacteria

Extracellular bacteria may be attacked by the alternative complement pathway or by antibodies and killed through the classical complement pathway. Antibodies and complement proteins also act as opsonins facilitating engulfment and killing by phagocytes. Intracellular bacteria, e.g. TB bacilli, *Salmonella* and *Brucella*, evade the immune system by surviving in host cells such as monocytes and macrophages. The immune system counteracts by mounting a cell-mediated immune (CMI) response to the infection and releasing cytokines such as IL-12 and IFNγ which enhance monocytes/macrophages killing of intracellular bacteria.

Immunity to viruses

Viruses replicate by infecting host cells and require a CMI response for eradication. The natural inhibitors of viral infection are IFNα and β. Antibodies can neutralize free virus (prevent its attachment to, and infection of, target cells) and enhance phagocytosis of the virus. When viruses infect, viral specific peptides become expressed on the cell surface in MHC molecules. These peptides act as targets on the host cells for cytotoxic T cells.

Immunity to fungi

The immune response to fungal infections (mycoses) is poorly understood. While antibodies may have some role in their eradication, immunity principally involves T cells and macrophages.

Immunity to protozoa

Protozoa infections such as malaria, trypanosomiasis, leishmaniasis and toxoplasmosis are a major threat to health in the tropics and in the developing world. Protozoa are difficult to immunize against and protection is thought to require both cellular and humoral immunity.

Immunity to worms

Immune protection against helminths (worms) is difficult to achieve because of their size and complexity. The response mechanisms include the production of antibodies especially IgE, and a cellular response including eosinophils, mast cells, macrophages and CD4 T cells. Degranulation of mast cells and eosinophils through IgE-antigen and IgA-antigen complexes results in acute inflammation and the release of cationic proteins and neurotoxins.

Related topics

Cytokine families (G2)	T helper cells (K3)
The acute inflammatory response (I)	The microbial cosmos (O1)
T cytotoxic cells (K2)	Deficiencies in the immune system (S1)

Immunity to bacteria

A summary of the main defense mechanisms against extracellular bacteria is shown in *Fig. 1*. Bacteria that avoid destruction by the classical or alternative complement pathways may be opsonized by acute phase reactants or specific anti-

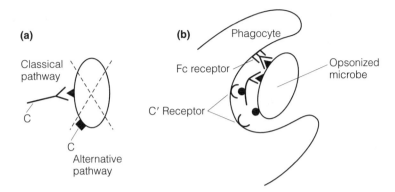

Fig. 1. Defense mechanisms against extracellular bacteria. Bacteria can be killed by
(a) complement-dependent lysis with or without antibodies and (b) phagocytosis following
opsonization with complement and/or antibody alone.

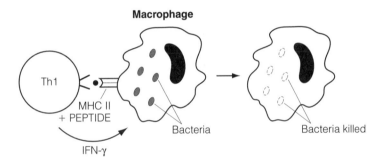

Fig. 2. Defense mechanisms against intracellular bacteria. Macrophages containing
intracellular bacteria present microbial peptides on their MHC class II molecules to specific
Th1 cells which produce IFNγ. This 'activates' the macrophage resulting in enhanced
intracellular killing.

bodies and engulfed by phagocytes expressing receptors for the Fc region of these
antibodies. Both PMNs and macrophages express receptors for IgG as well as IgA.
Inflammatory cytokines such as IFNγ can upregulate expression of these receptors
increasing their number dramatically. Some bacteria are intracellular parasites
invading cells and surviving in them. These include TB bacilli, *Listeria monocyto-
genes*, *Salmonella typhi* and *Brucella* species. Intracellular bacteria evade the
immune systems surveillance by surviving in host cells such as monocytes and
macrophages. The immune system counteracts them by mounting a cell-mediated
immune (CMI) response to the infection. Cells involved in the CMI response
include CD4 cells (Th1, Th2) subsets, CD8 cells, monocytes/macrophages and NK
cells. Th1 cells release IFNγ which make the monocytes/macrophages more
potent at killing intracellular bacteria as well as enhancing their antigen presenting capabilities. A summary of immune mechanisms against intracellular
microbes is shown in *Fig. 2*. The CMI response is important in the protection
against diseases such as TB, viral and fungal infections.

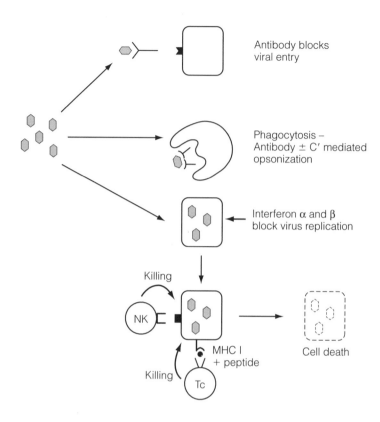

Fig. 3.   Defense mechanisms against viruses. Antibodies attach to viruses preventing their entry into cells and opsonize them for phagocytosis. Interferons α and β block viral replication in infected cells. NK cells can kill virus infected cells if they have little or no expression of MHC class I. Tc cells kill virus-infected cells expressing viral peptides in MHC class I.

Immunity to viruses

Natural immunity to viral infections is associated with interferons so called because of their interference with viral replication (Topic C4), although IFNγ does this through immune mediated mechanisms. Antibodies may also protect against viral infection. Viruses require attachment to host cells before they can replicate and cause infection. Circulating antibodies to a virus prevents attachment and represents an important defense mechanism against infection. These protective antibodies may be IgG or IgA as in the case of polio prevention. Viruses replicate in host cells where they are no longer exposed to circulating antibodies. However, virally infected cells usually express viral peptides in MHC class I on their surfaces rendering them targets for destruction by cytotoxic CD8 T cells. Cells infected by virus also become susceptible to being killed by NK cells (Topics B2 and M1). In this way, viral replication is prevented and the viral infection eliminated (*Fig. 3*).

Immunity to fungi

Fungal diseases (mycoses) are common but are most problematic when associated with immunocompromised individuals (Topic S1). The immune response to fungal infections is poorly understood. Neutrophils and other phagocytic cells are important in removing infections caused by some fungi and while antibodies may have some role in their eradication, it would appear that protective immunity is principally cellular, especially in those infections deep within the body. This is further suggested from studies in acquired immune deficiency syndrome (AIDS) patients where low T cell counts are commonly associated with fungal infections.

Immunity to protozoa

Protozoa infections such as malaria, trypanosomiasis, toxoplasmosis, leishmaniasis and amoebiasis are a major threat to health in the tropics and in particular in the developing world. Protozoa are difficult to immunize against and protection is thought to require both cellular and humoral immunity, although the humoral response, and in particular the IgG response, may be the most important. In malaria, antibodies appear to protect against infection by preventing the merozoites (blood stage) from gaining entrance to red cells. Moreover, immunity to one strain or species of malaria may not be protective against others.

Other innate or nonadaptive immune mechanisms help to protect against certain malaria infections. For example, individuals lacking the Duffy blood group antigen Fy (a-b-) are immune to *Plasmodium vivax* infection and the hemoglobin structure associated with sickle cell anemia appears to be inhibitory to the intracellular growth of *P. falciparum*. Trypanosomes continuously challenge the immune system by producing progeny with different antigenic coats. As the immune system develops a response to the new antigens on the parasite it again switches the antigenic coat. This leads to wave after wave of infection and response. *Toxoplasma* acquire protection from the immune system by coating themselves with laminin, an extracellular matrix protein, which prevents phagocytosis and oxidative damage. The cellular response to *Toxoplasma* appears to be most effective in combating infection, since patients with low T cell counts as in HIV infection are more at risk from infection with *toxoplasma*. Other protozoan diseases such as leishmaniasis have a predilection for infecting macrophages and require a cellular response for eradication. Moreover, a Th1 response seems to be essential for protection, since IFNγ appears to be the most important cytokine for parasite killing.

Immunity to worms

An immune response to worms (helminths) is not very effective and difficult to achieve, probably as a result of the size and complexity of the parasite. Thus, diseases such as those caused by *Schistosoma mansoni* (schistosomiasis) and *Wuchereria bancrofti* (lymphatic filariasis, elephantiasis) represent major problems in the developing world. Although PMNs, macrophages and NK cells may be involved, the main protective mechanism against helminths appears to be mediated by eosinophils and mast cells. While worms are too large to be phagocytosed, they can be coated with IgE, IgA and IgG antibodies. In the event that this happens, the major phagocytic cells as well as eosinophils and mast cells will bind to the parasites surface through their receptors for these molecules and release their toxic cellular contents. Both mast cells and eosinophils degranulate in the presence of IgE antigen complexes. When mast cells degranulate they release histamine, serotonin and leukotrienes. These vasoactive amines are neurotransmitters and cause neurovasculature as well as neuromuscular changes resulting in gut spasm diarrhoea and the expulsion of material from the intestine. Eosinophils also have IgA receptors and have been shown to release their granule contents when these receptors are cross-linked. On degranulation, eosinophils release powerful antagonistic chemicals and proteins including cationic proteins, neurotoxins and hydrogen peroxide, these also probably contribute to a hostile environment for worm habitation. Helminth infections usually direct the immune system towards a

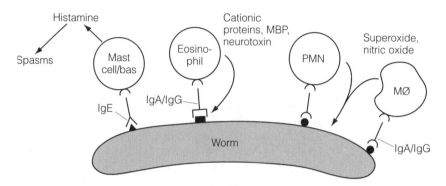

*Fig. 4.   Defense mechanisms against worms. Worms are usually too large to phagocytose.
IgE mediated degranulation of mast cells/basophils results in production of histamine which
causes spasms in the intestine where these worms are often found. Eosinophils attach to the
worm via IgG/IgA antibodies and release cationic proteins, major basic protein and
neurotoxin. PMNs and macrophages attach via IgG antibodies and release superoxide, nitric
oxide and enzymes which kill the worm.*

Th2 response and the production of IgE, IgA and Th2 cytokines as well as
the chemokine eotaxin. The Th2 cytokines IL-3, IL-4 and IL-5 as well as the
chemokine eotaxin are chemotactic for eosinophils and mast cells. *Fig. 4* summarizes the major immune mechanisms for removal of helminths.

O3 PATHOGEN DEFENSE STRATEGIES

Key Notes

The battle to stay ahead

In order for microbes to continue to be successful, they have developed strategies to avoid recognition by the host and to inactivate the immune mechanisms. Some pathogens avoid immune recognition by intracellular habitat, mimicking of self-antigens, encapsulation or by changing their surface antigens (antigenic variation). Other pathogens compromise effector mechanisms by inhibiting complement activation, phagocytosis and/or cytokine production, by release of superantigens or by overall immunosuppression.

Avoidance of recognition

The intracellular habitat of viruses, some bacteria and protozoa prevents recognition by innate and adaptive immune systems. Microbes can change their antigens by mutation (drift), by nucleic acid recombination (antigenic shift) and by switching genes controlling cell surface antigens. Some microbes express antigens very similar to self antigens (molecular mimicry), while others wear the antigens of the host they are infecting. Distraction of the lymphoid cells is achieved by poly- or oligoclonal activation by microbial products.

Inactivation of immune effector mechanisms

Some microbes can inhibit phagocytosis e.g. by encapsulation, a critical mechanism for killing extracellular microbes. Viruses such as hepatitis B inhibit the production of IFNα by infected cells. Low affinity antibodies are produced to some organisms, e.g. treponemes, while others inactivate the antibodies by production of proteases. Complement activation is also blocked by some viruses and bacteria. CD4$^+$ T cells are inactivated by HIV and some viruses decrease expression of MHC class I molecules by infected cells, blocking the activity of cytotoxic T cells. Other microbes produce endotoxins that channel the immune response toward one that is ineffective, e.g. inducing a humoral response when a cellular response is required for protection.

Related topics

The microbial cosmos (O1)
Immunity to different organisms (O2)

Mechanisms leading to the development of autoimmune disease (U3)

The battle to stay ahead

Immune defense against pathogens is dependent on first being able to recognize the intruder as a threat, and second being able to eliminate it. While the physical and mechanical barriers as well as the adaptive and nonadaptive immune systems are powerful in the prevention of infection, microbes have developed ways of both avoiding recognition and of inactivating components used for their elimination (*Table 1*). Some pathogens avoid immune recognition by intracellular habitat, mimicking of self-antigens, encapsulation or by changing their surface antigens

Table 1. Pathogen defense strategies

Avoidance of recognition	
Intracellular habitat	Viruses, mycobacteria, *Brucella*, *Legionella*
Antigenic variation	
Drift	Viruses can undergo mutation to alter antigens, e.g. influenza, HIV
Shift	Recombination with animal viral nucleic acids, e.g. influenza pandemics
Gene switching	Expression of a sequence of different surface antigens, e.g. *Borellia*, *Trypanosoma*
Disguise	
Molecular mimicry	Microbes have antigens in common with self, e.g. Streptococcus, bacteroides
Coating with self proteins	Covering of surface with serum proteins, e.g. *Schistosoma*, *Toxoplasma*
Immune distraction	Some microbes produce superantigens which stimulate many different B and T cells, diluting the effects of specific antigens e.g. Staphylococcal enterotoxins for T cells
Inactivation of host immune effector mechanisms	
Phagocytosis	Encapsulation by cell walls of some bacteria inhibits phagocytosis e.g. Pneumococci, *H. influenzae* and *E. coli.*
Cytokines	Inhibition of interferon production e.g. Hepatitis B
Antibodies	Low affinity antibody production e.g. treponemes
	Neutralization of antibody by large amounts of soluble antigens e.g. *Streptococcus pneumoniae*, *Candida* sp.
	Release of proteases that cleave IgA e.g. *Pseudomonas* sp., *Neisseria gonorrhoeae*, *H. influenzae*
	Production of proteins that bind to the IgG Fc region and prevent opsonization e.g. *Staphylococcus* protein A
Complement activation (classical pathway)	Inhibition by incorporation of host complement regulatory proteins into microbial cell wall e.g. HIV
T cells	CD4 T cells infected and killed e.g. HIV
Antigen processing and presentation	Inhibition of antigen processing e.g. Measles virus
Regulatory mechanisms	Endotoxins released by some microbes induce a Th2 response that is ineffective against intracellular microbes e.g. *Salmonella typhi*

(antigenic variation). Other pathogens compromise effector mechanisms of immunity by inhibiting complement activation, phagocytosis and/or cytokine production. They can release soluble neutralizing antigens, produce enzymes capable of destroying antibodies or complement, produce superantigens or induce overall immunosuppression.

Avoidance of recognition

Intracellular habitat

Viruses, some bacteria (e.g. mycobacteria, listeria, *Salmonella typhi* and *Brucella* species) and certain protozoa (i.e., malaria causing *Plasmodium falciparum, P. malariae, P. ovale* and *P. vivax*) are obligate intracellular organisms, thus evading the effects of the innate and adaptive immune systems.

Antigenic variation

Alteration of cell surface antigens through mutation is achieved by some viruses, e.g. influenza (**antigenic drift**). This makes it very difficult for the immune system to keep up, as a continuous primary response would need to be generated. The recombination of nucleic acids from human and animal viruses can lead to major **antigenic shifts**, and is known to be responsible for pandemics, e.g. influenza. Other organisms can produce continuous changes in their antigenic coat distracting the immune system, e.g. trypanosomes, *Borrelia recurrentis*. In the case of trypanosoma, at least 100 different surface coats can be expressed in sequence.

Disguise

Some microbes use antigens common or cross-reactive with self to try to look like self antigens so as to appear nonimmunogenic (molecular mimicry). For example, the hyaluronic acid capsule of some streptoccocal species is the same as that of host connective tissue. While this seems an excellent strategy, it can lead to the development of autoimmune disease (Topic U3). *Schistosoma* wears the antigens of the host that it infects, again trying to look like self. In other cases, specific T cells and B cells can be 'distracted' through poly- or oligoclonal activation by microbial products. For example, an enterotoxin of *Staphylococcus* activates large numbers of T cells ('superantigens'), independent of their specificity. Similarly, Epstein–Barr virus activates most B cells but results in low affinity IgM antibodies.

Inactivation of immune effector mechanisms

This approach involves creation of at least a partial immunodeficient/ immunosuppressed state in the host in order to allow survival of invading microbes.

Phagocytosis

This is a critical mechanism for killing extracellular microbes. Microbes use different strategies to inhibit several of the stages of phagocytosis (Topic B1). Virulent strains of *Pneumococcus*, *H. influenzae* and *E. coli* are encapsulated making them difficult to phagocytose. Once engulfed, microbes are normally killed in phagolysosomes through oxygen-dependent and oxygen-independent mechanisms. Some microbes have developed enzymes that inhibit the oxygen burst, an essential event leading to killing. Certain strains of staphylococci have a protein coat (protein A) that can also inactivate IgG and IgA antibodies by binding to their Fc fragment thereby preventing them from acting as opsonins.

Inhibition of cytokines

Some viruses inhibit the production of IFNα by infected cells. This is seen in hepatitis B infection of hepatocytes.

Antibodies

Some organisms, e.g. treponemes, induce low affinity antibodies, while others, e.g. *Streptococcus pneumoniae* and *Candida*, inactivate antibodies by releasing large amounts of soluble antigens. Another strategy is for microbes to produce proteases that destroy the antibodies. Bacteria associated with mucosal infections such as *Neisseria gonorrhoeae* and *Pseudomonas* species produce protease enzymes that can destroy IgA, the antibody associated with mucosal protection. Pseudomonas also produces an elastase that inactivates C3b and C5a inhibiting opsonization and chemotaxis.

The complement system

Some organisms block complement activation and the lytic effects of complement. For example, HIV incorporates host complement regulatory proteins in their outer membranes to counteract the activation of complement.

T cells

HIV targets CD4 T cells, infecting and destroying them, effectively disarming the immune system and leaving the host immunodeficient. Some viruses decrease the expression of MHC class I on infected cells thus making it difficult for cognate interactions and killing of the infected cell by CD8$^+$ cytotoxic T cells.

Antigen processing

Measles virus, as well as infecting human T cells, inhibits antigen processing required to generate an immune response against it.

Regulatory mechanisms

Microbes such as typhi produce endotoxins that predispose the immune system to develop a Th2 response and thus primarily humoral immunity to the pathogen. However, eradication of these organisms requires a cellular response.

P1 ORIGIN AND HOST DEFENSE AGAINST TUMORS

Key Note

Origin and host defense against tumors	While the etiology of most human tumors is still unknown, it is now clear that radiation as well as a variety of viruses and chemical carcinogens can induce tumors and that immune responses in tumor bearing patients can develop, or be induced to develop, against antigens associated with these tumors. These responses may be important in tumor regression. Promising therapeutic approaches based on these findings have recently been developed which are efficacious in the treatment of at least some tumors. Vaccines are also likely to become available for therapy of tumors.

Related topics Cytokine and cellular
immunotherapy of tumors (P5)

Immunotherapy of tumors with
antibodies (P6)

Origin and host defense against tumors

The origin and host response to tumors is currently the focus of extensive basic and clinical research. With regard to origin, a large number of environmental factors have been shown to be carcinogenic and/or mutagenic in animals. Several tumors have, in fact, been associated with exposure to certain substances (asbestos with mesotheliomas in shipyard workers, hydrocarbons with scrotal cancer in chimney sweeps). Viruses are also known to induce tumors in animals. In humans, the Epstein–Barr DNA virus is involved in Burkitt's lymphoma and nasopharyngeal carcinoma, and the hepatitis B virus in liver cancer. The human T cell leukemia virus (HTLV) is involved in certain forms of lymphocytic leukemia and human herpes virus 8 (HHV8) causes Kaposi's sarcoma. In many instances host immune responses develop against tumors and in some instances may be protective. Based on the development of a clearer understanding of tumor immunology, numerous immunotherapeutic approaches have been explored for the treatment of cancer. Although the results from the use of monoclonal antibodies (mAbs), derivatized mAb, lymphokine activated killer (LAK) cells, tumor infiltrating lymphocytes (TILs), cytokines, etc., have been less promising than hoped, much has been learned about these immunological approaches and how best to use them. In fact, several promising therapeutic approaches have recently been developed which are efficacious in the treatment of at least some tumors. It seems likely, therefore, that additional effective immunotherapeutic approaches will also soon be developed for the treatment of cancer.

P2 TUMOR ANTIGENS

Key Notes

Introduction	Tumor cells can be distinguished from normal cells by quantitative and qualitative differences in their antigens. Tumor specific antigens (TSA) are unique to tumor cells but are rare, whereas tumor associated antigens (TAA) are on normal cells and more common. Tumor antigens can be classified based on their origin or nature.
Virally or chemically induced tumor antigens	Oncogenic DNA and RNA viruses code for viral antigens which are expressed by the tumor, and are shared by all tumors induced by the same virus. However, because of random mutagenesis of DNA, chemically induced tumors often express antigens unique to the individual tumor.
Oncofetal antigens	Antigens such as carcinoembryonic antigen (CEA) and alpha-fetoprotein (AFP) are highly associated with gastro-intestinal (GI) derived tumors and hepatomas, respectively. They are not unique to tumor cells since they are also found in normal cells during embryonic development and at low levels in normal human serum.
Differentiation antigens	Since many tumors result from the expansion of a single cell, a tumor will express the normal antigens characteristic of the type and differentiation stage of the cell that became malignant. This has permitted a clearer understanding, classification and prognosis of tumors.
Related topics	Antigens (A4) Antibodies as research and diagnostic tools (V1)

Introduction

A number of properties distinguish tumor from normal cells, including their invasiveness, loss of growth contact inhibition and their lack of response to regulation. In addition, there is considerable evidence for quantitative and qualitative differences in antigens associated with normal vs tumor cells. These antigens can be divided into tumor specific antigens (TSA), those unique to tumor cells, or tumor associated antigens (TAA) those also found on some normal cells. Another classification system is based on the origin or nature of the antigens and includes viral, chemical, oncofetal and differentiation antigens.

Virally or chemically induced tumor antigens

In animal models, oncogenic DNA viruses (*Table 1*) code for both cell surface and nuclear antigens which become expressed by the tumor. RNA tumor viruses induce tumor cell surface antigens which are viral proteins (*Table 1*). Thus, these antigens are shared by all tumors induced by the same virus. On the other hand,

Table 1.   Virally induced/associated tumors

Tumor viruses	Human tumor
RNA	
Human T cell lymphotrophic virus-1 (HTLV)	Adult T cell leukemia/lymphoma
DNA	
Epstein–Barr (EBV)	B cell lymphomas, Hodgkins lymphoma, nasopharyngeal carcinoma
Human papillomavirus (HPV)	Cervical carcinomas
Hepatitis B virus (HBV)	Hepatocellular carcinoma

because of the random mutagenesis of DNA that occurs, chemically induced tumors express antigens which are unique to the individual tumor.

Oncofetal antigens   Although highly associated with some tumors, both on their cell surface and in the serum, oncofetal antigens are not unique to tumor cells since they are also found on cells during embryonic development and are found at very low levels in normal human serum (*Table 2*).

Carcinoembryonic antigen (CEA) and alpha-fetoprotein (AFP) are two such antigens. CEA is expressed (both on the cells and in the extracellular fluids) by many gastrointestinal (GI) derived tumors including colon carcinoma, and pancreatic, liver or gall bladder tumors as well as by breast cancers. It is also expressed by the gut, liver and pancreas of human fetuses (2–6 months). AFP is found in secretions of yolk sac and fetal liver epithelium as well as in the serum of patients with hepatomas (liver tumors). These oncofetal antigens are thus not TSA nor is their presence, even at high concentration, in the serum diagnostic of cancer, because high levels can result from non-neoplastic diseases including chronic inflammation of the bowel or cirrhosis of the liver. However, the quantitation of these molecules in the serum can be used to evaluate the tumor burden and effectiveness of drug treatment.

Differentiation antigens   Some normal cellular antigens are expressed at specific stages of cell differentiation. These differentiation antigens can also be found on tumor cells and can be detected using mAbs (Topic V3). Moreover, since most tumors result from the expansion of a single cell arrested at some point in its differentiation, mAb to differentiation antigens are used to determine the approximate stage of differentiation at which the malignant event occurred. This which in turn permits the most appropriate therapy based on a clearer understanding and classification of the malignancy. Using this approach, for example, it has been found that most T cell leukemias are derived from early thymocytes or prothymocytes. Similar approaches have been applied to B cell tumors and other malignant states (*Table 3*).

Table 2.   Examples of oncofetal antigens

Antigen	MW (kD)	Nature	Associated tumor
Carcinoembryonic antigen (CEA)	180	Glycoprotein	Gastrointestinal, breast
Alpha-fetoprotein (AFP)	70	Glycoprotein	Hepatomas

Table 3.   Differentiation antigens on lymphoid and myeloid malignancies*

| Acute | | Chronic | |
Disease	Markers	Disease	Markers
common ALL	CD10 (CALLA), CD19, TdT (n)	B-CLL	CD19, CD20, CD5
null ALL	CD19, TdT (n)	HCL	CD19, CD20, TRAP
Pre-B cell ALL	CD19, IgM (m;cyt)	PLL	CD19, CD20,
T cell ALL	CD7, CD3 (cyt), TdT (n)	Sezary	CD3, CD4
Myeloid leukemia	CD13, CD33, myeloperoxidase	T-CLL	CD3, CD8

* ALL, acute lymphocytic leukemia; CLL, chronic lymphocytic leukemia; Tdt, terminal deoxynucleotidyl transferase; (n), nuclear; (cyt), cytoplasmic; TRAP, tartrate resistant acid phosphatase; Sezary, *Mycosis fungoides*.

P3 IMMUNE RESPONSES TO TUMORS

Key Notes

Immune surveillance
That the immune system surveys constantly for neoplastic cells and destroys them is suggested by the observation of increased incidence of tumors of lymphoid or epithelial cells in immunodeficient animals and humans. NK cells have been proposed to search for and eliminate certain tumors early in their development.

Effector mechanisms
Specific antitumor immunity appears to develop in tumor-bearing patients in much the same way as it does to pathogens or foreign antigens. Both TSA and TAA associated with tumor cells appear to be processed and presented in association with MHC class I molecules, making them potential targets for cytotoxic T cells. NK cells kill tumor cells not expressing MHC class I. Antibody coated tumor cells can be killed by complement activation, by MØ and PMN mediated phagocytosis and/or by ADCC.

Tumor escape
Mechanisms by which tumor cells may escape killing by the immune system include: (i) Induction of tolerance to tumor antigens; (ii) Development of tumor cells lacking antigens to which the immune system has responded; (iii) Modulation of tumor antigen expression; (iv) Tumor suppression of antitumor immunity; (v) Poor immunogenicity of the tumor perhaps resulting from lack of expression of MHC class I; (vi) Expression of Fas ligand (FasL) on tumors, which may induce apoptosis of effector cells.

Related topics
Natural killer cells (B2)
The cellular basis of the antibody
  response (J1)
T cytotoxic cells (K2)

Peripheral tolerance (M3)
Deficiencies in the immune system
  (S1)

Immune surveillance
It is supposed, but difficult to prove, that the immune system surveys constantly for neoplastic antigens associated with a newly developing tumor and destroys the cells bearing them. Evidence supportive of this possibility comes from the observation of increased tumor incidence in immunodeficient animals or humans. However, congenitally athymic mice do not have high tumor rates, suggesting that the T cell system may not be involved in surveillance for most tumors. Moreover, congenitally immunodeficient and immunosuppressed patients have high rates of tumors only of lymphoid or epithelial cells. Thus, a less-specific tumor surveillance system, perhaps NK cells, may search for and eliminate certain types of tumor cells early in their development. The best evidence for a surveillance mechanism involving T cells comes from experimental mouse models with virus-induced tumors but here the response is essentially directed to viral antigens and not tumor antigens.

Effector mechanisms

If a tumor evades the surveillance system, it might then be recognized by the specific immune systems. In models of chemically and virally induced tumors, the tumor associated antigens are immunogenic and trigger specific cellular and antibody responses against the tumor. This immunity may be protective and can be passively transferred with immune cells. In tumor bearing patients as well, it is possible to demonstrate antitumor antibody, which may mediate some tumor cell lysis.

It is likely that antitumor immune responses develop in tumor-bearing patients in much the same way as they do to pathogens or foreign antigens. Thus, anti-tumor antibodies and T cells are generated and, along with more non-specific immune defense mechanisms, play a role in tumor immunity. More specifically, it is likely that both TSA and TAA are associated with tumor cells and, after their intracellular synthesis, are processed and presented in association with MHC class I molecules, making them potential targets for cytotoxic T cells. Overall, the potential effector mechanisms which may be involved in human tumor cell lysis *in vivo* are the same as those used in microbial immunity (*Table 1*).

Tumor escape

If tumors possess immunogenic antigens which eventually stimulate specific immune responses, how do they escape rejection? The various possibilities which may explain tumor cell escape from the immune system include:

- Tolerance to tumor antigens. This might happen if the antigen is a TAA and thus also associated with normal cells and/or if the antigen is presented in a form or under conditions such that T cells are rendered unresponsive to it.
- Selection for tumor antigen negative variants. If antigens associated with tumor cells are able to elicit strong effective immune responses, tumor cells bearing these antigens would be rapidly eliminated, and only those tumor cells lacking, or with decreased amounts of, these antigens would survive.
- Modulation of tumor antigen expression. Binding of antibody to antigens on the surface of tumor cells may result in rapid internalization of antibody and its loss from the cell surface, permitting the tumor cell to escape temporarily from further detection by antibody and thus from FcR bearing effector cells.
- The tumor may immunosuppress the patient. Tumors may release molecules such as TGF-β or IL-10 which have immunosuppressive properties.
- The tumor may have low immunogenicity. Tumor cells having little or no MHC class I on their surface are able to avoid recognition by cytolytic T cells. Although these tumor cells are more susceptible to NK cells, NK cells do not have memory and thus there may be insufficient expansion of these cells to deal with a large tumor burden.
- Tumor cells sometimes express Fas ligand (FasL). When FasL on the tumor interacts with Fas on T cells, T cell apoptosis may result.

Table 1.   Potential tumor immune effector mechanisms

Antibody and complement
Antibody dependent cellular toxicity (ADCC) mediated by MO, PMNS or lymphocytes with Fc receptors
Specific cytotoxic T cells recognizing TAA or TSA peptides associated with MHC class I
Activated macrophages
Natural killer (NK) cells have surface Fc receptors for Ig (FcγRIII). They are activated for: antitumor activity by interferon and/or IL-2 and kill antibody coated tumor cells or tumor; cells lacking, or with decreased expression of, MHC class I molecules.

P4 IMMUNODIAGNOSIS

Key Notes

Classification	MAbs to antigens associated with a particular differentiation state can sometimes be used to classify the origin of the tumor and its stage in normal cell differentiation. This information permits prediction of the likelihood of success of current therapy.
Monitoring	MAbs can sometimes be used to determine the rate of change of TAA (oncofetal antigens, PSA, CA-125, CA-19-9) within the serum of a patient as a measure of tumor progression and duration of remission. Using cytological analysis, mAbs to certain TAA (e.g. cytokeratin, MUC-1) can be used to search for micrometastases.
Imaging	Radioconjugated mAbs specific for an appropriate TAA can sometimes be used to locate and image metastases in a tumor-bearing patient.
Related topics	Hemopoieis – development of blood cells (E1) Antibodies as research and diagnostic tools (V1)

Classification

Numerous mAbs have been developed against tumor cells. As few, if any, of these antibodies are absolutely tumor specific, binding of these mAbs to tissues from a patient will not necessarily indicate the presence or location of a tumor. However, because tumors often appear to be monoclonal in origin (develop from a single cell which has undergone a malignant event) and to have characteristics of the cell of origin, mAbs to antigens associated with a particular differentiation state can be used to classify the origin of the tumor and the stage in normal cell differentiation most similar to that of the tumor cell (see Topic P2). One of the most prominent uses of this approach is in the subgrouping of leukemias (*Fig. 1*). In particular, mAbs have permitted the definition of a large number of markers associated with lymphoid and myeloid cell populations, and with different stages of their differentiation. Information obtained using panels of such mAb permits classification of some types of tumors, and as a result, it is possible to develop patterns of tumor cell progression and responsiveness to therapy for tumors subclassified in this way. Thus, it becomes possible to predict, for a particular tumor subtype, whether or not current therapy will be effective and the need for a different therapeutic approach.

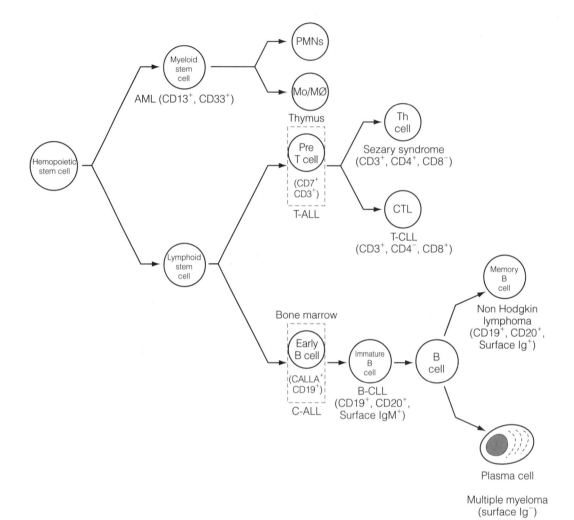

Fig. 1. Subgrouping of leukemias. AML, acute myeloid leukemia; T-ALL, thymic acute lymphoblastic leukemia; T-CLL, T-cell chronic lymphocytic leukemia; c-ALL, common acute lymphoblastic leukemia; B-CLL, B-cell chronic lymphocytic leukemia. Each myeloid or lymphoid tumor expresses a set of markers (molecules) typical of normal myeloid or lymphoid cells at a particular stage of their differentiation.

Monitoring

MAbs to TAA can sometimes be used to monitor the progression of tumor growth in a patient. Oncofetal antigens, because of their presence in serum, are useful for this purpose. That is, because they are normally only present at very low levels in normal human serum, the presence of large amounts of CEA and AFP may indicate a gastrointestinal or liver tumor, respectively. However, since conditions other than tumors elevate the level of these molecules in the serum, their levels are most useful in tumor bearing patients whose serum level of the oncofetal protein is known. Relapses or duration of remission can be followed by monitoring their rate of change (*Fig. 2*). In addition, quantitation of other TAA are used to monitor tumor presence and growth in patients with other tumor types. The serum levels of the mucins CA-125 and CA-19-9 (both high molecular weight proteoglycans) in a patient with ovarian cancer are useful in following the status and progression of this tumor. Prostate specific antigen (PSA) is similarly useful in prostate cancer.

Using cytological analysis, mAbs to certain TAA (e.g. cytokeratin) can be used to search for micrometastases in bone marrow or lymph node. Similarly, another mucin, MUC-1, is expressed on breast carcinomas in a pattern different from that on normal breast epithelium.

Imaging

By linking a radioisotope (e.g. ^{131}I) to a mAb specific for an appropriate TAA (e.g. CEA), and intravenously injecting this construct into a tumor bearing patient, it is possible to image tumor metastases using scintigraphy.

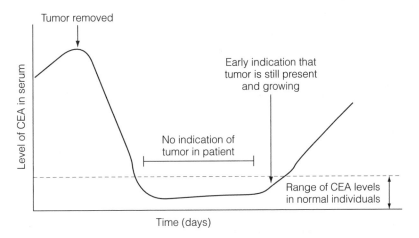

Fig. 2.   Monitoring serum levels of CEA in a cancer patient with a CEA expressing tumor.

P5 CYTOKINE AND CELLULAR IMMUNOTHERAPY OF TUMORS

Key Notes

Immunostimulation and cytokines	Nonspecific immunostimulants induce cytokine producing immune responses which activate effector cells, but have limited ability to mediate tumor cell lysis. Cytokines are critical to the development of immunity, but to be effective in tumor therapy, will probably need to be used in conjunction with specific immunotherapy.
Lymphokine activated killer (LAK) cells	Lymphocytes from a tumor bearing patient are cultured in IL-2 to expand and activate cytotoxic LAK cells, primarily NK cells. They are then infused into the patient with or without more IL-2.
Tumor infiltrating lymphocytes (TILs)	TILs are $CD8^+$ T cells isolated from patient tumor samples, some of which react with tumor antigens. After activation with IL-2, they are infused into the patient with or without more IL-2. As with LAK therapy there is significant toxicity if high doses of IL-2 are used.
Macrophage activated killer (MAK) cells	Monocytes isolated from peripheral blood of tumor-bearing patients are cultured *in vitro* with cytokines which activate these cells for enhanced cytotoxicity before reinjection into the patient.
Related topics	Molecules with multiple functions (G1)　　　　Cytokines in the clinic (G3)　　T cytotoxic cells (K2)

Immunostimulation and cytokines

Initially, immunotherapy in humans utilized nonspecific immunostimulants such as BCG and *C. parvum*, which have had limited success. These results probably reflect the development of strong immune responses involving production of cytokines capable of activating immune effector cells which mediated increased tumor cell lysis. When recombinant cytokines became available, they were tried, but again with limited success. Thus, although cytokines are critical to the development of specific immune responses, when used alone they primarily enhance nonspecific activation of immune cells (see Table 1, Topic G2). To be effective antitumor agents they will probably need to be used in conjunction with other more specific stimulation of immunity.

Lymphokine activated killer (LAK) cells

This approach involves expansion and activation of cytotoxic cells outside the body, which are then reinjected (*Fig. 1*). Peripheral blood lymphocytes from a tumor bearing patient are cultured in IL-2 to expand and activate cytotoxic LAK

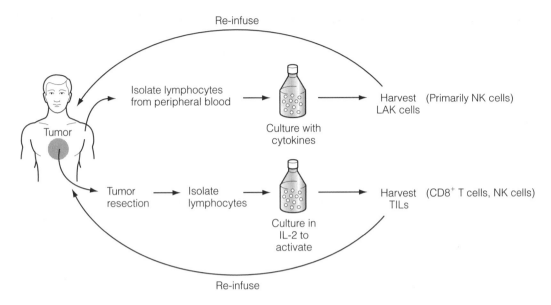

Fig. 1.   Therapy with LAK cells and TILs.

cells. These are primarily NK cells and thus do not have the specificity of T cells, but rather react with and kill tumor cells which express few or no cell surface MHC class I molecules. LAK cells may be infused back into the patient with or without more IL-2. Although some tumor regression occurs with this approach, significant toxicity is evident if high doses of IL-2 are used.

Tumor infiltrating lymphocytes (TILs)   As with LAK cells, TILs are obtained from tumor-bearing patients, expanded and activated with IL-2 (*Fig. 1*). In particular, TILs are lymphocytes isolated from patient tumor samples that are primarily CD8$^+$ T cells, at least some of which are thought to be specific for tumor antigens. They are also infused back into the patient with or without more IL-2. TIL therapy induces tumor regression in some patients and especially in patients with renal cell carcinoma. Again, there is significant toxicity if high doses of IL-2 are used to maintain the active status of the TIL cells *in vivo*.

Macrophage activated killer (MAK) cells   Another immunotherapeutic approach involves the use of cytokines and activated macrophages. Monocytes are isolated from peripheral blood of tumor-bearing patients and cultured *in vitro* with cytokines (e.g. IFNγ) which activate these cells for enhanced cytotoxicity before reinjection into the patient. Although these cells are highly cytotoxic and phagocytic, they are relatively nonspecific, and may require co-injection with antibody to TAAs to be most effective.

P6 IMMUNOTHERAPY OF TUMORS WITH ANTIBODIES

Key Notes

Specificity of antibodies to tumors	The vast majority of mAbs prepared against human tumors are not truly tumor specific. The TSAs which have been identified include: (i) idiotypes of antibody on a B cell tumor; and (ii) a mutant form of epidermal growth factor receptor (EGF-R) which has a deletion of an extracellular domain.
Tumor therapy with antibodies alone	MAbs kill tumor cells by apoptosis or through complement activation, ADCC or phagocytosis. Several humanized mAbs have demonstrated efficacy including an mAb to: (i) HER2/neu for treatment of breast cancer; and (ii) CD20 for therapy of B cell tumors. Thus, mAbs may be useful if they are human or humanized, react with an antigen highly expressed on the tumor are used to treat minimal disease and are used in patients whose immune system is fully functional.
Tumor therapy with immunotoxins (ITs)	ITs are mAbs to TAA that are linked to a toxin or radioisotope. MAbs coupled to toxin are internalized where they inhibit critical cellular processes. Radioisotope coupled mAbs mediate killing by DNA damage from decay and release of high energy particles.
Tumor therapy with bispecific antibodies (BsAbs)	BsAbs are molecules which have two different covalently linked specificities, one against a TAA, the other to a trigger molecule on a killer cell. *In vivo*, BsAbs bind to immune effector cells, arming them to seek out and kill tumor cells.
Purging of bone marrow for autologous transplants	The high doses of chemotherapy or irradiation necessary to cure some patients of their tumor are toxic to hemopoeitic stem cells. Thus, bone marrow transplants are sometimes used in which stem cell-containing blood or bone marrow is taken from the patient, after which the patient is treated with high doses of chemotherapy or irradiation. The patient is then rescued by infusion of their own stem cells, which have been purged of contaminating tumor cells using mAbs to antigens associated with the tumor.

Related topics   Hemopoiesis – development of   The transplantation problem
                            blood cells (E1)   (Q1)
                            Allotypes and idiotypes (F4)
                            Monoclonal antibodies (F6)

Specificity of antibodies to tumors

Considerable effort has been expended on the development of mAbs to TSA, since it was thought that only mAbs specific for tumor cells would be useful in the diagnosis and treatment of tumors. However, few if any mAbs prepared against human tumors have been found to be truly tumor specific. Examples of antigens which could be considered to be TSA include:

- The idiotype of the antibody on a B cell tumor (e.g. CLL). The first successful use of an mAb in tumor therapy involved treatment of a patient with anti-idiotype antibody prepared specifically against the patient's tumor. DNA coding for idiotypes is currently being explored as a potential way to immunize patients against their own B cell tumor (Topic P7).
- A mutant form of the epidermal growth factor receptor (EGF-R) which has a deletion of an extracellular domain. That this molecule is antigenic and uniquely expressed on tumors may be the basis for an antibody based therapeutic or for a vaccine to induce a CTL response.

Tumor therapy with antibodies alone

Although mAbs can cause tumor cell lysis through complement activation, by targeting NK cells, Mo, and/or MØ ADCC or phagocytosis, or by inducing apoptosis, the use of mAbs to treat human tumors has had, until recently, little success. To some extent these failures probably resulted from: (i) the lack of specificity of the mAb utilized; (ii) the presence of soluble forms of the antigen in the serum, which effectively interfered with the interaction of antibody with the tumor cell; (iii) modulation and loss of the antibody–antigen complexes from the tumor cell surface before antibody mediated killing could occur; (iv) outgrowth of (selection for) tumor cells not expressing the antigen; and (v) the use of mouse mAbs, which do not interface well with human effector cells (NK cells, macrophages, PMNs) and being foreign, induced a human anti-mouse antibody (HAMA) response which blocked the effectiveness of the mAb.

Nonetheless, the clearer appreciation that developed of how to use mAbs more effectively in cancer therapy has resulted in a renaissance in antibody therapy (*Fig. 1*). Many trials are with humanized mAbs (Topic V5) and some have already demonstrated efficacy (indicated by the long term survival of some patients), including: (i) a mAb to HER2/neu (Herceptin) which has been approved by the US FDA for treatment of breast cancer; (ii) a mAb to CD20 (Rituxan) a molecule expressed on B cells and B cell tumors, also approved by the US FDA; and (iii) mAb, 17-1A which reacts with an antigen associated with colorectal cancer. Thus, there is growing optimism that mAbs will be very useful tumor therapeutic agents, especially if they are human or humanized to permit long term use, the antigen to which they react is expressed at a high level on the tumor, the mAb is used to treat minimal disease and the patient's immune system is fully functional.

Tumor therapy with immunotoxins (ITs)

Many studies, including clinical trials, have used mAbs to which toxins or radioisotopes have been coupled (*Fig. 1*). Thus, when injected into a patient, ITs would not need to activate patient effector mechanisms. Rather, ITs would seek out and bind to tumor cell antigens, and mediate their own lethal hit. Toxins such as ricin are very potent inhibitors of critical intracellular processes, with a single molecule able to kill a cell. It is essential, however, that the targeting mAbs react with a TAA that is internalized on binding of IT.

Radioisotope coupled mAbs mediate killing by DNA damage from decay and release of high energy particles. This kind of IT will kill bystander cells (those nearby) which may result in killing of normal cells, but also of adjacent tumor cells

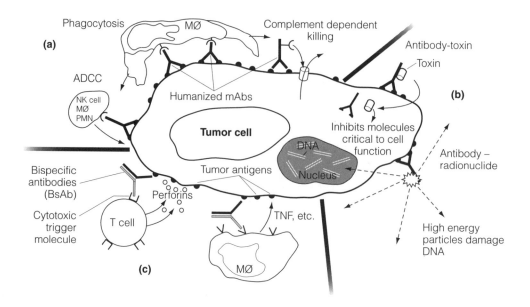

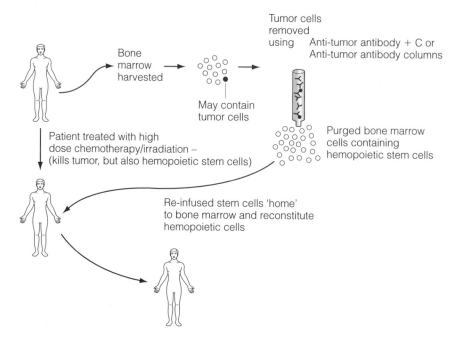

Fig. 1.   Antibody-based tumor therapy. (a) antibody alone; (b) antibody toxin/radionuclides constructs; (c) bispecific antibodies; (d) purging of tumor cells from bone-marrow or stem cell populations.

which do not express the targeted antigen. The development of useful ITs has taken more time than initially anticipated due to toxic side effects, but many of the problems have been solved and some ITs are now in late stage clinical trials.

Tumor therapy with bispecific antibodies (BsAbs)

Directing or redirecting immune effector cells is also being explored as a way to enhance the ability of a patient's own immune system to reject their tumor. BsAbs, consisting of the binding sites of two different covalently linked mAbs, have been prepared as anti-tumor therapeutics. One specificity of this BsAb is to a TAA (e.g. HER2/neu), the other to a trigger molecule on a killer cell (e.g. CD3 on T cells). When injected into a tumor-bearing patient, the BsAb binds to the immune effector cell thereby arming it to seek out, and kill tumor cells. Several BsAbs have shown considerable promise and are now in late stage clinical trials for therapy of different cancers.

Purging of bone marrow for autologous transplants

Much of cancer therapy involves the use of cytotoxic drugs and/or irradiation, both of which primarily target dividing cells. Although effective for many patients, a significant number are not cured and eventually succumb to their tumor, partly because the amount of chemotherapy or irradiation a patient can receive is limited by the toxicity of these agents to normal cells and especially hemopoeitic stem cells (cells that give rise to platelets, PMNs, lymphocytes, etc.). In order to be able to increase these dosages, bone marrow transplants are sometimes used in conjunction with chemotherapy and irradiation. In particular, stem cell-containing blood or bone marrow is first taken from the cancer patient. The patient is then treated with doses of chemotherapy or irradiation high enough to kill all tumor cells, but doses likely to kill all hemopoietic stem cells as well. The patient is then rescued by infusion of their own stem cells which repopulate the bone marrow (Topic E1). Autologous marrow is commonly given because donor marrow of identical MHC types is not often available (Topic Q2). However, because tumor cells may contaminate the stem cell populations harvested before therapy, mAbs to antigens associated with the tumor are used to purge the marrow so that these cells are not returned to the patient to reestablish the tumor. This approach has been successfully used in the treatment of some tumors, including myeloid leukemia.

P7 TUMOR VACCINES

Key Notes

Prophylactic vs therapeutic vaccines
The development of vaccines for treatment of cancer is a very active area of research. Prophylactic vaccines induce immunity to viruses associated with tumor development; other approaches are designed to enhance/induce effective immunity in tumor bearing patients.

Immunization with tumors and tumor antigens
Killed or irradiated patient tumor cells or appropriate TAAs and their peptides are being tested for induction of patient antitumor immunity to antigens that are primarily tumor associated. Immunizing with DNA for the TAA or peptide may induce a stronger CTL response.

Immunization with transfected tumors
Transfecting tumor cells with costimulatory molecules enhances their immunogenicity and ability to induce a CTL response. Tumor cells transfected with cytokine genes attract, expand and activate immune cells reactive to tumor antigens.

Immunization with APCs loaded with TAA
Since immature dendritic cells (DC) are best able to ingest antigen and mature DCs are best at presenting antigen, considerable effort is directed at determining optimal conditions for loading and maturing DCs so they induce strong CTL antitumor responses when introduced into the patient.

Related topics
T cytotoxic cells (K2)
Antigen preparations (R3)

Vaccines to pathogens and
tumors (R4)

Prophylactic vs therapeutic vaccines

Numerous approaches are being used to develop vaccines for use in the treatment of cancer. Prophylactic approaches focus on the use of vaccines that induce immunity to viruses known to be associated with the development of a tumor. Hepatitis B vaccines would prevent infection by this virus and reduce the incidence of liver cancer. Human papilloma virus (HPV) vaccines would prevent the development of cervical carcinoma. Vaccines developed against specific viral proteins of HPV are currently in clinical trials. In contrast, most other tumor vaccine approaches are designed to enhance or induce effective tumor immunity in patients who have already developed cancer.

Immunization with tumors and tumor antigens

A variety of approaches have been explored for inducing or enhancing a patient's immunity to their tumor. These include injecting killed or irradiated tumor cells from the patient, an approach which has had little success. The identification of appropriate TAAs (those expressed at low levels on normal cells and high levels on tumors), and their potentially immunogenic peptides has resulted in their use in vaccines to focus the patient's immune system to respond to antigens that are primarily tumor associated. As with immunization using whole cells, these antigens would most likely induce a T helper cell rather than a more desirable CTL response, as they would enter APCs by the exogenous pathway and be presented on MHC class II molecules. However, it is now clear that the APC presenting antigen to the CTL needs first to be conditioned by interaction with a T helper cell before it can effectively induce a CTL response. Moreover, antigens entering by the exogenous pathway may in some instances be presented on MHC class I molecules and initiate a CTL response.

Still another approach that is being very actively pursued involves immunizing with DNA encoding the TAA or peptide, either alone or in an appropriate expression vector. This DNA introduced into a cell would be integrated, expressed, and translated into proteins in the cytosol, some of which would be degraded to peptides for loading onto MHC class I molecules and thus potential induction of a CTL response.

Immunization with transfected tumors

Since most kinds of tumor cells do not express the costimulatory molecules (e.g., B7.1, B7.2) which are important to the induction of an immune response, studies were carried out to determine if transfecting tumor cells with these molecules would enhance their immunogenicity. In fact, B7 transfected tumor cells induced a strong CTL response against the tumor. Furthermore, these CTLs were sometimes able to lyse parent tumor cells not expressing B7, because once activated, CTLs do not need the B7 costimulatory signals to kill.

Another approach involves transfecting tumor cells from a patient with a cytokine gene, as certain cytokines expressed by the tumor may attract, expand and activate cells of the immune system and induce or enhance immunity to tumor antigens. In experimental models, tumor cells transfected with cytokine genes (e.g., IL-2, IFNγ, GM-CSF) are able to induce immunity to the tumor resulting in its regression or rejection. IL-2 may, for example, enhance the development of cytotoxic cells to TAAs from their precursors (e.g. in melanoma).

Immunization with APCs loaded with TAA

A very active area of tumor vaccine research at the present time involves loading of patient dendritic cells *in vitro* with TAA and reinjection of these cells into the patient. This approach has the benefit that potential APCs can be isolated from a patient's peripheral blood and manipulated such that their antigen presenting capabilities are optimal. Since immature DCs are best able to ingest antigen and mature DCs are best at presenting antigen, loading of immature DCs followed by cytokine induced differentiation of these cells to mature DCs is more readily accomplished *in vitro* than *in vivo*. These mature, loaded APCs are then reintroduced into the patient, fully able to stimulate T cells. Many groups are currently trying to define the optimal conditions for obtaining immature DCs, for loading and maturing them, and for their reintroduction into the patient.

Q1 THE TRANSPLANTATION PROBLEM

Key Notes

Historical perspective

Much of our early knowledge about transplantation rejection was gained during the Second World War when skin grafts were given to treat wounds. Animal experiments led to the first definition of antigens responsible for transplant rejection.

Types of grafts

Transplants are either from one part of the body to another (autografts), to a member of the same species (allografts), or across species (xenografts). Allografts that are commonly used clinically include blood, heart, kidney and liver.

The major problem of rejection

The major transplantation antigens are those of the ABO blood groups and the human leukocyte antigen (HLA) system which are polymorphic, i.e. are coded for by several possible alleles. Antibodies and cell mediated immunity (CMI) are responsible for graft rejection. The likelihood of rejection can be reduced by transplanting within families, tissue typing, and immunosuppression. Bone marrow transplantation can result in graft versus host reactions.

Related topics

The major histocompatibility antigens and antigen processing

and presentation (H4)
Transplantation antigens (Q2)

Historical perspective

Skin grafts were used to treat major wounds acquired during the Second World War, and it was from this experience that the early concept of transplantation rejection was founded. This led to the now widely known fact that transplantation of donor organs/tissues to another individual usually results in rejection, unless histocompatible tissues (based on specific tissue typing) and immunosuppression are used. Early experiments in mice in the 1950s and 60s defined the role of the major histocompatibility molecules in graft rejection. Transplantation is now common medical practice and many different organs/tissues are transplanted (*Table 1*).

Types of grafts

Tissues/organs are transplanted either from one part of the body to another (autograft), and since they are self are not rejected. Transplantation can be with tissue/organs from an individual within the same species (allograft) or from one

Table 1. Commonly transplanted organs/tissues

Allografts	Autografts
Kidney, pancreas, heart (heart/lung), skin, cornea, bone marrow, liver, blood	Skin, bone marrow

species to another (xenograft). Human transplants are usually allografts but xenografts are now being considered as an alternative due to inadequate supplies of human donor organs/tissues.

The major problem of rejection

That the immune system is responsible for the rejection process has been demonstrated in animal models and in humans. The immune mechanisms used for rejection are the same as those used in immune responses to invading microbes and are essentially adaptive immune responses. The cause of the problem is genetic polymorphism, and in particular that the transplantation antigens are mainly polymorphic gene products, e.g. blood groups and major histocompatibility complex (MHC) molecules, which vary among different individuals within the same species. Rejection can be minimized by using familial donors, tissue typing and immunosuppressive drugs. Bone marrow transplantation given to provide stem cells can result in graft versus host reactions.

Q2 TRANSPLANTATION ANTIGENS

Key Notes

The blood group antigens	The major blood group antigens are those of the ABO system. These carbohydrate antigens are present on erythrocytes and some other tissues. Most individuals have antibodies (isohemagglutinins) which recognize these antigens. Thus, blood group A individuals have antibodies to blood group B, and blood group B individuals antibodies to blood group A. Blood transfused from one group to the other would be rejected.
The major histocompatibility complex antigens	The main tissue transplantation antigens are encoded by the polymorphic MHC locus (HLA in man). The inheritance of two alleles (out of many possible) at six different loci (A,B,C, DP,DQ,DR) means that the chance of all HLA antigens of two individuals being exactly the same is very low (1 in 10 million).
Minor histocompatibility antigens	Minor transplantation antigens include non-ABO blood groups and antigens associated with the sex chromosomes. These are usually 'weaker' than the MHC antigens, and are probably the antigens targeted by the immune system in late onset rejection.
Related topics	Basic structure (F1) The major histocompatibility antigens and antigen processing	and presentation (H4) Genes, T helper cells and cytokines (N3)

The blood group antigens

The major blood group ABO antigens are mainly present on the surfaces of erythrocytes and the genes encoding them are polymorphic, i.e. there is more than one allele coding for the gene product. This is in contrast to most proteins, e.g. albumin, which are coded for by nonpolymorphic genes or genes which lack allelic variation. The major blood group alleles A and B, code for enzymes which create different sugars on proteins and lipids on the surface of erythrocytes. Blood group O is a null allele and does not add sugars. These alleles are inherited in a simple Mendelian inheritance pattern and are codominantly expressed (i.e. both allelic products are expressed on the erythrocyte surface, *Table 1*). An individual can either be homozygous (the same) or heterozygous (different) for the inherited alleles.

The major problem with transplanting blood is that all of us have antibodies (isohemagglutinins) to these blood group antigens (*Table 1*). The reason for

Table 1.   Blood group antigens and isohemagglutinins

Blood group	A	B	AB	O
Genotype	AA or AO	BB or BO	AB	OO
Isohemagglutinins	Anti-B	Anti-A	None	Anti-A and B

development of these antibodies is unclear, but is probably due to cross-reactivity of AB antigens with those of certain ubiquitous microbes. Transplantation of blood to a recipient who has serum isohemagglutinins can result in a severe transfusion reaction mediated by a type II hypersensitivity reaction (Topic T3).

The major histocompatibility complex antigens

These are the major barrier to transplantation of nucleated cells. As previously described, MHC molecules are expressed on all nucleated cells of the body and their physiological function is to direct T cells to carry out their function. However, like the locus coding for the major blood group antigens and unlike the majority of other gene products, genes coding for MHC molecules are polymorphic. In contrast to the ABO system, each MHC locus can encode for a very large number of different allelic forms and to further increase the complexity, there are six different loci. In humans, this locus is found on chromosome 6 (*Fig. 1*) and encodes HLA, since the antigens were first discovered in humans on leukocytes.

The combinations of the many different allelic forms which are codominantly expressed means that the chances of two individuals having a completely identical set of alleles is extremely remote (1 in 10 million). Thus the different allelic products of the donor organ/tissue will be foreign to the recipient who does not have them and will therefore generate an immune response to them. An example of alleles that might be expressed by donors/recipients is shown in *Table 2* and the

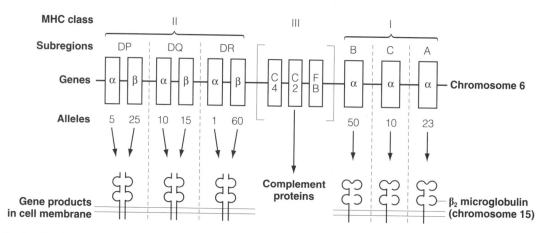

Fig. 1. The human major histocompatibility locus. Class I and Class II human leukocyte antigens (HLA) are encoded by three (A, B and C) and six genes (DP, DQ and DR), respectively. Each gene can be coded by many different alleles, the products of which, if different from self, are recognized as transplantation antigens. Thus, there are millions of different combinations of the different allelic products. The class III HLA locus encodes complement proteins.

Table 2.   Human leukocyte antigens (HLA) alleles of a hypothetical donor and recipient

Locus	Donor	Recipient	Alleles to which the recipient's immune system responds
HLA-A	A2/A2	A6/A2	None*
HLA-B	B21/B26	B23/B8	B21, B26
HLA-C	C5/C8	C9/C4	C5, C8
HLA-DR	DR4/DR6	DR8/DR3	DR4, DR6
HLA-DP	DP3/DP1	DP2/DP1	DP3
HLA-DQ	DQ3/DQ3	DQ4/DQ2	DQ3

* The recipient's immune system sees A2/A2 as self.

target of the recipient 's immune system would be the products of the mismatched alleles.

Minor histocompatibility antigens
There are a number of minor transplantation antigens that include non-ABO blood groups and antigens associated with the sex chromosomes. These are usually 'weaker' than the MHC antigens, and are probably the antigens targeted by the immune system in late onset rejection (Topic Q3).

Q3 REJECTION MECHANISMS

Key Notes

Rejection is an adaptive immune response	Transplants given to recipients that have previously rejected a graft having the same transplantation antigens, are rejected more rapidly. This is due to a specific memory response to these antigens, a property of the adaptive immune system.
Mechanisms of rejection of allografts	The adaptive immune system recognizes the mismatched HLA allelic products expressed on donor tissues and is responsible for rejection. Both antibody and T cell mediated (CMI) rejection occurs depending on the source of tissue for the transplant, e.g. skin, mainly CMI and kidney, antibodies and CMI. The number of mismatches between donor and recipient (i.e. transplantation antigens) usually determines the strength of rejection.
Xenotransplant rejection	Due to the inadequate supply of human donors, animals are being considered as an alternative source of organs/tissues. The pig is deemed appropriate, since the size of many of its internal organs is comparable with that of man. Hyperacute rejection problems have arisen due to the presence in the pig of cell surface sugars to which humans have natural hemagglutinins, similar to those against ABO antigens.
Donor rejection of host tissues	In addition to donor rejecting graft tissue, T cells in bone marrow grafts are stimulated by mismatched host HLA leading to a graft versus host reaction. Care to avoid this response is required in using bone marrow as a source of stem cells in cases of anemia, metabolic diseases of the newborn, primary immunodeficiency and some tumors, especially leukemias.
Related topics	The cellular basis of the antibody response (J1) Prevention of graft rejection (Q4) Cell mediated immunity (K1) Deficiencies in the immune system (S1)

Rejection is an adaptive immune response

The immune system treats mismatched transplants in the same way as microbes. Thus, if a patient rejects a transplant through transplantation antigens, it will reject a second graft carrying the same or shared transplantation antigens much faster. This 'second set' rejection in due to the sensitization by the first graft and a memory response on subsequent exposure. This is a property of the adaptive immune system.

Mechanisms of rejection of allografts

Graft rejection is mediated by both cell mediated (T cell) and humoral immune mechanisms (antibodies). Furthermore, the number of mismatched alleles also determines the magnitude of the rejection response. The more mismatches, the larger the number of antigens to which an immune response can be made. Thus in Topic Q2, *Table 2* above, the recipient's immune response could respond to eight different donor transplantation antigens. Although both T cell mediated responses and antibodies can be generated against the foreign antigens, the rejection of particular types of graft may be preferentially mediated more through antibodies than through T cell mediated immune (CMI) responses and vice versa (*Table 1*). In general, immune responses against transplantation antigens mediated by preformed antibodies result in a rapid rejection (hyperacute).

Allografts can show three main types of rejection patterns. The best studied transplant being the kidney (*Table 2*).

Table 1.   *Main mechanisms of rejection of different kinds of grafts*

Organ/tissue	Mechanism(s)
Blood	Antibodies (isohemagglutinins)
Kidney	Antibodies, CMI (T cell)
Heart	Antibodies, CMI (T cell)
Skin	CMI (T cell)
Bone-marrow	CMI (T cell)
Cornea	Usually accepted unless vascularized, CMI (T cell)

- Hyperacute rejection occurs within a few minutes or hours and is believed to be mediated by pre-existing circulating antibody in the recipient to antigens of the donor. Unlike other transplants, the kidney has ABO coded sugar antigens expressed on the endothelial cells of the blood vessels. Thus, if the donor has a different blood group from the recipient, the antibodies will result in a type II hypersensitivity reaction in the kidney graft (Topic T3). Graft recipients might also have some memory responses to HLA through rejection of a previous graft. In addition, multiparous women recipients may have been sensitized to paternal HLA expressed by their child's cells. This could occur during pregnancy and at parturition when small amounts of blood of the newborn may get into the maternal circulation. Prior transfusion with blood containing some leukocytes of a recipient can also result in priming to HLA alleles.
- Acute rejection occurs within the first weeks or months following transplantation. The graft shows infiltrates of activated lymphocytes and monocytes. Antibody may be a factor in the process, but the effector mechanism is primarily through cytotoxic T cells or helper/delayed type hypersensitivity T cells (Topic T5) and monocytes/macrophages.
- *Chronic rejection* is the gradual loss of function of the grafted organ occurring over months to years. The lesion often shows infiltration with large numbers of mononuclear cells, predominantly T cells. The mechanism of rejection is not clear but following transplantation, memory (and primary) responses which generate antibody and cellular immunity to HLA may take some time, especially since the patient will be immunosuppressed to improve graft 'take' (see later) and there might be only a limited number of mismatched alleles. Furthermore, minor transplantation antigens may eventually produce a significantly large immune response to result in rejection.

Table 2.   *Kidney graft rejection*

Type of rejection	Time to rejection	Cause
Hyperacute	Within hours	Preformed antibodies (anti-ABO and/or anti-HLA)
Acute	Weeks to months	Cell-mediated ($CD8^+$, $CD4^+$ T cells)
Chronic	Months to years	Cell-mediated ($CD8^+$ T cells), antibodies to tissue antigens

Xenotransplant rejection

The inadequate supply of donor organs/tissues has led to consideration of animals as donors. In particular, the pig appears to be a suitable source of transplantable tissues since the size of many of the internal organs is comparable with that of man. However, a major unforeseen problem is that pig cells have sugars which are not found on human cells and to which humans have serum IgM hemagglutinating antibodies (similar to the ABO isohemagglutinins, *Table 1*, Topic Q2). Thus, pig organs will be rejected through a hyperacute mechanism due to preformed hemagglutinins which activate complement resulting in lysis of the grafted cells. Strategies planned to prevent this include:

- Trying to inactivate the gene encoding the glycosyltransferase responsible for the sugar residues.
- Introducing genes into the pig which code for molecules which inhibit the lytic component of complement activation (see Topic M1, *Fig. 3*).

Even if these strategies are successful, there is still the problem of the MHC molecules expressed by pig tissues. The use of nonhuman sources of grafts have additional problems. These include ethical issues and the possibility of transferring unknown viruses that, in the long-term, could enter the germ-line.

Donor rejection of host tissues

Although most transplant rejection is the result of the immune system of the recipient recognizing and responding to the donors' HLA (host versus graft response), in the case of bone marrow transplants there is an additional problem in that the graft (the bone marrow) contains viable active lymphocytes. In particular, T cells may recognize recipient cells as foreign and produce a graft versus host reaction (*Table 3*). More specifically, donor T cells may recognize mismatched HLA alleles and respond to them.

Table 3. Host versus graft and graft versus host reactions

Host versus graft reaction	Graft versus host reaction
Response to donor HLA by host immune system	Response to recipient HLA by donor T cells

This often results in skin rashes and gastrointestinal problems and may be quite serious. The pathology is probably mediated by inflammatory cytokines released from the donor T cells. In some cases it can be alleviated by cyclosporin A treatment. Bone marrow stem cells are given for a number of clinical conditions to provide functional genes. These conditions include some primary immunodeficiency diseases, anemias, tumors and metabolic diseases (*Table 4*). Other conditions in which bone marrow grafts are being tested are for breast cancer and rheumatoid arthritis following heavy chemotherapy/irradiation to remove the tumor and lymphoid cells, respectively.

Table 4. Clinical conditions for which bone marrow grafts are given

Anaemias	Metabolic diseases	Immunodeficiency diseases	Tumors
Fanconi's anemia	Gaucher's disease	Reticular dysgenesis	Acute lymphoblastic leukemia
	Thalassemias	Severe combined	Acute myeloid leukemia
Aplastic anemia	Osteopetrosis	Chronic granulomatous disease	Chronic myeloid leukemia
		Wiskott-Aldrich syndrome	Chronic lymphocytic leukemia

Q4 PREVENTION OF GRAFT REJECTION

Key Notes

Familial grafting	Due to the inheritance pattern of the HLA genes, transplantation within families reduces greatly HLA mismatches. Transplants from parents to siblings have at least a 50% match of HLA alleles, whilst sibling to sibling grafts have a 25% chance of having identical HLA alleles.
Tissue typing	Typing of the HLA of both transplant donor and recipient can be done by antibodies or 'typing' cells. Molecular genetic based techniques are also now used by some laboratories.
Cross-matching	Cross-matching is used to test for preformed antibodies in the recipient directed to donor tissues. This is measured by mixing serum from the recipient with blood lymphocytes from the donor.
Immunosuppression	Suppression of the immune system by drugs is usually necessary to aid in maintenance of the graft. The drugs used include corticosteroids, cytotoxic drugs (e.g. azathioprine) and cyclosporin A.
The special case of the 'fetal transplant'	The fetus is an allograft, and yet in most cases it is not rejected due to the body itself suppressing the rejection process. There are probably several mechanisms involved including lack of expression of conventional HLA on the trophoblast, absorption of potental anti-HLA antibodies in the placenta and immunosuppressive molecules produced in the placenta.
Related topics	Functions (F5) Rejection mechanisms (Q3) Molecules with multiple functions (G1)

Familial grafting

Transplantation within families significantly reduces allele mismatches because of the inheritance patterns of HLA (*Fig. 1*). In general, there is little crossover within the locus and the whole locus is usually inherited *en bloc*. Thus, if parents donate grafts to their children there is equal to or greater than (due to chance) 50% match of the HLA alleles. If siblings (brothers and sisters) donate to each other there is a one in four chance of a complete match. Thus, if you need a transplant, make sure you come from a family with lots of brothers and sisters! Other tissue antigens that trigger far less vigorous rejection responses (minor histocompatibility antigens) are encoded outside the MHC locus and include male specific antigens. In fact, mismatches of minor transplantation antigens can be important in determining the fate of grafts between HLA matched donor and recipient, especially as it relates to chronic rejection over a longer period of time.

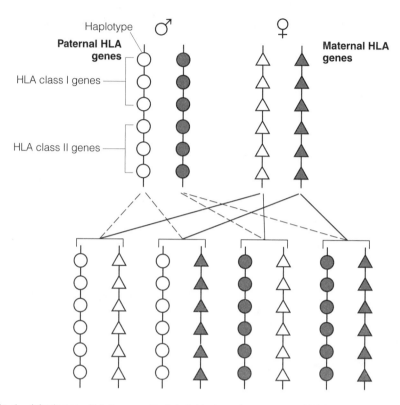

Fig. 1.   *Inheritance of HLA genes. Each individual receives one set of HLA genes from each parent (i.e. they receive one haplotype from each parent). Because of their position on the chromosomes, alleles are inherited en bloc. Grafts from parents to siblings and vice versa have at least 50% of matched alleles whilst sibling to sibling grafts have a 1 in 4 chance of a complete match.*

Tissue typing   If a familial donor is not available, then the extent of the mismatches between alleles must be determined by tissue typing, in order to best match donor and recipient. In this context, one of the most useful assays involves cytotoxic antibodies (usually mAbs) to individual HLAs. The principal of the antibody method depends on the surface expression of the HLA. Donor and recipient blood for typing are enriched for B cells (they express both class I and II HLA) and specific cytotoxic antibodies are added. Binding of the antibody to a surface HLA in the presence of complement results in the direct killing of the B cells (*Fig. 2*). These can be microscopically scored. Using a panel of antibodies, it is possible to HLA type for the majority of alleles.

Many HLA typing labs are now turning to identification of the HLA genes inherited via molecular genetics based tests that utilize the restriction fragment length polymorphism (RFLP) or polymerase chain reaction (PCR) amplification techniques. These technologies determine the nucleotide sequence of the HLA genes in question and give unequivocal results. Outside its use in tissue typing for transplants, this technology has been particularly important in identifying minor polymorphisms within the HLA-D regions which might be associated with susceptibility to particular kinds of diseases (Topic U2).

Typing can also be done using the 'mixed lymphocyte' reaction, which primarily identifies HLA-D class II antigens. In this case, 'typing cells' (usually cell lines

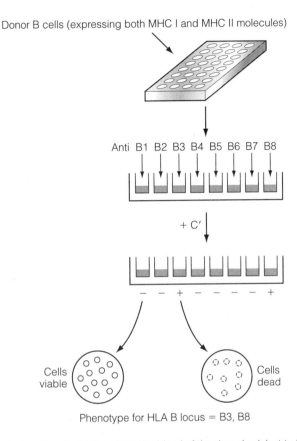

Donor B cells (expressing both MHC I and MHC II molecules)

Anti B1 B2 B3 B4 B5 B6 B7 B8

+ C'

− − + − − − − +

Cells viable

Cells dead

Phenotype for HLA B locus = B3, B8

Fig. 2.   Tissue typing. B cells obtained from the blood of the donor/recipient to be typed are placed in microplates and antibodies to the different MHC allelic products added together with complement. These include antibodies to HLA A, B and C loci and some D antigens. Only antibodies to B1 to B8 are shown here to illustrate the concept. Following incubation at 37°C, lysis (cell death) of the B cells occurs in those wells where antibodies have attached to the B cells. Thus, in this example, lysis of the B cells indicated that the donor was heterozygous for the B locus – B3 and B8.

carrying specific homozygous HLA-D allelic products) are treated with a drug to inhibit their proliferation. They are then mixed with the potential recipient's blood lymphocytes and cultured for 3–5 days. If the recipient's T cells do not carry the typing cell's HLA, they will proliferate in response to 'foreign' HLA since they will not have been eliminated by negative selection in the thymus (Topic M2). By using panels of typing cells, it is possible to determine the HLA type of the donor and recipient.

Matching of HLA for liver transplants does not appear to be of major advantage, probably due to the weak expression of HLA by hepatic cells.

Cross-matching   Cross-matching is used to check that there are no preformed antibodies to donor HLA in the recipient. Blood lymphocytes from the donor are mixed with serum from the recipient (*Fig. 3*). Anti-donor antibodies are detected by lysis of the cells (mediated by complement) or by using fluorescent staining and flow cytometry. The presence of such antibodies is contraindicatory to the use of the tissues from that donor. Cross-matching for blood groups is also important for renal transplants (Topic Q3).

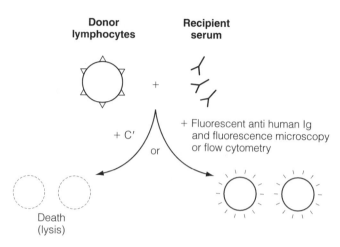

Donor lymphocytes

Recipient serum

+

+ C'

or

+ Fluorescent anti human Ig
and fluorescence microscopy
or flow cytometry

Death
(lysis)

Fig. 3.   Cross-matching. Serum from the potential recipient is mixed with donor lymphocytes and is evaluated for lysis (see Fig. 2), in the presence of complement, or stained with fluorescent antibodies to human immunoglobulin (Topic V3 Figure 2) and assayed by fluorescence microscopy or flow cytometry. Dead cells or positive fluorescence signifies the presence of antidonor antibodies which could lead to a hyperacute rejection of the graft. This is contraindicatory to the use of this donor/recipient combination. This assay identifies HLA antibodies in the recipient serum. Cross-matching for blood groups is also carried out for renal transplants.

Immuno-suppression

In the vast majority of cases, there will be some allelic mismatches and some donor minor histocompatibility antigens, therefore the immune system of the recipient has to be suppressed to avoid rejection. The mainstay drug treatment is a mixture of corticosteroids, synthetic cytotoxic drugs and cyclosporin A (a fungal nonapeptide). The mechanisms of immunosuppression by these and other drugs used are shown in *Table 1*. Not surprisingly, a major problem with these drugs is that by inhibiting the immune response against the graft they can also lead to increased susceptibility to infections (see Topic S1). In fact, infection and rejection are the main reasons for the failure of kidney grafts to be maintained. Other drugs, e.g. anti-lymphocyte antibodies, which kill the recipient's lymphocytes, are also used by some transplant teams.

Table 1.   Drugs used to suppress graft rejection

Drug	Mechanism(s) of immunosuppression
Corticosteroids	
Prednisone	Blocking of migration of neutrophils: Inhibition of IL-1, IL-6 and IL-2 production
Cytotoxics	
Azathioprine	Kills cells at division
Methotrexate	
Cyclophosphamide	
Immunophilins	
Cyclosporin A	Inhibits IL-2 production and/or responses to IL-2
FK506	
Rapamycin	

The special case of the 'fetal transplant'

The fetus is a chimera carrying HLA alleles from both parents. It is therefore effectively an allograft in close apposition to maternal tissues. The mechanism(s) by which rejection is prevented (i.e. it is tolerated) are still under intensive research. However, there are several possibilities including:

- Classical HLA molecules are not expressed by the trophoblast, the outermost layer of the fetus which comes into direct contact with the maternal tissue in the placenta. These nonclassical HLAs might also act to suppress the activity of NK cells (which infiltrate the placenta) and also T cells.
- Any anti-HLA antibodies produced against paternal antigens would be absorbed on the fetal side of the placenta (sink) so that they could not enter the general fetal circulation. Effects of anti-HLA may also be inhibited by over-expression of complement regulatory proteins (Topic M1).
- A number of immunosuppressive molecules have been isolated from the placenta that may play a role in suppressing the induction of an immune response to the paternal antigens. The placenta has high levels of a tryptophan-degrading enzyme, depleting tryptophan essential for T cell activation and growth.

R1 PRINCIPLES OF VACCINATION

Key Notes

Principles of vaccination	The primary goal in vaccination is to provide protective immunity by inducing a memory response to an infectious microorganism using a non-toxic antigen preparation. It is important to produce immunity of the appropriate kind: antibody and/or cellular immunity.
Antibody mediated protection	Antibodies produced as a result of immunization are effective primarily against extracellular organisms and their products, e.g. toxins. Passively administered antibodies have the same effect as induced antibodies.
Cell-mediated immunity	Cell-mediated immunity (T cells, macrophages) induced by vaccination is important particularly in preventing intracellular bacterial and viral infections and fungal infections.
Related topics	The cellular basis of the antibody response (J1) Cell mediated immunity (K1)

Principles of vaccination

Edward Jenner, a country physician in England, noticed that dairymaids who frequently contracted cowpox often were immune to the ravages of smallpox, leading him to develop an approach whereby cowpox was used to vaccinate people against smallpox. The term vaccination is derived from the Latin word 'vaccinus' meaning 'from cows'. Vaccination eventually resulted in the complete eradication of smallpox (in 1980) and has been generalized as a reliable method of protection against many pathogens.

The aims of vaccination are to induce memory in T and/or B lymphocytes through the injection of a nonvirulent antigen preparation. Thus, in the event of an actual infection, the infectious agent and/or its toxin is met by a secondary rather than a primary response. The ideal vaccine would protect the individual and ultimately eliminate the disease, but most vaccines simply protect the individual. A more or less standard set of vaccines are now in use worldwide, some of which are (or should be) given to everyone and others to those particularly at risk (*Table 1*). The timing of vaccination depends on the likelihood of infection; vaccines against common infections being given as early as possible, allowing for the fact that some vaccines do not work properly in very young infants.

Antibody mediated protection

Antibodies either produced as a result of immunization or passively introduced into the host are very effective means of preventing infection. They will be ready and able to bind the infectious agent at the time of infection instead of waiting for the host's immune system to respond. Antibodies can either block viral or

Table 1. Vaccine recommendations.

Recommended for	Vaccine	When given/to whom
All	Measles Mumps Rubella	From 1 year (6 months in tropics) boost at 10–14 yrs
	Diphtheria Tetanus Pertussis	From 2–3 months old dip/tet boost at 5 yrs
	Polio (Sabin) (or *Salk)	2–6 months (oral) parenterally
All, unless Mantoux +	BCG	10–14 yrs (at birth in tropics)
Those at risk	Hepatitis B	1–6 months/12 intervals (childhood in tropics)
	Hepatitis A Influenza Rabies	Institutions, nurses etc., annual boost needed Travel, post-exposure: vaccine + antibody
	Meningococcus Pneumococcus Haemophilus Varicella-zoster	Epidemics Elderly Children Children with leukaemia
At risk (travel)	Typhoid Cholera Yellow fever	Travelers Travelers Travelers: boost 10 intervals

* The Salk is the polio vaccine of choice in Holland and Scandinavia.

bacterial antigens from entering host cells by preventing adherence or prevent damaging effects on other cells by neutralizing toxins such as those produced by *Diphtheria* or *Clostridium* species (Topic O2). IgA plays an important role at the mucosal surfaces where it helps to prevent viral or bacterial access to the mucosa lining cells. This is the mechanism by which polio vaccination works.

IgG antibodies are usually effective in the blood. Antibodies can also be transferred across the placenta to provide **passive immunity**. Mothers transfer their preformed IgG antibodies across the placenta to their newborn in order to protect them during the first months of life. This passive transfer can be of a disadvantage in that the presence of the maternal antibody inhibits effective immunization. Thus, immunization has to be delayed until after most of the maternal antibodies have been metabolized.

In pre-antibiotic days, it was common to treat or prevent infection by injecting antibody preformed in another animal, usually a horse or a recently recovered patient. This principle is still in use for certain acute conditions where it is too late to induce active immunity by vaccinating the patient (see Topic T4).

Cell-mediated immunity

While antibodies may play a major role in combating infections, cell-mediated immunity is essential for eradicating certain bacteria, fungi and protozoa (Topic K1): vaccination should therefore be aimed at inducing both cellular and humoral responses to the infectious agent. In certain instances not only are CD4 and CD8 lymphocyte responses desired but it may be more advantageous to specifically target Th1 or Th2 responses e.g., infections with helminths might favour a Th2 type immunity via induction of IgE antibodies, whereas protection against mycobacterial infections may be better obtained by a Th1 response, by producing macrophage activation factors. CD8 cytotoxic T lymphocytes find and kill infected cells which are making proteins that are components of pathogens. The cell that is targeted is determined by the presence of the foreign protein in association with MHC class I molecules. The CD8 T cells lyse the infected cell; hopefully before progeny infectious organisms are fully developed. The CD4 cells are basically the directors of the immune response. These cells interact with foreign antigen expressed with MHC class II molecules and then provide soluble or membrane bound signals for B cells, macrophages or CD8 T cells to help them obtain their full effector cell functions: Ig production by B cells, killing by macrophages and CD8 T cells. Some diseases only require an antibody response for protection or clearance, while others require a cell-mediated immune response. Still other diseases are only resolved if both forms of protection are present. Some infections will self-resolve and the immune response is not necessary and can complicate the infection.

R2 IMMUNIZATION

Key Notes

Passive immunization	Passive immunization is the administration of preformed antibodies either intravenously or intramuscularly. It is used to provide rapid protection in certain infections such as diphtheria or tetanus or in the event of accidental exposure to certain pathogens such as hepatitis B. It is also used to provide protection in immune compromised individuals.
Active immunization	Active immunization is the administration of vaccines containing microbial products with or without adjuvants in order to obtain long term immunological protection against the offending microbe.
Systemic immunization	At present the normal route of vaccination in most instances is either intramuscularly or subcutaneously.
Mucosal immunization	Oral immunization is the method of choice for polio and *Salmonella typhi* vaccines. However, there is an increasing awareness that this route of immunization may be the best for most immunizations since nearly all infectious agents gain entrance through the mucosal surfaces.
Related topics	Mucosa-associated lymphoid tissues (D3) Immune-complex mediated (type III) hypersensitivity (T3) Cytokine families (G2) Antigen preparations (R3)

Passive immunization

Passive immunization is the administration of preformed antibodies, usually IgG, either intravenously or intramuscularly. These antibodies may be derived from individuals who have high titres to particular microbes and are used to provide rapid protection in certain infections such as *Diphtheria*, *Clostridium* species, rabies etc., or in the event of accidental exposure to certain pathogens such as hepatitis B. Passive immunization is also used to provide protection in immune compromised individuals who are unable to make the appropriate antibody response or in some instances incapable of making any antibody at all, i.e., severe combined immunodeficiency. Antibodies given to immune deficient patients are usually IgG-derived from pooled normal plasma. These antibodies have to be given on a continuous basis, ideally every three weeks, since they are being continuously catabolized and only effective for a short period. Antibodies preformed in animals, notably horses, are also administered for some diseases. However, it is important that with repeated injections of horse antibody, there is the danger of immune complex formation and serum sickness (Topic T4). Antisera are usually injected intramuscularly, but can be given intravenously in extremely acute conditions. Indications for the use of passive immunization by the injection of pre-formed antibody are shown in *Table 1*.

Active immunization

Active immunization is the administration of vaccines containing microbial products with or without adjuvants in order to obtain long term immunological protection against the offending microbe.

Systemic immunization

Systemic immunization is the method of choice at present for most vaccinations. This is usually carried out by injecting the vaccine subcutaneously or intramuscularly into the deltoid muscle. Ideally all vaccines would be given soon after birth, but some are deliberately delayed, for various reasons. The common systemic vaccines for measles, mumps and rubella are usually given at 1 year of age because, if given earlier, maternal antibody would decrease their effectiveness. The carbohydrate vaccines for *Pneumococcus*, *Meningococcus* and *Haemophilus* infections are usually given at about 2 years of age as before this age they respond poorly to polysaccharides unless they are associated with protein components that can act to recruit T cell help for the development of anti-polysaccharide antibody.

Mucosal immunization

Recent vaccination approaches have focused on the mucosal route as the site of choice for immunization either orally or through the nasal associated immune tissue (NALT: Topic D3). This is because most infectious agents gain entry to the systemic system through these routes and the largest source of lymphoid tissue is at the mucosal surfaces. Moreover, if successful it would obviate the need for, in some instances, painful injections and allow for the self-administration of certain vaccines such as those used for immunization against influenza. Adjuvant vaccines and live vectors have been used to target the mucosal immune system with some success. Attenuated strains of salmonella can act as a powerful immune stimulus as well as acting as carriers of foreign antigens. This approach has been used to immunize mucosal surfaces against herpes simplex virus and human

Table 1. Passive immunization

Infection	Source of antiserum	Indications
Tetanus	Immune human; horse	Post exposure (plus vaccine)
Diphtheria	Horse	Post-exposure
Gas gangrene	Horse	Post-exposure
Botulism	Horse	Post-exposure
Varicella-zoster	Immune human	Post-exposure in immunodeficiency
Rabies	Immune human	Post-exposure (plus vaccine)
Hepatitis B	Immune human	Post-exposure Prophylaxis
Hepatitis A	Pooled human Ig	Prophylaxis
Measles	Immune human	Post-exposure in infants
Snakebite	Horse	Post-bite
Some autoimmune diseases	Pooled human Ig	Acute thrombocytopenia and neutropenia

papilloma virus. Furthermore, bacterial toxins, e.g. those derived from cholera, *E. coli* and *Bordetella pertussis*, have immunomodulatory properties and are thus being exploited in the development of mucosally active adjuvants. Pertussis toxin has been shown to augment the costimulatory molecules B-7 on B cells and CD28 on T cells (Topic L1) as well as increasing IFNγ production. Hopefully, oral and nasal vaccines may soon be available to obviate the need for the invasive techniques that are currently in use.

R3 ANTIGEN PREPARATIONS

Key Notes

Antigen preparations
Protection against pathogenic microorganisms requires the generation of effective immune mechanisms. Thus, vaccines must be capable of targeting the immune system appropriately i.e. cellular and/or humoral mechanisms. Most vaccines consist of either attenuated organisms, killed organisms, inactivated toxins, or subcellular fragments and more recently genes for antigens in viral 'vectors', and DNA itself.

Adjuvants
Nonliving vaccines, especially those consisting of small molecules require the inclusion of agents to enhance their effectiveness. These adjuvants include microbial, synthetic and endogenous preparations having adjuvant activity, but at present only aluminium or calcium salts are generally used in humans. Adjuvants should enable antigens to be slowly released, preserve antigen integrity, target antigen presenting cells and induce cytotoxic lymphocytes.

DNA vaccines
The use of DNA encoding antigens as vaccines as distinct from bacteria or bacterial proteins has shown potential. Intramuscular injection of circular DNA results in DNA uptake by muscle cells, expression of the encoded protein and induction of both humoral and cell-mediated immunity.

Recombinant vaccines
Using molecular genetics, selective recombinant proteins of defined epitopes can be prepared that protect the host. This approach overcomes the problem of disease complications which might occur with modified live vaccines.

Cytokines
Cytokines can be added at the time of immunization to skew the immune response to a Th1 or Th2 type depending on which is associated with protection. The cytokines can be added either as purified protein made from recombinant technology, or they can be cloned into the vectors (virus or bacterial vaccine) to be delivered at the time of vaccination. Cytokines that might be useful are IL-12 or IFNγ that favour a Th1 response, or IL-4 and IL-10 that favour a Th2 response.

Related topics

Molecules with multiple functions (G1)

The cellular basis of the antibody response (J1)
Cell mediated immunity (K1)

Antigen preparations

The protective immune response to pathogenic microorganisms requires the generation of specific T and B cell responses and appropriate effector mechanisms. In order to do this, vaccines must be capable of targeting the immune system appropriately. In principle anything from whole organisms to small peptides can be used, but in practice most vaccines consist of either attenuated organisms, killed organisms, inactivated toxins, or subcellular fragments (*Table 1*).

There is a also a fundamental distinction between live and dead vaccines. Living and nonliving vaccines differ in many important respects, notably safety and effectiveness. Live ones consist of organisms (nearly always viruses) that have been attenuated by growth in unfavourable conditions, forcing them to mutate their genes; mutants that have lost virulence but retain antigenicity are repeatedly selected. Nowadays, mutation is usually 'site-directed' by recombinant DNA technology. Such organisms, which are essentially new strains, can sometimes regain virulence by back-mutation, and can also cause severe disease in immunocompromised individuals. On the other hand they often induce stronger and better localized immunity, do not often require adjuvants or 'booster' injections and provide the possibility of 'herd' immunity in that mutated nonvirulent virus could be transferred to nonimmunized individuals in a local community. Moreover, the immunity induced is usually more appropriate for protection against the pathogenic strain of the organism, e.g. Th1 vs Th2 responses.

Killed organisms or molecules derived for these organisms are used when for some reason stable attenuated organisms cannot be produced. These antigens may however induce weak and/or inappropriate (e.g. antibody vs CTL) responses. Immune memory may be variable or poor, but they are usually safe if properly inactivated. In only one case (polio) is there a choice between effective live and killed vaccines. Recently, it has been shown that the genes for one or more antigens can be inserted into a living vaccine (usually virus) 'vector', and experi-

Table 1.   Antigen preparations used in vaccines

Type of antigen	Examples	
	Viruses	Bacteria
Normal heterologous organism	Vaccinia (cowpox)	
Living attenuated organism	Measles Mumps Rubella Polio: Sabin Yellow fever Varicella-zoster	BCG Typhoid (new)
Whole killed organism	Rabies Polio: Salk Influenza	Pertussis Typhoid Cholera
Subcellular fragment Inactivated toxin (toxoid)		Diphtheria Tetanus Cholera (new)
Capsular polysaccharide		*Meningococcus* *Pneumococcus* *Haemophilus* Typhoid (new)
Surface antigen	Hepatitis B	

ments are being performed with totally synthetic peptides, the idiotype network, and even DNA itself.

Adjuvants

Nonliving vaccines, especially those consisting of small molecules, are not very strong antigens, but can be made stronger by injecting them along with some other substance such as aluminium hydroxide, aluminium phosphate, calcium phosphate or hen egg albumin; such substances are called adjuvants. The properties of adjuvants should include the following: (i) the ability to enable antigens to be slowly released so as to prolong antigen exposure time to the immune system; (ii) preserve antigen integrity; (iii) target antigen presenting cells; (iv) induce cytotoxic lymphocytes; (v) produce high affinity immune responses; and (vi) have the capacity for selective immune intervention. A variety of microbial, synthetic, and endogenous preparations have adjuvant activity, but at present only aluminum and calcium salts are approved for general use in man.

Combinations of macromolecules (oils and bacterial macromolecules) are commonly used as adjuvants in experimental animals to promote an immune response. The oil in the adjuvants increases retention of the antigen, causes aggregation of the antigen (promoting immunogenicity), and inflammation at the site of inoculation. Inflammation increases the response of macrophages and causes local cytokine production, which can modulate the costimulatory molecules, needed for T cell activation. Microparticles have also been used as adjuvants in the experimental model; these include latex beads and poly (lactide-co-glycolide) microparticles. Adjuvants are now being designed and tested to determine how to selectively drive Th1 or Th2 responses. Some experimental adjuvants currently under investigation are shown in *Table 2*.

DNA vaccines

A few years ago an exciting discovery was made when it was shown that 'naked' cDNA that encoded the hemagglutinin of the flu virus could be inoculated into muscle tissue to stimulate both antibody production and a CTL response that was specific for the flu protein. The potential for this is still unknown, but if this can become a routine method of immunization, then the cost of generating and transporting vaccines should be very low. Other uses of recombinant DNA technology are the cloning of defined epitopes into viral or bacterial hosts. Typically well characterized infectious agents such as vaccinia, polio, or *Salmonella* are used. DNA sequences are cloned into the genome of these agents and are expressed in target structures that are known to be immunogenic for the host. This way the antigen is presented for optimal recognition by the host. Inclusion of cytokines with the vaccine vectors may prove to be an efficient method for ensuring the correct cytokine environment to steer the immune response accordingly. DNA vaccines have potentially a number of advantages over

Table 2.   Experimental adjuvants currently undergoing assessment.

Experimental, but likely to be approved
Liposomes (small synthetic lipid vesicles)
Muramyl dipeptide, an active component of mycobacterial cell walls
Immune-stimulating complexes (ISCOMS) (e.g. from cholesterol or phospholipids)
Bacterial toxins (*E. coli*, pertussis, cholera)

Experimental only
Cytokines: IL-1, IL-2, IFNγ
Slow-release devices; Freunds adjuvant
Immune complexes

traditional methods of vaccination. These include specificity, the induction of potent Th1 and cytotoxic T lymphocyte responses similar to those observed with attenuated vaccines but without the potential to revert to overt infection.

Recombinant vaccines

Advances in molecular virology and bacteriology have provided the immunologist with many new targets for vaccine development. The last 20 years of study of viral and bacterial pathogenesis have identified the components of the immune system that are protective for many infectious agents. The use of defined epitopes that are protective for vaccines is now possible. The idea is that certain parts of an infectious disease causing organism, such as herpes virus glycoprotein D (glyD), stimulate CTL that are protective. If the host is inoculated with the defined peptide of glyD, they develop CTL responses to the epitope and do not have to worry about resulting disease from vaccination with a modified live vaccine. This approach is also possible for protection to infectious agents that is provided by antibody. In this scenario, both a B cell epitope (the site that the antibody binds to on the infectious agent) and a T cell epitope (the peptide that binds to the MHC Class II to stimulate the CD4 helper cells) must be present, so as to select the appropriate B cells, and to stimulate the specific T cell help.

Cytokines

The effects of cytokines can influence the function of professional antigen presenting cells (APC) enabling these cells with much greater efficiency. Thus, IFNγ and IL-4 causes increased levels of class II molecules to be expressed thereby enhancing their antigen presentation abilities. The use of such effector cytokines is being considered as a useful adjunct in vaccination, as polarization of the immune system to a Th1 or Th2 response may be preferable in some instances, e.g. a Th1 response is the preferred response in tuberculosis whereas a Th2 response is important in protecting against polio. Since Th1 and Th2 responses are mutually inhibitory manipulation of these responses may open up avenues of selective intervention.

R4 VACCINES TO PATHOGENS AND TUMORS

Key Notes

Bacterial vaccines

Bacterial vaccines have been developed to many different types of bacteria: *Escherichia*, *Haemophilus*, *Pneumococcus*, *Vibrio*, *Helicobacter* (ulcer causing bacteria) and Lyme's disease spirochete to name a few. Perhaps more familiar is the diphtheria, pertussis and tetanus (DPT) vaccine that many young children receive to protect them from often fatal childhood diseases.

Viral vaccines

Vaccines have been developed to viruses that infect the respiratory tract (flu, adenovirus), the gastrointestinal tract (polio, roto), the skin (yellow fever, La Crosse fever) and some that infect the reproductive tract (herpes). As with bacteria, viral vaccines are either modified, live, killed, or subunit.

Vaccines to other infectious agents

Protozoan parasites, such as those that cause malaria (*Plasmodium*), African sleeping sickness (*Trypanosoma*) and *Schistosomiasis* are major diseases mostly of the Third World. The ability to vaccinate people and animals to protozoan diseases will allow people to live in areas that are endemic (where the organism is always present) for the disease.

Tumor vaccines

Vaccination strategies against cancer are currently being investigated. Vaccines containing tumor antigens such as those associated with prostate cancer (prostate specific antigens) as well as those associated with the breast, colon and ovarian cancers such as HER2/neu offer hope for the future.

Related topics

T cell activation (L2)	Immunity to different
B cell activation (L3)	organisms (O2)
	Tumor vaccines (P7)

Bacterial vaccines

Bacterial vaccines have been developed to many different types of bacteria: *Escherichia*, *Haemophilus*, *Pneumococcus*, *Vibrio*, *Helicobacter* (ulcer causing bacteria) and Lyme's disease spirochete to name a few. Perhaps more familiar is the diphtheria, pertussis and tetanus (DPT) vaccine that many young children receive to protect them from often fatal childhood diseases. Some bacterial vaccines are specific for proteins on the bacteria that are required for their attachment and subsequent invasion of the host. Vaccines can be used to induce immunity to endo- or exotoxins. Vaccines, as typified by BCG (*Mycobacterium tuberculosis*) can be developed that clear bacterial-infected cells. Modified, live, killed, and subunit vaccines have been developed for various bacteria. The difference in the forms will be discussed below. T-independent vaccines to carbohydrates such as the capsule of *Pneumococcus* or *Haemophilus* are in use. These vaccines are effective but have limitations because T cell help is not provided for affinity maturation and isotype switching.

Viral vaccines

Vaccines to viruses that infect the respiratory tract (flu, adenovirus), that infect the gastrointestinal tract (polio, roto), that infect the skin (yellow fever, La Crosse fever) and some that infect the reproductive tract (herpes) have been developed. As with bacteria, viral vaccines are either modified-live, killed, or subunit. The recent emergence of HIV virus as a world-wide health hazard has focused the world's attention on viral vaccine development. In fact, some viral vaccines have been developed for viruses that are in the same genetic classification group as HIV. These have proven to be effective, but why not for HIV? This question highlights an important issue in vaccine development. What is a good vaccine? They must be safe, effective, cheap to make and distribute, stable for long-term storage or transport, be insensitive to major changes in temperature and they should provoke an immune response that lasts for a long period of time.

Vaccines to other infectious agents

Protozoan parasites, such as those that cause malaria (*Plasmodium*), African sleeping sickness (*Trypanosoma*) and *Schistosomiasis* are very important diseases mostly of the Third World. The ability to vaccinate people and animals to protozoan diseases will allow people to live in areas that are endemic (the organism is always present) for the disease. Parasites express many antigens which are usually immunogenic, but most do not consistently stimulate protective responses. Of note, parasites have evolved defense mechanisms that allow a continual evolution of the immunogenic epitopes. This is best typified by *Plasmodium* that continually and rapidly develops variants with different surface proteins so that the current immune response is no longer effective. Parasites have also developed mechanisms to shift the focus of the immune response by altering the cytokine profile during the induction phase to one that is not protective (e.g. from Th1 to Th2 as in the case of *Mycobacterium lepri*) (Topic O3).

Tumor vaccines

These vaccines are in their infancy. In principle, the immune system should be able to recognize tumors which may have foreign antigens associated with them through immune surveillance. This works in part, but most tumor associated antigens are either absent or weakly immunogenic through being expressed at low levels. In experimental animals, tumors that are induced by chemicals are more likely to have new or neo-antigens that are immunogenic and are characteristic of the individual tumors. Most new approaches to both direct therapy and vaccines is through targeting the overexpressed products of proto-oncogenes which have been found in a variety of tumors. For example, the HER2/neu antigen is overexpressed by many prostate and breast tumors. The major challenge for immunologists is to optimize the routes of delivery of these antigens to maximize induction of protective immunity (Topic P7). Clearly of importance is the role of CTLs in immunity to tumors and recently immunogenic peptides have been isolated from class I molecules expressed on myeloma tumor cells which are effective at inducing tumor specific immunity.

S1 DEFICIENCIES IN THE IMMUNE SYSTEM

Key Notes

Components of the immune system

Each of the four components of the immune system (T cells, B cells, phagocytes, and complement) has its domain of function important to protection against certain pathogens. These components are intimately integrated into a program of immune defense that could be severely compromised if even one were absent or deficient.

Defects in specific immune components

The occurrence of repeated or unusual infections in a patient is a primary indication of immunodeficiency. Although a deficiency may compromise several components of the immune system, in most instances the deficiency is more restricted and results in susceptibility to infection by some but not all microbes. For example, defects in T cells tend to result in infections with intracellular microbes, whereas those involving other components result in extracellular infections.

Classification of immunodeficiencies

Immunodeficiencies are either primary (mostly congenital/inherited), or secondary (acquired as the consequences of other diseases and their treatments). These can be defined on the basis of the specific immune component that is abnormal.

Related topics

Phagocytes (B1)
Innate molecular immune defence
  against microbes (C1)
Hemopoiesis – development of
  blood cells (E1)

Molecules with multiple functions
  (G1)
Cell mediated immunity (K1)

Components of the immune system

The multiple interactive cellular and molecular components making up the immune response usually provide sufficient protection against bacterial, viral or fungal infections. However, any situation that results in impaired immune function may contribute to a spectrum of disorders referred to as immunodeficiency diseases. In particular, immunodeficiency is defined as an increased susceptibility to infection. It is evident from a consideration of the disorders and infections in individuals with selective immunodeficiency that each component of the immune response (T cells, B cells, phagocytes and complement) has its domain of function. These four systems, although somewhat independent, are intimately integrated into a program of immune defense that could be severely compromised if even one were absent or deficient. In particular, the requirements for cell cooperation, the importance of chemotactic stimuli and activating factors emphasize the interdependence of these systems and the potential consequences of an abnormality in any of these systems. However, although the absence of, or an abnormality in, one domain may compromise the individual, they need not be life threatening if other components of the immune system can compensate for this deficiency.

Defects in specific immune components

The occurrence of repeated or unusual infections in a patient is a primary indication of abnormalities in immune function and of immunodeficiency. A variety of circumstances may be involved in this impairment of immune function including genetic, tumors, irradiation, cancer chemotherapy, malnutrition, ageing, etc. Although it is possible that the deficiency could be global and thus effect several components of the immune system (e.g. as in the case of severe combined immunodeficiency), in most instances the deficiency is restricted to a single component. Such deficiencies result in susceptibility to infection by some but not all microbes. For example, diseases involving defects in T cells predispose to infections with intracellular organisms including mycobacteria, some fungi and viruses, whereas those involving the other three systems tend to result in many bacterial infections which have an extracellular habitat. In other words, infections with particular microbes are a reflection of which components of the immune system are defective. Moreover, it is often possible to define the abnormal immune component in an immune deficiency disease and in the process, discover a considerable amount about the importance of that component in normal immune defense and in its interrelationships with the other components of the immune system. Furthermore, it is important to recognize such abnormalities and to pinpoint them as accurately as possible since correction, if possible, must be tailored to the specific abnormality.

Classification of immuno-deficiencies

The immunodeficiency diseases can be classified as either primary – usually **congenital** (the result of a failure of proper development of the humoral or cellular immune systems), or secondary – **acquired** (the consequences of other diseases and their treatments). A large number of specific congenital or acquired abnormalities in the immune system have been identified which contribute to patient susceptibility to recurrent infectious problems. These abnormalities range from those that affect the immune system at a very early level, and thus compromise the immune response to many antigens, to those that affect the final stages of differentiation of particular immune cells and hence lead to very selective abnormalities. The primary diseases are very rare whilst the secondary diseases are relatively common. A more pathophysiological description characterizes the specific immune component that is abnormal. Thus, one notes quantitative or qualitative abnormalities of the cells (lymphocytes, phagocytes) and/or molecules (antibodies, cytokines, complement components) of the immune system.

S2 PRIMARY/CONGENITAL (INHERITED) IMMUNODEFICIENCY

Key Notes

Complement	Patients deficient in certain complement components (especially C3) are prone to recurrent infections with encapsulated organisms (*Pneumococcus* and *Streptococcus*) and *Neisseria*. Opsonization of these pathogens by C3b is important for their removal by phagocytosis. Deficiencies in membrane attack complex (MAC) components and in complement regulatory molecules also result in increased susceptibility to certain infections or to inflammation, respectively.
Phagocytes	Intrinsic defects include those associated with differentiation, chemoattraction, and intracellular killing of the microbe. Extrinsic or secondary defects (not an inherent phagocytic defect) may result from antibody or complement deficiency or suppression of phagocytic activity.
Humoral immunity	Primary antibody deficiency may result from abnormal development of B cells or from lack of T helper activity. Patients suffer from recurrent extracellular bacterial infections. Patients with severe combined immunodeficiency (SCID) and Bruton's disease have few or no B lymphocytes and no antibodies. In hyper-IgM syndrome, CD40 signaling is defective and there is no class switch from IgM. Common variable immunodeficiency (CVID) may result from lack of B cell terminal differentiation or absence of T cell help.
Cellular immunity	Most T cell deficiencies result in severely compromised humoral as well as cellular immunity. These patients have recurrent life threatening viral, fungal, mycobacterial, and protozoan infections. In Di George syndrome, thymus embryogenesis is defective and few T cells develop. SCID may result from defects in the cytokine receptor γ chain or adenosine deaminase enzyme or purine nucleoside phosphorylase deficiency.

Related topics	Hemopoiesis – development of blood cells (E1)	The acute inflammatory response (I)
	Cytokine families (G2)	Cell mediated immunity (K1)
		B cell activation (L3)

Complement

Primary immune deficiencies of the complement system have been described for many of the 21 different complement components and their inhibitors, some in terms of specific gene mutations. Patients with deficiency of certain of these complement components (especially C3) are prone to recurrent infections with both encapsulated organisms such as *Pneumococcus* and *Streptococcus*, as well as with *Neisseria* (*Table 1*). The attachment of complement to the surface of some of these organisms is clearly important for their removal by phagocytic cells. Deficiencies in the later complement components and in the regulatory molecules of the complement system also result in increased susceptibility to certain infections (by meningococcus e.g. *Neisseria*) or to inflammation, respectively.

Phagocytes

Defects in phagocytic function can be classified as either intrinsic (related to the inherent properties of the phagocyte) or extrinsic (not the result of an inherent phagocytic defect). Intrinsic disorders related to different stages of phagocyte differentiation and function have been identified, including those associated with stem cell differentiation, chemoattraction to the site of microbial assault, and to intracellular killing of the microbe (*Table 2*). Extrinsic defects may result from: (i) deficiency of antibody or complement, i.e. other primary defects; or

Table 1. *Complement deficiencies*

Component deficient	Disease caused/common infections seen
Regulatory components	
C1q inhibitor	Hereditary angiedema (continuous complement activation and consumption)
Decay accelerating factor DAF (CD55)	Paroxysmal nocturnal hemoglobulinuria (lysis of red blood cells)
Complement components	
C1, C2 or C4	Immune complex disease (unable to remove Ag-Ab complexes); C2 deficiency associated with SLE
C3	The most serious; repeated infections with pyogenic bacteria
MAC complement component deficiencies (C5–8)	Meningococcal infections, e.g. Neisseria

Table 2. *Phagocytic defects*

Defect	Disease/ mechanism
Stem cell differentiation/early development	Neutropenia: too few neutrophils
Lack of adhesion to endothelium for margination	Leukocyte adhesion deficiency (LAD); due to a lack of expression (through specific gene mutation) of the critical surface adhesion molecule CD18, a leukocyte function associated (LFA) molecule.*
Defective phagocytosis	Chediak-Higashi syndrome: lack of fusion of phagosome with lysosomes
Defective intracellular killing	Chronic granulomatous disease: defect in genes coding for NADPH oxidase, involved in oxygen dependent killing within the phagolysosome
Defects in IFNγ or IL-12 receptors	Mycobacterial infections; failure to activate NADPH oxidase

*CD18, with CD11 is also part of the C3bi receptor (CR3) and is necessary for binding C3b and thus for binding opsonized microbes, a critical step in the cell's attempt to engulf a bacterium. LFA molecules are present on all effector cell populations (including cytotoxic T cells) and are important in linking effector and target cells as an initial step in cytotoxicity or phago-cytosis. Thus, the function of more than just phagocytes is affected by this defect. NADPH, reduced nicotinamide adenine dinucleotide phosphate.

(ii) suppression of phagocytic activity (e.g. by glucocorticoids or autoantibodies), i.e. secondary defects to be discussed later.

Humoral immunity   Primary antibody deficiency mainly results from abnormal development of the B cell system. Any of the steps involved in B cell maturation may be blocked or abnormal (*Table 3*). The overall lack of antibodies means that the patients suffer from recurrent bacterial infections, predominately by *Pneumococcus*, *Streptococcus* and *Haemophilus*. Patients with severe combined immuno-deficiency and Bruton's disease have few or no B lymphocytes and therefore few if any antibodies in their circulation. Thus, they are unable to coat the surface of (opsonize) bacteria for which phagocytosis is the primary defence.

Although some of these disorders are related to basic biochemical abnormalities of the B cell lineage, others are the result of defective regulation by T cells. Thus, humoral immune deficiency may result from the absence of T helper activity. This is seen as one form of common variable immunodeficiency (CVID). Another form of CVID involves B cells that do not respond to signals from other cells. It is also possible that monocyte presentation and/or IL-1 (or other cytokine) production abnormalities may contribute to, or be responsible for, some of these disorders. Moreover, since different classes of immunoglobulin are regulated by different T helper cell subpopulations (e.g. Th1 cells help IgG1 and IgG3 responses; Th2 cells help IgA and IgE responses) selective antibody class (IgA or IgG) deficiencies may result from abnormalities in the number or activities of these T cell subpopulations.

Table 3.   B cell deficiencies

Stage of differentiation/maturation	Disease
Lack of stem cells	Severe combined immunodeficiency (SCID), also affects T cell development
B cells fail to develop from B cell precursors	Bruton's disease: congenital agammaglobulinemia mostly X-linked (XLA); due to a defective gene coding for a tyrosine kinase (btk) involved in activation of the pre-B cell to immature B cell (see Topic E3); patients have normal T cells
B cells do not switch antibody classes from IgM	Hyper-IgM syndrome: increased IgM but little or no IgG in the circulation, due to defective gene coding for either CD40 on B cells or CD40L on activated T cells (see Topic J2)
Common variable immunodeficiency (CVID)	IgG/IgA deficiency 1) B cells do not undergo terminal differentiation; IgA deficiency most common (1/700 people) 2) B cells normal; T cell signaling defective
Transient hypogammaglobulinemia	B cells normal; no CD4$^+$ T cell help early in life

Cellular immunity   Deficiencies caused only by the loss of cellular immunity are very rare, as most T
cell deficiencies result in severely compromised humoral immunity as well. T cell
defects occurring during development are shown in *Table 4*. Deficiencies in
cellular immunity may relate to T effector cells (e.g., cytotoxic T cells), whereas the
T helper population may be normal. Children have also been described with an
inability to produce or respond to IFNγ. In general, children with T cell
deficiencies have recurrent viral, fungal, mycobacterial and protozoan infections.

Table 4.   T cell deficiencies during development

T cell deficiency	Disease
Lack of a thymus	Di George syndrome; defect in thymus embryogenesis
Stem cell defect	SCID; 50% have a defect in γ chain used by many cytokine receptors including the IL-2 receptor
Death of developing thymocytes	SCID; 25% have adenosine deaminase enzyme deficiency or purine nucleoside phosphorylase deficiency; toxicity due to build up of purine metabolites which inhibit DNA synthesis

S3 SECONDARY (ACQUIRED) IMMUNODEFICIENCY

Key Notes

Factors causing acquired immunodeficiency	Secondary or acquired immunodeficiency, mainly affecting phagocytic and lymphocyte function, is the most common immunodeficiency. It may result from infection (HIV), malnutrition, aging, cytotoxic therapy, etc.
HIV and AIDS	Acquired immune deficiency syndrome (AIDS) is caused by human immunodeficiency virus (HIV)-1 or HIV-2. The virus enters the body via infected body fluids and exhibits trophism for monocytes/MØ (primary reservoir for the virus) and helper T cells, gaining entry through the CD4 molecule on these cells. Chemokine receptors are also involved in HIV gp120 binding to these cells and critical to infection. Loss of CD4+ T cells eventually compromises the ability of the immune system to combat opportunistic infections.
Immune senescence: consequences of aging	With ageing, memory T cells increase but become less able to expand. Moreover, fewer new (naive) T cells enter the pool due to thymic involution, diminishing the immune repertoire and the quality of T and B cell responses. B cell development in the bone marrow may also decrease. As a result of this reduction in immune capability, the elderly respond less well to vaccination.
Trauma	Patients suffering trauma (e.g., associated with burns or major surgery) are less able to deal with pathogens, perhaps as a result of the release of factors that dampen immune responses.
Related topics	Phagocytes (B1) T cells are produced in the thymus (E2)	The cellular basis of the antibody response (J1) T helper cells (K3)

Factors causing acquired immunodeficiency

Secondary or acquired immunodeficiency is by far the most common immunodeficiency and contributes a significant proportion to hospital admissions. Factors causing secondary immunodeficiency mainly affect phagocytic and lymphocyte function and include the following (*Table 1*).

HIV and AIDS

Acquired immune deficiency syndrome (AIDS) is caused mainly by the retrovirus human immunodeficiency virus (HIV)-1 but also by HIV-2. The virus enters the body via infected body fluids and exhibits tropism for T cells, in particular the

Table 1. Factors causing secondary immunodeficiency

Factor	Components affected
Malnutrition	Protein–calory malnutrition and lack of certain dietary elements (e.g. iron, zinc); world-wide the major predisposing factor for secondary immunodeficiency
Tumors	Direct effect of tumors on the immune system by effects on immunoregulatory molecules or release of immunosuppressive molecules, e.g. TGFβ
Cytotoxic drugs/irradiation	Widely used for tumor therapy, but also kills cells important to immune responses, including stem cells, neutrophil progenitors and rapidly dividing lymphocytes in primary lymphoid organs
Aging	Increased infections; reduced responses to vaccination; decreased T and B cell responses and changes in the quality of the response
Trauma	Increased infections probably related to release of immunosuppressive molecules such as glucocorticoids
Other diseases, e.g. diabetes	Diabetes is often associated with infections but the mechanism is unclear
Immunosuppression by microbes	Examples include malaria, measles virus but especially HIV; mechanisms involve decreased T cell function and antigen processing/presentation

CD4$^+$ T helper population. It binds and gains entry into T cells and monocytes (the primary reservoir for the virus) through the CD4 molecule on these cells. Other accessory receptors (chemokine receptors – see Topic G2) are involved in viral gp120 binding to T lymphocytes and monocytes, and individuals lacking functioning chemokine receptors do not progress from HIV infection to AIDS. The development of AIDS is defined as the occurrence of opportunistic infections (e.g. pneumocystis) or Kaposi's sarcoma (caused by HHV8) in an individual who has been infected with HIV. This is a direct result of the loss of CD4$^+$ helper cells. Damage to the pivotal CD4$^+$ T cell has major effects on the functions of other cells of the immune system (*Fig. 1*). Infection of monocytes and antigen presenting cells is also likely to be important in the speed of progression of the disease.

Immune senescence: consequences of aging

As one ages there are some striking changes in immune status. Reduced responses to vaccination and increased risk of infectious disease in the elderly are the result of reductions in immune function. Perhaps one of the most striking features as one ages is the involution of the thymus. By the age of 60, thymus tissue is almost completely replaced by fat and intrathymic T cell education is all but lost. Thus, the host is dependent on the pool of T cells generated earlier in life. As one ages, the number of memory T cells (CD45R0+ T cells (memory phenotype)) increase, suggesting that there is an accumulation of activated T cells and limited numbers of naïve cells entering the pool. In addition to a restricted repertoire, it appears that the ability of 'old' T cells to expand is limited. Thus, upon antigenic stimulation, 'old' T cells cannot clonally expand as effectively as 'young' T cells and this diminishes cell-mediated immune responses. Therefore, diminished heterogeneity and function of the T cell compartment contributes to the immune senescence.

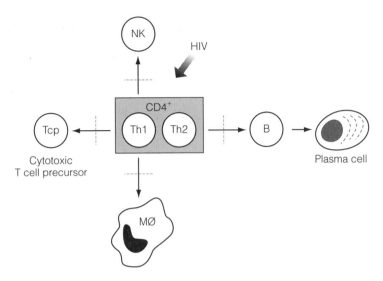

Fig. 1.   HIV infection of CD4$^+$ Th cells compromises their ability to help other immune cell populations.

There is also an age-associated reduction in humoral immunity. This is manifested as a change in the quality of the antibody response. The changes observed include shifts in:

● Antibody specificities from foreign to autoantigens.
● Antibody isotypes from IgG to IgM.
● Antibody affinities from high to low.

It is believed that these alterations in humoral immunity may be due to the impaired capacity of T cells to induce the maturation of B cells to produce high affinity, isotype-switched antibody. Therefore, the immune system shifts from an adaptive immune system (that produces high affinity, isotype-switched immunoglobulin) to a system more dependent on natural antibody-mediated immune responses (low-affinity, polyreactive, IgM antibodies). In addition to this impaired T cell function which is at the root of immune senescence, it is also believed that there is a reduction in the production of B cell development in the bone marrow which limits B cell diversity. Nutritional deficiency that comes with age also contributes to reduced immunocompetence.

Trauma

After significant trauma including that associated with burns or major surgery, the immune system seems less able to deal with pathogens. Although the basis for this apparent immunodeficiency is not understood, it is possible that these traumatic events induce release of other immunomodulatory factors (e.g. glucocorticoids), which dampen immune responses (Topic N5).

S4 DIAGNOSIS AND TREATMENT OF IMMUNODEFICIENCY

Key Notes

Family history	Since defective genes can be inherited, an investigation into the family history is especially important in the diagnosis of primary immunodeficiencies.
Evaluation of specific immune components	Evaluation of the nature of the immunodeficient components in a patient is important for determining appropriate treatment. This may be achieved by assay of: Ig classes and B cell numbers for antibody-mediated immunity; T cell and T cell subset numbers and their cytokine production for cell-mediated immunity; overall lytic ability and individual components for complement activity; granulocyte and monocyte counts and their ability to phagocytose opsonized particles, kill bacteria, and respond to chemotactic and activation signals for phagocytosis.
Antibiotics and antibodies	Antibiotic therapy is the standard treatment for infections. In addition, antibodies from a pool of donors are used for antibody deficiencies.
Bone marrow transplants and gene therapy	Replacement of faulty cells/organs with cells from normal individuals is used when MHC compatible donors can be found and has been used to reconstitute normal phagocytic function in chronic granulomatous disease (CGD) and B and T cells in SCID. Fetal liver and thymus grafts have also been successfully used. Treatment for these defects may eventually involve replacing faulty genes, once identified, in the patient's stem cells with a normal gene.
Related topics	Hemopoiesis – development of blood cells (E1) Cell mediated immunity (K1) Rejection mechanisms (Q3) Immunization (R2) Primary/congenital (inherited) immunodeficiency (S2) Antibodies as research and diagnostic tools (V1)

Family history

Since defective genes can be inherited, e.g. defective CD40 and/or CD40 ligand in hyper-IgM syndrome (Topic S2, *Table 3*), it is important to establish any history of family members with similar recurrent episodes of infection. This information on family history is especially important in the diagnosis of primary immunodeficiencies and is valuable for genetic counseling.

Evaluation of specific immune components

Recognizing immune defects and pinpointing them is critical, since correction must be tailored to the abnormality. Although the nature of an infection or disorder will provide clues to which immune component is at a disadvantage, in

Table 1. *Evaluation of the different components of the immune system.*

Evaluation of antibody mediated immunity

Serum immunoelectrophoresis
Quantitate antibodies in serum and secretions by ELISA or radial immunodiffusion
Assay for specific antibodies:
  Assay by agglutination for IgM antibodies to blood group substances A and B
  Before and after immunization with killed vaccines
Quantitate circulating B cells by flow cytometry with mAbs to surface Ig
Evaluate induction of B cell differentiation *in vitro*
Evaluate the presence of B cells and plasma cells in lymph nodes (biopsy)

Evaluation of cell-mediated immunity

DTH skin tests to common antigens – candida, streptokinase, streptodornase
Determine:
  Total lymphocyte count (60–80% of blood lymphocytes are T cells)
  T cell number in blood (using mAb to CD3 and flow cytometry)
  T cell subpopulation percentages (using mAbs to CD4 and to CD8)
Evaluate lymphocyte proliferation to lectins (PHA, Con A) and alloantigens (MLR)
Analyse T-lymphocyte function:
  Lymphokine production: IFNγ, IL-2, etc
  Helper cell activity and cellular cytotoxicity

Evaluation of the complement system

Assay for total hemolytic complement – CH_{50}, a functional assay
Quantitate individual complement components by immunoassay
Assay neutrophil chemotaxis using C in patient's serum as a chemoattractant

Evaluation of phagocyte function

Determine total granulocyte and monocyte count
Assay for:
  Chemotaxis – using a Boyden chamber
  Phagocytosis – using opsonized particles
  Superoxide generation using nitroblue tetrazolium (NBT) reduction
  Bacterial killing
  Individual enzymes and for cytokines (IL-1 and IL-12)
  Response to activation by IFNγ, GM-CSF, etc
Evaluate ability to process and present antigen

PHA, phytohemagglutinin; Con A, concanavalin A; MLR, mixed lymphocyte reaction.

many instances it is not clear which subcomponents are compromised. It is important, therefore, to apply a systematic evaluation of immune function to individuals suspected of immune abnormalities.

Humoral immunity may be initially evaluated by determining the presence and levels of the different antibody classes and subclasses in the serum of a patient using serum immunoelectrophoresis, radial immunodiffusion and/or radio-immunoassay (Topics V2 and V3). Detection of specific antibodies can be determined using skin tests (Topic T5), by agglutination (e.g. for IgM antibodies to blood group substances A and B) and/or enzyme-linked immunosorbent assay (ELISA) (e.g. for specific antibodies after immunization with killed vaccines). It is also important to determine B cell numbers and functional properties using mAbs to surface immunoglobulin and B cell differentiation assays, respectively. Lymph node biopsy is used to determine the presence and numbers of B cells and plasma cells in the tissues.

Cell-mediated immunity is often evaluated by skin tests (delayed type hypersensitivity, DTH, Topic T5) to common antigens (e.g. candida, streptokinase, streptodornase). Total lymphocyte, T cell ($CD3^+$) and T cell subpopulation ($CD4^+$ or $CD8^+$) numbers are also useful in evaluating the potential for cell mediated immune responses (Topic V3). However, normal numbers of T cells and T cell subpopulations in a patient do not mean that they function normally. Thus, lymphocyte proliferation to lectins (PHA and Con A) and alloantigens (MLR), lymphokine production (e.g. IFNγ, IL-2) and helper and killer cell activities may also need to be carried out.

The complement system can be evaluated for its overall functional activity in red cell lysis assays that determine total hemolytic complement (CH_{50}). Immunoassays can then be used to determine the concentration of individual complement components including those associated with the alternative pathway. Neutrophil chemotaxis assays using complement from a patient's serum as a chemoattractant can be used to evaluate complement chemotactic factors (Topics C2 and F5) such as C5a.

Cells of the phagocyte system are able to respond to chemotactic stimuli and migrate toward a pathogen, recognize the pathogen and mediate its phagocytosis and/or killing. These cells are involved in immune defense both as a result of their own recognition of microbe molecular patterns (Topic H1) and as a result of direction by the humoral, cellular and/or complement systems. Total granulocyte and monocyte blood counts permit determination of their presence in normal numbers. Chemotaxis assays (using Boyden chambers) evaluate their response to chemotactic molecules such as C5a. Assays for phagocytosis (using antibody and/or complement opsonized particles), for superoxide generation (using the reduction of nitroblue tetrazolium (NBT) test), and for bacterial killing are important in determining the functional capability of these cells. Assays for individual enzymes and for cytokines (IL-1 and IL-12) indicate their ability to produce molecules critical to microbe killing and in recruiting other cells and immune mechanisms. Their response to activation by IFNγ, GM-CSF, etc., indicates their ability to be induced to a higher level of cytotoxic ability. Finally, as many of these cells (monocytes, macrophages, dendritic cells) process and present antigen, it may be important to assay their ability to trigger T cells and thus to initiate specific immune responses.

One of the best ways to evaluate immune function involves looking at both the afferent (initiation) and efferent (effector) limb of the immune system of an individual. This can be done by injecting antigen into an individual and determining if a normal response develops. If it does, all of the T and B cell systems are probably intact. Another even more definitive evaluation procedure might be to use a live attenuated vaccine, e.g. polio virus, as this would permit evaluation of the immune response in a very real setting. However, this would never be done as even an attenuated live pathogen could cause a lethal infection in an immunodeficient individual (Topic R3).

Antibiotics and antibodies

Antibiotic therapy is the standard treatment for infections. Children whose immune system produces no antibodies begin to experience recurrent infections after maternal antibody from placental transfer *in utero* has been depleted. These individuals are treated with antibiotics and intravenously with periodic injections of pooled immunoglobulins from normal human serum. Contamination of immunoglobulin preparations with viruses including HIV and hepatitis B and C must be excluded.

Bone marrow transplants and gene therapy

Replacement of faulty cells/organs with cells from normal individuals is now commonly used when MHC compatible donors can be found. In particular, bone marrow transplantation has been successfully used for reconstitution of normal phagocytic function in chronic granulomatous disease (CGD) and of B and T cells in SCID. Fetal liver and thymus grafts have also been successfully used. Such transplants carry the risk of rejection (Topic Q3). A number of genes have already been identified as faulty (Topic S2, *Tables 2–4*) in patients with primary immunodeficiency diseases.

The ultimate treatment for many of these defects may well be gene replacement therapy, in that faulty genes will be replaced in the patient's stem cells with a 'normal' gene. This approach has already been tried for adenosine deaminase (ADA) deficiency and is currently being tried for several of other disorders for which a faulty gene has been identified. The difficulty thus far appears to be in appropriately expressing the normal gene.

T1 DEFINITION AND CLASSIFICATION

Key Notes

Introduction

Damage to host tissue can occur as an overreaction by the immune system to a variety of both inert antigens and infectious organisms. This hypersensitivity occurs only after antigen sensitization of the host and is therefore the effect of the adaptive immune system. Overreaction to microbial antigens can occur in the natural immune system although these reactions are not currently classified as hypersensitivity reactions.

Classification

Hypersensitivity reactions have long been classified into four types, with an additional type recently added. Types I, II, III and V depend on antibodies, alone or with complement, and because they are evident within hours, are termed immediate hypersensitivities. Type IV is mediated by T cells and the cytokines they produce when activated. As this response requires at least a day to develop, it is termed delayed hypersensitivity.

Related topics   Complement (C2)   Cell mediated immunity (K1)
Functions (F5)

Introduction

The immune system normally responds to a variety of microbial invaders with little or no damage to host tissues. However, in some situations, immune responses (especially to some antigens) can lead to more severe tissue damaging reactions (immunopathology). This 'overreactivity' by the immune system to antigens is often referred to as hypersensitivity and is by no means restricted to antigens of microbial origin since it also includes both inert and self antigens (autoimmunity). Hypersensitivity reactions are antigen specific and occur after the immune system has already responded to an antigen (i.e. the immune system has been primed). The adverse reactions are therefore mainly the result of antigen-specific memory responses. It is important to note that these responses are part of normal immune defense mechanisms and occur daily as immune cells and molecules come in contact with antigens and/or pathogens that had previously induced an immunity. What is unusual about hypersensitivities is that these normal responses become clinically evident because they are localized and/or involve interactions between large amounts of antigen with antibodies or immune cells. In addition, genetics plays a role in some types of hypersensitivity reactions. Moreover, some antigens can induce more than one type of tissue damaging reaction (hypersensitivity) and penicillin can induce types I, II, III and IV reactions.

Classification

Hypersensitivity reactions occur at different times after coming into contact with the offending antigens, within a few minutes (i.e. immediate), minutes to hours (intermediate) or after many hours (delayed). Generally, the delayed responses are mediated by the cellular components of the immune system (i.e. T cells) whilst the former are the result of the humoral arm of the immune response which includes antibodies and the complement system. The original classification by Gell and Coombs was into four main types, a fifth has since been added. *Table 1* summarizes the main immune system components which contribute to tissue damage. It should be stressed that more than one of these mechanisms can contribute to any one particular disease process.

Table 1. Classification of hypersensitivities

Time of appearance	Type	Immune mechanism
2–30 min (immediate)	I	IgE antibodies (enhancement of acute inflammatory response)
5–8 h (cytotoxic)	II	Antibody and complement
2–8 h (immune complex)	III	Antibody/antigen complexes
24–72 h (delayed)	IV	T cell mediated (can be granulomatous)
(Stimulatory)	V	Antibody mediated

T2 IgE-MEDIATED TYPE I HYPERSENSITIVITY: ALLERGY

Key Notes

Introduction	This most common type of hypersensitivity is mediated by IgE and causes mild (hayfever) to life threatening (bee sting) clinical situations. Some individuals (atopic) have a genetic predisposition to make high levels of IgE. Skin tests can be used to test for sensitivity to allergens.
Sensitization phase	Sensitization to a particular antigen is dependent on stimulation of IgE antibody production. This requires CD4+ Th2 cells to induce class switching of antigen specific B cells and to secrete IL-4 for B cell growth and differentiation.
Effector phase – IgE-mediated mast cell degranulation	IgE antibodies produced following initial contact with the specific antigen, bind to IgE receptors on mast cells and basophils. Cross-linking by antigen of the IgE and the receptors with which it is associated results in rapid degranulation and release of pharmacological mediators (e.g. histamine) causing local inflammation (anaphylaxis). In the case of systemic release, systemic anaphylactic reactions are produced requiring treatment with adrenaline (epinephrine) to restore blood pressure.
Common antigens causing type I hypersensitivity	These include grass and tree pollens, insect venoms, nuts, drugs and animal dander. Fungal and worm antigens also induce this type of hypersensitivity.
Drugs and immunotherapy (desensitization)	Drugs used to counteract Type I hypersensitivity inhibit production or release of inflammatory mediators (nonsteroidal anti-inflammatory drugs (NSAIDs), such as aspirin and indomethacin, glucocorticoids and cromolyn) or inhibit the action of inflammatory mediators which then relieve symptoms (benadryl, dramamine, glucocorticoids). Epinephrine is used to counteract mediator effects such as low blood pressure and bronchospasm. The aim of desensitization is to induce an IgG immune response and/or divert the immune response away from production of IgE. This approach has been used successfully for only a few allergens (e.g. bee venom).
Related topics	Mast cells and basophils (B3) Genes T helper cells and Antibody classes (F2) cytokines (N3) The acute inflammatory response (I) Immunoassay (V3)

Introduction   Allergy affects about 17% of the population through mild (hayfever) to life threatening conditions (bee sting allergy). It is mediated by IgE which is normally found in very small amounts in the circulation (Topic F2) and probably evolved to protect us against worm infestations (Topics I1 and O2). Allergic reactions can occur to normally harmless antigens (such as pollen or foodstuffs) and microbial antigens (fungi, worms). Some individuals in the population are genetically predisposed to respond to certain antigens by producing IgE to these antigens and are said to be atopic. Testing for allergy (Prausnitz-Kustner test) involves introduction of the allergen intradermally. A positive skin test occurs in the form of a wheal (fluid accumulation) and flare (redness) reaction at the site of injection.

Sensitization phase

Sensitization to a particular antigen is dependent on stimulation of IgE antibody production. Thus, B cell antigen receptors specific for the allergen bind, internalize, process and present the antigen in MHC class II molecules. CD4+ Th2 cells recognize the antigen presented by these B cells and induce class switching of antigen-specific B cells. These T cells also secrete IL-4 which is important for B cell growth and differentiation (Topics G2, J2 and K3) (*Fig. 1*). Why certain individuals become sensitized to particular antigens by producing IgE is unclear, but the possibilities include: (i) the genetics of the individual; (ii) environmental factors (pollution) that condition mucosal tissues of the immune system to produce IL-4 which then predisposes a Th2 response; and (iii) that regulation of the response through Th1 cells is defective (Topics K3 and N3).

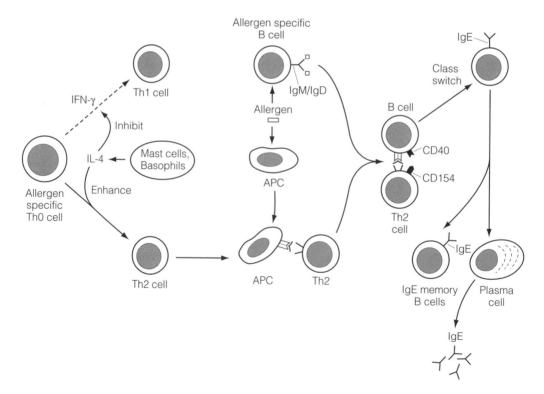

Fig. 1. IL-4 induces IgE responses. In an environment high in IL-4 (perhaps from mast cells) relative to IFNγ, an allergen-specific Th0 cell differentiates into a Th2 cell rather than a Th1 cell. APCs present allergen peptides to this Th2 cell, inducing its activation and proliferation. An allergen specific B cell which has internalized allergen then presents allergen peptides in MHC class II to this Th2 cell. The Th2 cell stimulates antibody class switch (through triggering of B cell CD40 by CD154 on the T cell) and releases IL-4 which induces class switch to IgE antibodies. The IgE producing B cell proliferates and differentiates into IgE expressing B memory cells and IgE producing plasma cells.

Effector phase – IgE-mediated mast cell degranulation

Specific IgE antibodies produced as a result of previous contact with antigen (allergen) diffuse throughout the body, eventually coming in contact with mast cells and basophils. These cells have high affinity receptors for the Fc region of IgE and therefore bind to these antibodies. This does not have any effect on the mast cells directly until the specific antigen (allergen) comes into contact with the mast cell bearing the IgE antibodies in sufficient numbers to cross-link the antibodies on the cell surface (*Fig. 2*). The mast cells now immediately release granules (degranulate) which contain large amounts of pharmacological mediators (*Table 1*). These substances have a direct effect on nearby blood vessels causing vasodilation and an influx of eosinophils, which in turn release mediators that cause a prolonged 'late phase' reaction. Locally, e.g. in the nose, mediator release results in the symptoms of redness, itching and increased secretions by mucosal epithelial cells leading to a runny nose. Systemic release of histamine and other substances released by mast cells can lead to severe vasodilation and vascular collapse resulting in life-threatening systemic anaphylactic reactions which require treatment with epinephrine to restore blood pressure.

Leukotrienes, histamine, prostaglandins and platelet activating factor released from mast cells are key mediators of type I hypersensitivity. One way of classifying this growing body of inflammatory mediators is by their effects on target cells and tissues (*Table 1*).

Common antigens causing type I hypersensitivity

There are many antigens which can cause allergic (type I hypersensitive) reactions (*Table 2*). The most common allergic response is probably to pollens (allergic rhinitis: hayfever). Antigens from some invading organisms can also give rise to allergic reactions. These include fungal spores, viruses and worms. Systemic release of worm antigens from hydatid cysts binding to serum IgE can cause anaphylaxis

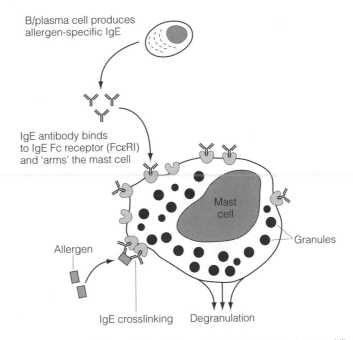

B/plasma cell produces allergen-specific IgE

IgE antibody binds to IgE Fc receptor (FcεRI) and 'arms' the mast cell

Mast cell

Granules

Allergen

IgE crosslinking   Degranulation

Fig. 2.   IgE-mediated mast cell degranulation. Allergen binds to and crosslinks cytophilic (cell bound) IgE, signaling FcεR to trigger mast cell activation and degranulation with release of histamine, leukotrienes, etc.

Table 1. Inflammatory mediators classified by their effects on target cells

Mediators with pharmacologic effects on smooth muscle and mucous glands

1. *Histamine*. Binds to two types of receptors on target cells, H1 and H2 receptors. Acting on H1 receptors, histamine contracts smooth muscle (e.g. in airways), increases vascular permeability and mucous secretion by goblet cells. Via H2 receptors, histamine increases gastric secretion, and feeds back to decrease mediator release by basophils and mast cells
2. *Slow reacting substance of anaphylaxis (SRS-A)*. These cysteinyl-leukotrienes (LTC_4, LTD_4, LTE_4), are potent constrictors of peripheral airways (i.e., bronchoconstrictors) and also cause leakage of post capillary venules, leading to edema. Leukotrienes are derived from the membrane fatty acids of mast cells, neutrophils and macrophages
3. *Prostaglandins*. A variety of effects are manifested by this large family of related compounds. Prostaglandin D_2 is produced by mast cells and causes bronchial constriction. Prostaglandin I_2 is produced by endothelial cells and probably synergizes with LTB_4 to cause edema
4. *Platelet activating factor (PAF)*. A low molecular weight lipid which causes platelet aggregation with release of vasoactive mediators (serotonin) and smooth muscle contraction
5. *Kinins*. Bradykinin (a nonapeptide) and lysyl-bradykinin (a decapeptide) cause increased vascular permeability, decreased blood pressure and contraction of smooth muscle

Mediators which are pro-inflammatory by chemotactic properties

1. *Eosinophil chemotactic factors of anaphylaxis (ECF-A)*. Includes histamine and tetrapeptides from mast cell granules
2. *Neutrophil chemotactic factor of anaphylaxis (IL-8)*. A granule-derived protein of mast cells which attracts and activates neutrophils
3. *Late-phase reactants of anaphylaxis*. Mediators that cause delayed inflammatory cell infiltration
4. *Leukotriene B_4 (LTB$_4$)*. Derived from membrane fatty acids, a potent chemotactic factor for PMNs, eosinophils and macrophages, causes adhesion of leukocytes to post capillary venules, degranulation and edema

Mediators which cause tissue destruction

1. *Toxic oxygen and nitrogen radicals*. (e.g., superoxide and nitric oxide). Released from PMNs, macrophages and mast cells.
2. *Acid hydrolases*. From mast cells
3. *Major basic protein*. A very destructive protein from the larger eosinophil granule.

leading to vascular collapse and death if left untreated. Allergic asthma is an important disease which can be triggered by a number of different environmental antigens and is mediated by IgE in its early stages.

Drugs and immunotherapy (desensitization)

Drugs used to counteract immediate hypersensitivity act at one of two levels: (i) inhibitors of the production or release of inflammatory mediators. These include nonsteroidal anti-inflammatory drugs (NSAIDs) such as aspirin and indomethicin, synthetic steroids (glucocorticoids) such as dexamethasone and prednisolone, and the inhibitor of histamine release, cromolyn. (ii) Inhibitors of mediator action such as histamine receptor antagonists. Benadryl, dramamine, chlortrimaton and dimetane are representative H1-blocking agents, which are most useful for relief of the sneezing, rhinorrhea (runny nose) and itching eyes associated with hay fever. They are not useful for bronchial asthma or systemic anaphylaxis, where mediators other than histamine play a more important role. Glucocorticoids also inhibit some of the actions of inflammatory mediators. Other drugs such as **epinephrine** and theophyline are used to counteract mediator effects such as low blood pressure and bronchospasm.

Desensitization is used to divert the immune response away from a predomi-

Table 2. Allergens

Pollens	Insect venoms	Microbes	Animals and foods	Drugs
Grass	Bee	Mold	Serum	Penicillin
Timothy	Wasp		Vaccines	Salicylates
Rye	Ant		Nuts	Anesthetics
Ragweed			Seafood	
			Hair	
Tree			Danders	
Plane				
Birch				

nantly Th2 driven IgE antibody response and toward a Th1 driven IgG response. This involves injection or ingestion of allergen in low and increasing amounts. Success has been achieved with only a few allergens e.g. venom. An IgG response, which would be driven by Th1 cells, could have two significant effects: (i) Larger amounts of IgG would be produced than IgE and this excess IgG antibody would bind and remove the antigen before it could bind IgE on the mast cells or basophils and trigger degranulation; (ii) IgG would also remove antigen before it could bind to and stimulate Th2 driven IgE producing B cells, thus decreasing the amount of antigen specific IgE produced (*Fig. 3*).

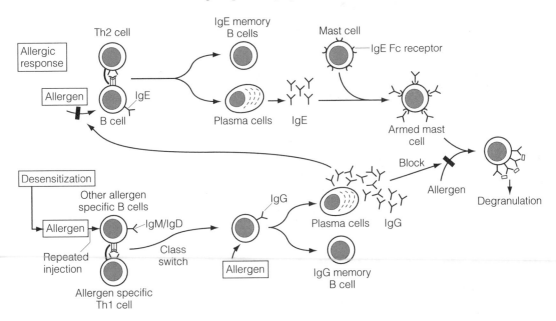

Fig. 3. Desensitization. In an individual with IgE antibody to an allergen, there are memory cells which respond to allergen by differentiating into plasma cells which produce allergen specific IgE (Topic T2, Fig. 1). This IgE binds to IgE Fc receptors on mast cells which degranulate when allergen is reintroduced and crosslinks IgE on these cells. Repeated injections of allergen is intended to induce an IgG response by stimulating allergen specific B cells which have not yet undergone a class switch. In particular, allergen specific Th1 cells would provide help to these B cells inducing class switch to IgG. This IgG would be produced in larger quantity than IgE and compete effectively for the allergen when it is reintroduced, preventing the allergen from stimulating IgE memory B cells and removing the allergen before it can bind IgE on mast cells.

T3 IgG AND IgM-MEDIATED TYPE II HYPERSENSITIVITY

Key Notes

Introduction	Antibody (IgM or IgG) directed mainly to cellular antigens (e.g. on erythrocytes) or surface autoantigens can cause damage through opsonization, lysis or antibody dependent cellular cytotoxicity. Also called cytotoxic hypersensitivity.
Rhesus incompatibility	Pregnant mothers who are rhesus D (RhD) antigen positive can respond to RhD antigen inherited from the father. Sensitization occurs either through prior blood transfusion with RhD+ erythrocytes or at parturition when fetal erythrocytes pass into the maternal circulation. During subsequent pregnancies, small numbers of fetal erythrocytes stimulate a memory response with the result that IgG antibodies to RhD antigen pass across the placenta and destroy the fetal erythrocytes (hemolytic disease of the newborn).
Transfusion reactions	Natural antibodies (isohemagglutinins) to major blood group antigens (A, B) bind to transfused erythrocytes carrying the target antigens resulting in massive hemolysis. This is now rare due to blood group typing.
Autoantigens	Antibodies to a variety of self antigens such as basement membranes of lung and kidney (Goodpasture's syndrome), the acetylcholine receptor (Myasthenia gravis) and erythrocytes (hemolytic anemia) can result in tissue damaging reactions.
Drugs	Drugs such as penicillin can attach to erythrocytes and cause IgG-mediated damage to erythrocytes.
Stimulatory hypersensitivity	A variant of type II hypersensitivity (sometimes called type V), this results in binding to a receptor and acting as the natural ligand e.g., in Graves disease antibodies are present which react with the thyroid stimulating receptor, stimulating hyperthyroidism.
Related topics	Functions (F5) autoimmune disease (U2) Transplantation antigens (Q2) Disease pathogenesis-effector Factors predisposing and/or mechanisms (U4) contributing to development of

Introduction Antibody alone or together with complement can cause hypersensitive reactions. These reactions can be against foreign (often erythrocytes) or autoantigens and usually result in the direct lysis or removal of cells. Type II hypersensitivity is therefore also termed cytotoxic hypersensitivity. Diseases caused by this type of hypersensitivity often involve erythrocytes (anemias) and self cells (autoimmune diseases). Cell death (or lysis) is mediated through normal mechanisms by which antibodies and complement carry out their function including phagocytosis, lysis and antibody dependent cellular cytotoxicity.

Rhesus incompatibility

Rhesus D (RhD) antigen is carried by erythrocytes. Children born to RhD− mothers and RhD+ fathers may express RhD on their erythrocytes. Prior to pregnancy, the mother can become sensitized to RhD antigen through blood transfusion and during pregnancy and especially at birth, the baby's RhD+ erythrocytes come into contact with the mother's immune system. Some pass across the placenta but most are released into the maternal circulation during placental shedding. Since RhD is not present in the mother, her immune system responds to it as a foreign antigen and makes antibodies (*Fig. 1*). This is usually not a problem during the first pregnancy but in subsequent pregnancies small amounts of erythrocytes passing across the placenta stimulate a memory response leading to specific anti-RhD antibody production. IgG antibodies pass across the placenta and bind to the fetal erythrocytes leading to their opsonization and lysis. This results in

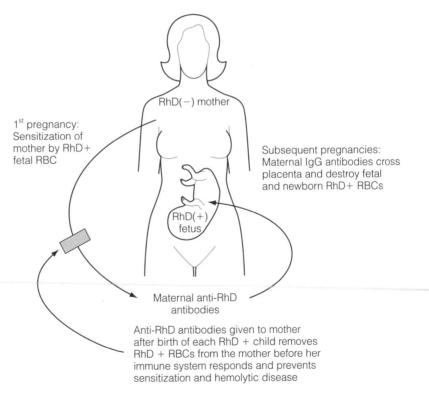

Fig. 1. RhD antigen and hemolytic disease of the newborn. RhD− mothers who give birth to RhD+ infants become immunized at birth with RhD antigen on fetal red blood cells (RBCs) which pass into the mother's circulation. This results in IgG antibodies to RhD which cross the placenta during subsequent pregnancies and destroy fetal and newborn RhD+ RBCs. This can be prevented by giving the mother anti-RhD antibodies immediately after birth of each RhD+ infant or during pregnancy in order to destroy RhD+ RBCs before they stimulate an active immune response in the mother.

hemolytic anemia of the newborn if not prevented. Generally, mothers at risk are detected during early stages of pregnancy and monitored thereafter. At termination of each pregnancy with an RhD+ fetus, RhD(−) mothers are given antibodies to RhD which is thought to remove the fetal erythrocytes from the blood stream and suppress the development of a subsequent immune response.

Transfusion reactions

It is common practice to give blood transfusions in cases of severe blood loss. The major blood group antigens A and B are expressed at the surface of erythrocytes and we have natural antibodies (mostly IgM) to these antigens (isohemagglutinins Topic Q2). Individuals who are blood group A have antibodies to B antigens, those who are blood group B will have anti-A antibodies and those who are AB will have neither. Those who are blood group O will have both antibodies. It is therefore important to do blood group typing on transfusion donors and recipients. In most cases, this is done accurately but occasionally accidents occur whereby blood is given to a recipient who has the reactive isohemagglutinins. This can result in a transfusion reaction which manifests itself as (a complement mediated) massive intravascular life-threatening hemolysis.

Autoantigens

Antibodies can be made to self antigens when there is breakdown of tolerance to self (Topics M3 and U3). These autoantibodies can cause tissue damaging reactions. In Goodpasture's disease, autoantibodies to the lung and kidney basement membranes cause inflammation and hemorrhage at the site of antibody binding. Antibodies to the acetylcholine receptor cause loss of receptors (*Fig. 2*) reducing conduction of nerve impulses across the neuromuscular junctions (myasthenia gravis). Autoantibodies to erythrocytes result in autoimmune hemolytic anemias.

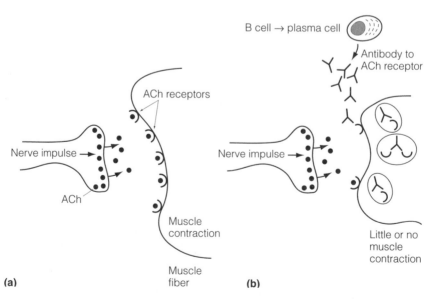

Fig. 2. *Myasthenia gravis. (a) Normal stimulation of muscle contraction. Nerve impulses trigger release of acetylcholine (ACh) from the nerve ending. The ACh then binds to ACh receptors on muscle cells triggering their contraction. (b) Autoantibodies to the ACh receptor bind to these receptors on muscle cells and cause their internalization and degradation so that when ACh is released as the result of a nerve impulse, there are few ACh receptors with which to bind. Thus, muscle contraction does not occur or is diminished.*

Drugs

Penicillin, as well as inducing an immediate type hypersensitivity through IgE can also stimulate an IgG response. IgG can then bind to penicillin attached to erythrocytes which induces hemolysis. This disappears when the drug is removed.

Stimulatory hypersensitivity

Since this relatively newly described type of hypersensitivity is antibody mediated it can be considered as a variant of type II hypersensitivity. In this case, the autoantibodies are directed to hormone receptor molecules and function in a stimulatory fashion, like the natural ligand i.e. the hormone itself. The classical example is Graves' disease where antibodies to the thyroid stimulating receptor result in overactivity of the thyroid (*Fig. 3*).

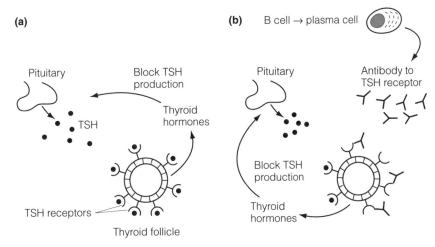

Fig. 3.   Graves' disease. (a) The pituitary makes thyroid stimulating hormone (TSH) which binds to TSH receptors on cells of the thyroid follicle and triggers them to make thyroid hormones. In turn, these thyroid hormones inhibit production of TSH by the pituitary as a form of normal feedback regulation of TSH production by thyroid hormones. (b) Autoantibodies to TSH receptor bind TSH receptors and trigger the thyroid follicle cells to release thyroid hormones which stop the pituitary from making TSH. However, they have no effect on production of the autoantibody which continues to stimulate thyroid follicle cells to make thyroid hormones, thus causing hyperthyroidism.

T4 IMMUNE-COMPLEX MEDIATED TYPE III HYPERSENSITIVITY

Key Notes

Introduction	Immune complexes can form to serum products as well as microbial and self antigens, either in local sites or systemically, leading to phagocytic and complement mediated damage.
Mechanisms of type III hypersensitivity	Tissue damage is caused mainly by complement activation and release of lytic enzymes from neutrophils. Local damage (Arthus reaction) can be seen in pulmonary disease resulting from inhaled antigen. Systemic antibody complexes with microbial or autoantigens result in immune complex deposition in blood vessels (vasculitis) or in the renal vessels (glomeruli) of the kidneys leading to glomerulonephritis.
Diseases associated with type III hypersensitivity	Pulmonary diseases result from inhalation of bacterial spores (Farmer's lung) or avian serum/fecal proteins (bird fancier's disease). Systemic disease can occur from streptococcal infections (streptococcal nephritis), autoimmune complexes (e.g. systemic lupus erythematosus (SLE)) or drugs (e.g. penicillin) or antisera made in animals.
Related topics	Antibody classes (F2) The acute inflammatory response (I)	Disease pathogenesis-effector mechanisms (U4) Precipitation and agglutination (V2)

Introduction

Normally, immune complexes are removed by phagocytic cells and there is no tissue damage. However when there are large amounts of immune complexes and they persist in tissues, they can cause damage which may be localized within tissues (Arthus reaction) or systemic. The antigens leading to this type of hypersensitivity can be microbial antigens, autoantigens and foreign serum components.

Mechanisms of type III hypersensitivity

Much of the tissue damage is the result of complement activation leading to neutrophil chemoattraction and release of lytic enzymes by the degranulating neutrophils. Local deposition of immune complexes results in an Arthus reaction (*Fig. 1*). Immune complexes (usually small) can also cause systemic effects such as fever, weakness, vasculitis, arthritis and edema and glomerulonephritis. An example of this is when passive antibodies are given to patients to protect them against microbial toxins such as tetanus toxin. An antibody response can develop (serum sickness) against the horse antitetanus toxin and forms immune complexes with them. Serum immune complexes can deposit in blood vessels (vasculitis) or can become trapped in the blood vessels of the kidneys leading to glomerulonephritis.

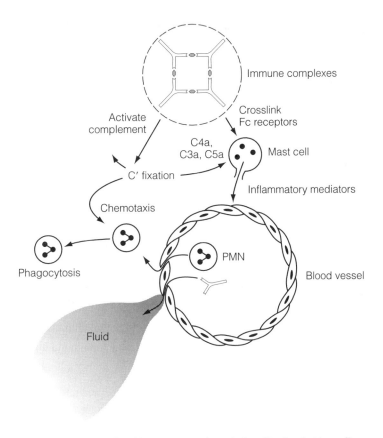

Fig. 1.   The Arthus reaction. Small immune complexes in the skin directly trigger Fc receptors and activate complement resulting essentially in an acute inflammatory response mediated through mast cells. Small immune complexes can also lodge in blood vessels and induce vasculitis or glomerulonephritis in the kidney.

Diseases associated with type III hypersensitivity

A list of some diseases mediated by type III hypersensitivity is shown in Table 1. IgG antibodies complexed with inhaled antigens cause local damage in the airways of the lung (which also includes pneumonitis and alveolitis). Immune complexes made against antigens encountered systemically cause a variety of symptoms and in particular kidney damage through deposition.

Table 1.   Diseases mediated by type III hypersensitivity

Site of reaction	Antigens	Disease
Localized (inhaled)	Bacterial spores	Farmer's lung
	Fungal spores	
	Pigeon serum / fecal proteins	Bird fancier's disease
Systemic	Microbes including Streptococcus	Streptococcal nephritis
	Hepatitis B	
	Epstein–Barr virus	
	Malaria	
	Autoantigens e.g. DNA	Systemic lupus erythematosus
	Drugs – penicillin, sulphonamides	Drug allergy

T5 DELAYED-TYPE TYPE IV HYPERSENSITIVITY

Key Notes

Introduction	This occurs from 24 h after contact with an antigen and is mediated by T cells together with dendritic cells, macrophages and cytokines. The persistent presence of the antigen e.g. chronic mycobacterial infections, results in granulomas. Skin contact with a number of small molecules (chemicals and plant molecules) can also result in delayed hypersensitivity.
The tuberculin reaction	This is a 'recall' response to purified mycobacterial antigens and is used as the basis of a skin test for an immune response (not necessarily curative) to TB.
The production of granulomas	The inability to kill all mycobacteria in macrophages by T cells often results in a chronic stimulation of the mycobacterial specific T cells. The cytokines produced are responsible for 'walling off' the macrophages containing the persistent antigens and thus the production of granulomas. This also occurs as a response to shistosomula worms and is seen in some clinical conditions with, as yet, undefined antigens.
Contact sensitivity	Contact with a number of small molecular weight chemicals (e.g. nickel in a watch strap buckle) and molecules from some plants (poison ivy) can penetrate the skin, bind to self proteins and induce a specific CD4+ T cell response. The resulting cytokines induce a local redness and swelling which usually disappears on removal of the antigen.

Related topics	Phagocytes (B1)	Genes, T helper cells and
	Dendritic cells (B4)	cytokines (N3)
	Cell mediated immunity (K1)	Immunity to different organisms (O2)

Introduction

This hypersensitivity reaction, the only type transferable by cells rather than antibodies, was shown to begin at least 24 h after contact with the eliciting antigen. It was first associated with T cell mediated immune responses to *Mycobacterium tuberculosis* (MTb) and was therefore initially termed 'bacterial hypersensitivity'. Such responses often lead to the production of granulomas some weeks later. This type of hypersensitivity now covers a range of T cell mediated responses including those induced by small molecules coming into contact with the skin – contact hypersensitivity. In addition to T cells, the key players in this type of sensitivity are dendritic cells, macrophages and cytokines.

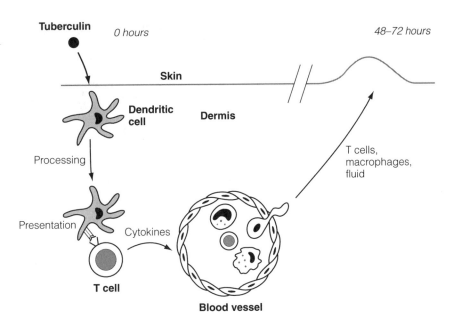

Fig. 1. *The tuberculin reaction (delayed-type hypersensitivity). Tuberculin protein introduced into the dermis is processed and presented by dendritic cells to T cells via MHC class II molecules. Cytokines produced by the T cells alter local endothelial cell adhesion molecules allowing monocytes to enter the site of injection and develop into macrophages. T cells and macrophage products result in edema (fluid) and swelling. A positive skin test shows up as a firm red swelling which is maximal at 48–72 h after injection.*

This type of hypersensitivity also plays a role in several clinical situations where there is persistence of antigen which the immune system is unable to remove, leading to chronic inflammation.

The tuberculin reaction

Initial experiments by Koch showed that patients with tuberculosis (TB) given subcutaneous injection of mycobacterial antigens derived from MTb, resulted in fever and sickness. This 'tuberculin reaction' is now the basis of a 'recall' test to determine if individuals have T cell mediated reactivity against TB. In this test (Mantoux test) small amounts of the purified protein derivative (PPD) of tuberculin derived from MTb organisms is injected into the skin and the site examined up to 72 h later. A positive skin test shows up as a firm red swelling which is maximal at 48–72 h after injection and is mediated by dendritic cells and an influx of both T cells and macrophages into the site of injection (*Fig. 1*).

The production of granulomas

We now know that CD4+ T cells control intracellular microbial infections such as mycobacteria and some fungi (Topic K3). The problem is that mycobacteria, in addition to some other intracellular infections, have escape mechanisms to prevent their elimination (Topic O3). Thus, the macrophage activation factors produced by CD4+ T cells are not always effective (*Fig. 2*). Antigen therefore persists and leads to the 'chronic' stimulation of CD4+ T cells and continuous production of cytokines. These mediate fusion of the macrophages containing the microbes and fibroblast proliferation, finally resulting in a 'walling off' of the offending microbes in a granuloma. This chronic inflammatory state is seen in both TB and in the tuberculoid type of leprosy caused by *Mycobacterium leprae* (Topic O2).

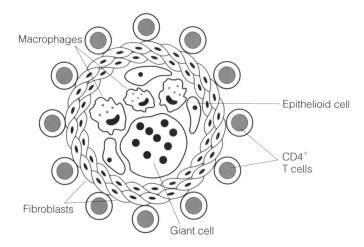

Fig. 2. Granulomas. Immune granulomas are formed in response to chronic stimulation of
CD4+ T cells by persistent nondegradable antigens including mycobacteria. They consist of
epithelioid cells, macrophages and giant cells which are 'walled off' by fibroblasts surrounded
by an outer layer of CD4+ T cells. Cytokines produced by the different cells all contribute to
the granuloma formation which is the immune system's way of isolating the nondegradable
microbes from the rest of the body.

Granulomatous reactions also occur with shistosomula infections and in some
clinical situations where the antigens have not yet been defined (e.g. sarcoidosis
and Crohn's disease).

**Contact
sensitivity**

A number of small molecules penetrating the skin can give rise to contact
sensitivity, seen clinically as dermatitis. Some chemical agents and plant products
shown to produce contact sensitivity are listed in *Table 1*. Classical examples of
contact sensitivity include reactions against metal fasteners on watch straps and
rashes seen in response to poison oak. Removal of contact with the agent usually
results in resolution of the hypersensitivity.

Sensitization against these molecules is thought to be mediated through binding to skin proteins and through the powerful antigen presenting properties of
skin dendritic cells, Langerhans cells, which present antigen on MHC class II molecules to CD4+ Th1 cells (*Fig. 3*). The subsequent contact sensitivity reaction
involves presentation of the antigens to memory CD4$^+$ T cells which release
cytokines causing vasodilation, traffic into the site of non-specific CD4$^+$ T cells
and activated macrophages, and localized pustule formation.

Table 1.   Agents causing contact sensitivity

Chemicals: nickel, turpentine, some cosmetics, formaldehyde

Plants: poison ivy, poison oak

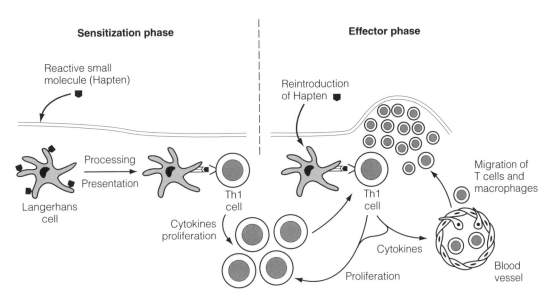

Fig. 3. Contact sensitivity mediated through Langerhans cells. In the sensitization phase, reactive small molecules, haptens (e.g. pentadecacatechol associated with poison ivy), which come in contact with the skin, bind to self proteins (including those on Langerhans cells) and are internalized, processed and presented by Langerhans cells to T cells. These proliferate to form clones of Th1 cells specific for hapten modified self peptide. When hapten is reintroduced, the modified self peptide is again presented on Langerhans cells in MHC class III. Memory T cells eventually find and respond to these antigens by releasing cytokines (e.g. IFNγ) which attract primarily Th1 cells and monocytes to this area and upregulate expression of adhesion molecules on endothelial cells that result in passage of Langerhans cells into the tissues.

U1 THE SPECTRUM AND PREVALENCE OF AUTOIMMUNITY

Key Notes

Autoimmunity and autoimmune disease	Autoimmunity is an acquired immune reactivity to self antigens. Autoimmune diseases occur when autoimmune responses lead to tissue damage.
Spectrum of autoimmune conditions	Autoimmune diseases may be organ specific, e.g. diabetes mellitus where the pancreas is the target organ, or systemic (nonorgan specific), e.g. systemic lupus erythematosus (SLE), where multiple organs may be involved. Pathogenesis associated with these diseases may be mediated primarily by antibody, by T cells or a combination thereof.
Prevalence	In the general population, approximately 3.5% of individuals have autoimmune disease, 94% of which are accounted for by Graves' disease/hyperthyroidism, type I diabetes, pernicious anemia, rheumatoid arthritis (RA), thyroiditis, vitiligo, multiple sclerosis (MS) and SLE. Women are 2.7 times more likely than men to develop autoimmune disease.
Related topics	Peripheral tolerance (M3) Antigen preparations (R3)

Autoimmunity and autoimmune disease

The immune system has the capacity to mount an immune response to virtually all molecules and/or cells. Although the capacity to respond to self antigen is present in all of us, in most instances such responses result in tolerance or anergy (Section M), indicating that mechanisms must exist to prevent or subdue autoimmune responses. Moreover, autoreactive T and B cells as well as autoantibodies are found in people who do not have autoimmune diseases, demonstrating that immunological autoreactivity alone is not sufficient for the development of disease. The mechanisms currently thought to prevent/dampen autoimmune responses include inactivation or deletion of autoreactive T and B cells, active suppression by cells or cytokines, idiotype/anti-idiotype interactions, and the immunosuppressive adrenal hormones, the glucocorticoids. When dampening mechanisms fail or are overridden, a response directed against self-antigen can occur, resulting in autoimmune diseases that range from those which are organ specific (diabetes and thyroiditis) to those which are systemic (non-organ specific) such as systemic lupus erythematosus and rheumatoid arthritis.

Several important cofactors in the development of autoimmune disease have been identified and include genetics (e.g. HLA associations), gender, and age. Characteristics of the antigen and how it is 'presented' to the immune system are also important. For example, injection of animals with chemically modified thyroid protein or with normal protein plus Freund's adjuvant (Topic R3) can give rise to severe thyroiditis that is due to immune recognition of normal thyroid proteins. Infection by organisms including Epstein Barr virus (EBV) or mycoplasma can provoke autoantibody production in otherwise normal persons. In addition, certain drugs such as procainamide which is used to treat cardiac arrhythmias, or toxic substances such as mercuric chloride and polyvinyl chloride can induce autoimmune pathology (Section T). Moreover, the attack by immune effectors on virus or drug antigens that results in inappropriate tissue damage, may also be considered an autoimmune-like disease (Section T).

Spectrum of autoimmune conditions

That autoimmune diseases involve immune recognition of specific antigens is evidenced by organ-specific diseases including thyroiditis, diabetes mellitus, multiple sclerosis (MS) and inflammatory bowel disease. Antigens shared by multiple tissue sites are apparently involved in systemic autoimmunity in diseases such as SLE, RA, systemic vasculitis and scleroderma. It is also clear that a given individual may develop autoimmune disease of more than one type (e.g. thyroid autoimmune disease is sometimes associated with gastric autoimmunity). Furthermore, the pathogenesis associated with autoimmune disease may be mediated primarily by antibody (e.g. hemolytic anemia), primarily by cellular immunity (e.g. MS) or by a combination of antibody and cell mediated immunity (e.g. RA).

Prevalence

Autoimmune diseases are quite prevalent in the general population, where it is estimated that approximately 3.5% of individuals are afflicted. The most common are Graves' disease/hyperthyroidism, type I diabetes, pernicious anemia, RA, thyroiditis, vitiligo, MS and SLE, which together account for 94% of all cases. Overall, women are 2.7 times more likely than men to develop an autoimmune disease, but the female:male ratio can be as high as 10:1 in SLE.

U2 FACTORS CONTRIBUTING TO THE DEVELOPMENT OF AUTOIMMUNE DISEASE

Key Notes

Autoimmune diseases are multifactorial	Autoimmune diseases arise as the result of a breakdown in self-tolerance. Factors predisposing and/or contributing to the development of autoimmune diseases include age, genetics, gender, infections and the nature of the autoantigen. Combinations of these factors are probably important in the development of autoimmune disease.
Age and gender	Autoantibodies are more prevalent in older people and women have a greater risk than men for developing an autoimmune disease. In SLE and Graves' disease, there is a female/male bias of 10:1 and 7:1, respectively. Evidence of a higher incidence in female mice is consistent with hormones playing an important role in autoimmune diseases.
Genetic factors	Antigen-specific autoimmune phenomena cluster in certain families. Particular HLA genes are associated with certain autoimmune diseases and particular HLA haplotypes predict the relative risk of developing a particular autoimmune disease. Gene polymorphisms and or mutations also play a role, as evidenced by the findings that Fas deficient Lpr mice develop SLE-like autoimmunity and that mutations in genes for certain complement components lead to an increased risk of SLE.
Infections	Many infectious agents (EBV, mycoplasma, streptococci, klebsiella, malaria, etc.) have been linked to particular autoimmune diseases and may be important in their etiology.
Nature of the autoantigens	Target antigens are often highly conserved proteins such as heat shock proteins (HSPs), stress proteins, enzymes, or their substrates. For example, in coeliac disease the enzyme tissue transglutaminase (tTG) is an autoantigen and its substrate, gliadin (a wheat protein), is the inducer of the disease. In this particular case, removal of the 'inducer' results in loss of response to tTG even though it is still present.
Drugs and autoimmune reactions	Certain drugs can initiate autoimmune reactions by unknown mechanisms. For example, patients receiving procainamide develop SLE-like symptoms and have antinuclear antibodies which disappear following discontinuation of the drug.

Immunodeficiency	A deficient immune response may allow persistence of infection or inflammation, which can lead to an increased incidence of autoimmune disease. For example, patients deficient in the complement components C2, C4, C5 or C8 have an increased incidence of autoimmune diseases, perhaps because of inefficient clearance of immune complexes.
Related topics	Genes, T helper cells and cytokines (N3) Primary/congenital (inherited) immunodeficiency (S2)

Autoimmune diseases are multifactorial

Autoimmune diseases arise as the result of a breakdown in self-tolerance. Moreover, autoimmune diseases are multifactorial in that their development, in most cases, probably results from combinations of predisposing and/or contributing factors. The factors known to predispose and/or contribute to the development of autoimmune diseases include (*Table 1*): genetics – inheritance of a particular HLA haplotype increases the risk of developing disease; gender – more females than males develop disease; infections – EBV, mycoplasma, streptococci, klebsiella, malaria, etc., have been linked to particular autoimmune diseases; the nature of the autoantigen – highly conserved enzymes and heat shock proteins (HSPs) are often target antigens and may be cross-reactive with microbial antigens; drugs – certain drugs can induce autoimmune-like syndromes; and age – most autoimmune diseases occur in adults.

Age and gender

Autoantibodies are more prevalent in older people and animals, perhaps due to less stringent immunoregulation by the ageing immune system. Few autoimmune diseases occur in children, the majority being in adults. Women have a greater risk than men for developing an autoimmune disease. In SLE and Graves' disease, there is a female/male bias of 10:1 and 7:1 respectively, whereas ankylosing spondylitis is almost exclusively a male disease. Taken together, these facts suggest that the neuroendocrine system plays an important role in the development of these diseases. This is supported by animal studies where it has been shown that female mice of a particular strain spontaneously develop SLE. This can be prevented by removing their ovaries (estrogen source) or by treating them with testosterone. Similarly, male mice that are more resistant to developing the disease lose this resistance if castrated.

Genetic factors

Antigen-specific autoimmune phenomena cluster in certain families. For example, thyroid-reactive antibodies are much more common in genetically related family

Table 1. Summary of factors contributing to development of autoimmune diseases

Genetics	Some diseases are HLA associated
Gender	Females generally more prone than males
Infections	Some common infections e.g. EBV, streptococcus, malaria, etc.
Nature of autoantigen	Often conserved antigens e.g. heat shock proteins and enzymes
Drugs	Some drugs e.g. procainamide, hydralazine induce SLE-like symptoms
Age	Higher incidence in aged population

Table 2. Some autoimmune diseases showing HLA association (Caucasians)

Disease	HLA	Risk*
Ankylosing spondylitis	B27	90
Reiter's disease	B27	36.0
Systemic lupus erythematosus	DR3	15
Myasthenia gravis	DR3	2.5
Juvenile diabetes mellitus (insulin dependent)	DR3/DR4	25
Psoriasis vulgaris	DR4	14
Multiple sclerosis	DR2	5
Rheumatoid arthritis	DR4	4

*Based on a comparison of the incidence of the autoimmune disease in patients with a given HLA type with the incidence of the autoimmune disease in patients without this HLA type.

members of a person with autoimmune thyroid disease than in the population at large. The role of the MHC (presumably in presenting autoantigenic peptides) is evidenced by the strong association between HLA type and incidence of certain autoimmune diseases. The possession of particular HLA haplotypes predicts the relative risk of developing a particular autoimmune disease (Table 2). Polymorphisms and/or mutations of many other genes involved in lymphocyte activation or suppression are also likely to play a crucial role. For example, in Lpr autoimmune mice, an autosomal recessive mutation in the Fas apoptosis gene leads to progressive lymphadenopathy and hypergammaglobulinemia, with production of multiple SLE-like autoantibodies. Complement deficiency due to mutations in genes for C2, C4, C5 and C8 results in increased risk of SLE, demonstrating the importance of complement in the clearance of immune complexes.

Infections

Many infectious agents (EBV, mycoplasma, streptococci, klebsiella, malaria, etc.) have been linked to particular autoimmune diseases. Lyme arthritis, for example, is initiated by chronic infection with spirochetes of the genus *Borrelia* (e.g. *Borrelia burgdorferi*) which are transmitted by deer ticks from deer and rodents to people. Some microbial antigens also have structures similar to self-antigens and induce autoimmune responses through 'antigenic mimicry' (see below).

Nature of the autoantigens

Target antigens for autoimmune disease can be cell surface, cytoplasmic, nuclear or secreted molecules (Table 3). They are often highly conserved proteins such as HSPs, stress proteins, enzymes or their substrates (Table 4). Of importance, the primary immune response to microbial infections includes a strong response to HSPs, followed by a response to a microbe specific component. Since HSPs are highly conserved, a dominant immune response to these antigens may confer on the host an ability to respond generally to other microbial infections. However, microbial and human HSPs have high sequence homology as well. Thus, an immune response to microbial HSP may induce a cross reactive response to human HSP. Target autoantigens are often enzymes (Table 4). For example, in coeliac disease the enzyme tissue transglutaminase (tTG) is an autoantigen and its

Table 3. Antigens targeted in autoimmune disease.

Organ specific diseases		Nonorgan specific diseases	
Disease	Antigen(s)	Disease	Antigen(s)
Addison's disease	Adrenal cortical cells (ACTH receptor and microsomes)	Ankylosing spondylitis	Vertebral
Autoimmune hemolytic anemia	RBC membrane antigens	Chronic active hepatitis	Nuclei, DNA
Graves' disease	TSH receptor	Multiple sclerosis	Brain/myelin basic protein
Guillain–Barré syndrome	Peripheral nerves (gangliosides)	Rheumatoid arthritis	IgG (rheumatoid factor) connective tissues
Hashimoto's thyroiditis	Thyroid peroxidase thyroglobulin/T4	Scleroderma	Nuclei, elastin, nucleoli, centromeres, topoisomerase 1
Insulin-dependent diabetes mellitus (IDDM)	β cells in the pancreas (GAD, tyrosine phosphatase)	Sjogren's syndrome	Exocrine glands, kidney, liver, thyroid
Pemphigus	Epidermal keratinocytes	Systemic lupus erythematosus	Double stranded DNA, nuclear antigens
Pernicious anemia	Intrinsic factor		
Polymyositis	Muscle (histidine tRNA synthetase)		
Several organs affected			
Goodpasture's syndrome	Basement membrane of kidney and lung (type IV collagen)		
Polyendocrine	Multiple endocrine organs (hepatic-cytochrome p450; intestinal-tryptophan hydroxylase)		

Table 4. Enzymes as autoantigens

Enzyme	Disease
Pyruvate dehydrogenase	Primary billiary cirrhosis
Glutamic acid decarboxylase	Insulin dependent diabetes
Myeloperoxidase	Glomerulonephritis
Thyroid peroxidase	Autoimmune thyroiditis
17α and 21 hydroxylase	Addison's disease
Proteinase 3	Wegener's granulomatosis
Tyrosinase	Vitiligo
Transglutaminase	Coeliac disease

substrate, gliadin (a wheat protein), is the inducer of the disease. Antibodies to both wheat proteins and tTG are found in patients with this disease. However, removal of the wheat protein from the diet leads to the removal of the immune response to tTG as well as to the wheat proteins, although tTG is still present.

Drugs and autoimmune reactions

Certain drugs can initiate autoimmune reactions by unknown mechanisms. For example, antinuclear antibodies appear in the blood of the vast majority of patients receiving prolonged treatment with procainamide for ventricular arrythmias, and nearly 10% develop an SLE-like syndrome which resolves following discontinuation of the drug.

Immunodeficiency

A deficient immune response may allow persistence of infection or inflammation. This possibility is supported by the observation that immune deficiency syndromes are associated with autoimmune abnormalities. For example, patients deficient in the complement components C2, C4, C5 or C8 have an increased incidence of autoimmune diseases (see Genetic factors). There are also diseases where paradoxically immunodeficiency and autoimmunity coexist. An example of this is in common variable immune deficiency (Topic S2) where autoantibodies to platelets are sometimes found.

U3 AUTOIMMUNE DISEASES – MECHANISMS OF DEVELOPMENT

Key Notes

Breakdown of self-tolerance	The mechanisms that lead to autoimmunity are unclear but may include molecular mimicry, defective regulation of the anti-self response through Th1 and Th2 cells, polyclonal activation, modification of self antigens through microbes and drugs, changes in availability of self antigen and dys-regulation of the idiotype network.
Molecular mimicry and the T cell bypass	An immune response may be generated against an epitope that is identical, or nearly identical, in both a microbe and host tissue, resulting in attack on host tissue by the same effector mechanisms activated to eliminate the pathogen. For example, a cross-reactive antigen between heart muscle and Group A *Streptococci* predisposes to the development of rheumatic fever as a result of inducing autoantibodies to heart muscle.
Defective regulation mediated via Th cells	Microbial infection induces either Th1 or Th2 cytokines. The Th1 response leads to the production of the pro-inflammatory cytokines, while the Th2 response is associated with anti-inflammatory cytokines and antibody formation. Predominance of Th1 or Th2 responses occurs in some autoimmune diseases and changes in the relative contribution of these subsets (e.g. as seen in pregnancy) can influence disease activity in RA and SLE.
Polyclonal activation via microbial antigens	Some microbes or their products activate lymphocytes independently of their antigenic specificity, i.e. are polyclonal activators, e.g. LPS and EBV. Patients with infectious mononucleosis produce IgM antibodies to several autoantigens including DNA. Since a switch to production of IgG autoantibodies (which requires Th cells) does not occur, T cells are probably not involved or are inhibited in their action.
Modification of cell surfaces by microbes and drugs	Foreign antigens, e.g. viruses and drugs, may become adsorbed onto the surfaces of cells or react chemically with surface antigens in a hapten-like manner to alter their specificity. For example, thrombocytopenia and anemia are relatively common in drug-induced autoimmune disease. Thrombocytopenia is also common in children following viral infections, and may involve association of viral antigens or immune complexes with the surface of platelets.

Availability of normally sequestered self-antigen	Since tolerance induction occurs mainly during embryonic development, antigens which are absent or anatomically separated (sequestered) from the immune system during this period are not recognized as self. Such antigens include the lens proteins of the eye, and molecules associated with the central nervous system, the thyroid and testes.
Dysregulation of the idiotype network	Anti-idiotypic antibodies resulting from an immune response to a hormone could interact with the receptor for the hormone, and thus initiate disease. Animal experiments have verified the existence of this mechanism. Clinical examples include those resulting from development of antibodies to insulin and acetylcholine receptors.
Related topics	Antigens (A4) Other control mechanisms Peripheral tolerance (M3) (N5) Genes, T helper cells and Pathogen defense strategies cytokines (N3) (O3)

Breakdown of self-tolerance

The mechanisms that lead to autoimmunity are unclear and involve many factors. In an ideal immune response only foreign antigens activate immune effector mechanisms, the foreign antigens are selectively cleared without damage to the host and immune effector mechanisms are turned off when they are no longer needed. Thus, the immune response may require the orderly interaction of at least four distinct cell types (antigen presenting cells, CTLs, Th cells, and B cells; Topics H4, J1, K2 and K3) that communicate by direct cell to cell contact and through cytokines. Although these interactions are usually well controlled, a defect could result in specific adaptive immune responses to self antigens which cause autoimmune disease. The various mechanisms which may explain breakdown of tolerance to self and how reactions may be initiated to autoantigens include molecular mimicry, defective regulation of the anti-self response through Th1 and Th2 cells, polyclonal activation, modification of self antigens through microbes and drugs, changes in the availability of self antigen and dysregulation of the idiotype network.

Molecular mimicry and the T cell bypass

The adaptive immune response continuously monitors microbial infections and responds accordingly. In some cases, however, a response may be generated against an epitope that is identical, or nearly identical, in both a microbe and host tissue, resulting in attack on host tissue by the same effector mechanisms which are activated to eliminate the pathogen. One example is rheumatic heart disease, which is due to an epitope that is common to heart muscle and Group A *Streptococci* (*Fig. 1*). In this case, previously anergized anti-self B cells (which also cross-react with *Streptococci*) may be reactivated by receiving co-stimulatory signals from microbe-specific T cells. The B cell interacts with the microbial antigen through its antigen receptor and presents microbial peptides to anti-microbial T cells which then provide help and activate the anti-self B cells (*Fig. 2*). Self reactive B cells also become activated if the self antigen forms a complex with a microbial antigen. In this event, the self reactive B cell can endocytose microbial antigens along with the self antigen and present microbial peptides to T cells. The microbe specific T cell in this instance will provide help to the self reactive B cell in the form of co-stimulatory molecules and cytokines leading to breakdown in tolerance (Topic M3).

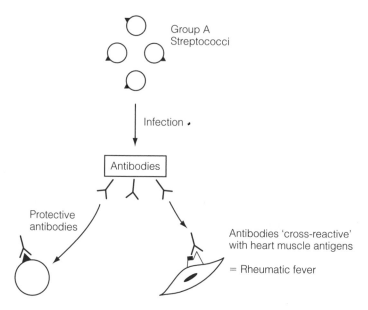

Fig. 1. *Group A streptococci and rheumatic fever. Antibodies to a streptococcal antigen 'cross-react' with heart muscle antigen leading to damage and rheumatic fever. Disease abates when the bacteria are eliminated and antibody production ceases.*

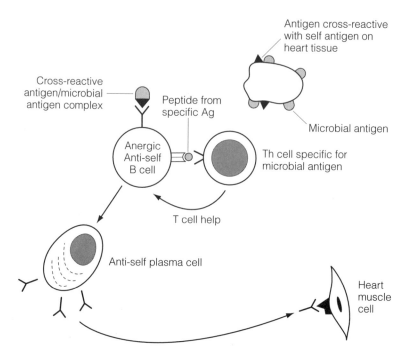

Fig. 2. *Activation of anergic anti-self B cells. The BCR on an anti-self B cell binds to self/microbial Ag complex. The B cell presents the microbial component of the complex to a T cell and receives T cell help for activation (second signal). This is also called the 'T cell bypass' mechanism of autoimmunity since T cell help for self is bypassed by presentation via a nonself antigen.*

Defective regulation mediated via Th cells

The initial response to a microbial infection is usually associated with predominantly either Th1 or Th2 cytokines (Topic N3). The Th1 response leads to the production of the pro-inflammatory cytokines IFNγ, IL2, and TNFα, followed by the release of the anti-inflammatory cytokines TGFβ, IL-4 and IL-10 from Th2 cells. The Th2 response is associated with anti-inflammatory cytokines and antibody formation. That polarized Th1 or Th2 responses may be involved in autoimmune pathogenesis is suggested by the observation that during pregnancy, a period when Th2 cytokines predominate, the Th1 autoimmune disease RA is decreased, whereas the Th2 autoimmune disease SLE is exacerbated.

Polyclonal activation via microbial antigens

Some microbes or their products activate lymphocytes independently of their antigenic specificity, i.e. are polyclonal activators. An example of this is endotoxin or lipopolysaccharide (LPS), which is produced mainly by Gram-negative bacteria. Another example involves EBV, which has been linked to autoimmunity in a small subset of infected individuals. Most patients with infectious mononucleosis, which is caused by EBV, develop IgM autoantibodies against several cellular antigens including DNA (*Fig. 3*). Since a switch to production of IgG autoantibodies, which requires Th cells, does not occur, T cells are probably not involved or are inhibited in their action. Moreover, on recovery, when the strong EBV stimulus is removed, autoantibodies disappear. Clearly, multiple factors are important for maintenance of long term tolerance to self, and a defect or impairment of immunoregulation following infection can result in activation and expansion of autoreactive clones.

Modification of cell surfaces by microbes and drugs

Foreign antigens may become adsorbed onto the surfaces of cells or react chemically with surface antigens in a hapten-like manner to alter their immunogenicity. Thrombocytopenia (low platelet levels) and anemia (low red blood cell levels are relatively common examples of drug-induced autoimmune disease. Thrombocytopenia is also common in children following viral infections, and may involve

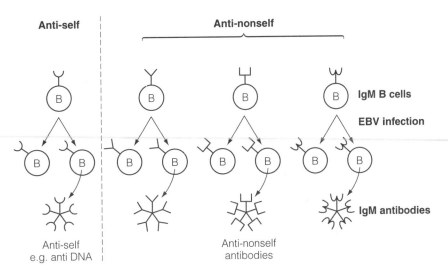

Fig. 3. Autoantibodies produced through polyclonal activation of B cells. B cells of all specificities including self, which have not been eliminated by central tolerance mechanisms, may be polyclonally activated (e.g. by EBV infection) to synthesize and release the antibodies they are programed to produce, perhaps including some autoantibodies. Transient production of the antibodies normally subsides after the microbe is eliminated or controlled.

association of viral antigens or virus–antibody immune complexes with the surface of platelets. Similarly, an autoimmune-like situation may result when microbial antigens become actively expressed on the surfaces of infected or transformed cells, especially during viral infection. Although the immune response that subsequently develops normally results in removal of these infected cells, in some cases the tissue destruction associated with elimination of these antigens may result in immunologically mediated disease which is much more serious than the infection itself. For example, mice infected *in utero* or at birth with lymphocytic choriomeningitis virus (LCMV) become tolerant to the virus and harbor it for life without overt disease symptoms. However, if normal adult mice are exposed to LCMV, the infection is invariably fatal. In X-irradiated or neonatally thymectomized (i.e. immunosuppressed) mice, the viral infection is not lethal. Thus, lethal neurological damage results, not from the virus itself, but from the immune response to LCMV-infected cells.

Availability of normally sequestered self antigen

Since tolerance induction occurs mainly during embryonic development, antigens which are absent or anatomically separated (sequestered) from the immune system during this period are not recognized as self. These antigens are either present in too low amounts to stimulate autoimmunity or are sequestered in immunologically privileged sites. In later life, these antigens may be released as a result of trauma or infection. They may then stimulate lymphocytes that have escaped tolerance, and induce the development of autoimmune disease. Antigens which fit this model include those found in the lens of the eye, central nervous system, thyroid and testes. For example, after vasectomy blocks the release of sperm through spermatic ducts, antibodies to spermatozoa are produced. In addition, trauma to the lens in one eye results in autoantibodies that can damage the nontraumatized eye.

Dysregulation of the idiotype network

Another mechanism by which autoantibodies may arise is through a failure of idiotype/anti-idiotype control (Topics M3 and N5). Anti-idiotypic antibodies resulting from an immune response to a hormone could interact with the receptor

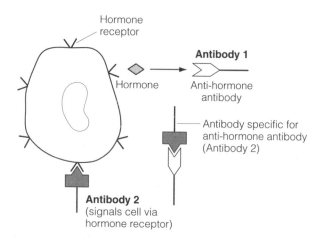

Fig. 4.   Antireceptor anti-idiotypic antibody in the development of autoimmune disease. Antibody 1 is directed towards the receptor-binding region of a ligand (e.g. a hormone). Antibody 2 is directed towards the idiotype of antibody 1. Antibody 2 can thus bind the receptor, potentially resulting in autoimmunity.

for the hormone, and thus initiate disease (*Fig. 4*). Many animal experiments have verified the existence of this mechanism. Possible clinical examples include those resulting from development of antibodies to insulin and acetylcholine receptors (Topic T3).

U4 DISEASE PATHOGENESIS – EFFECTOR MECHANISMS

Key Notes

Tissue damaging reactions in autoimmune diseases	Once autoantibodies have been produced, their mechanisms of tissue destruction are the same as the mechanisms that lead to protective responses – phagocytosis, complement activation and interference with molecular function. Both T and B cells may be involved as well as inflammatory cytokines, immune complexes, phagocytes and complement components. In this case they are considered as hypersensitivity reactions to self antigens. The main difference between anti-microbial and autoimmune responses is that, in autoimmune disease, autoantigen is always present and cannot be removed from the body. Removal of the autoantigen results in eventual loss of autoantibodies.
Autoantibodies can directly mediate cell destruction	Autoantibodies can bind to self cells and, either alone or with complement, cause damage mediated mainly through opsonization via Fc and C3 receptors on phagocytic cells. For example, IgG autoantibodies bind to red blood cells in autoimmune hemolytic anemia (AIHA) or to platelets in immune thrombocytopenia purpura (ITP) and mediate phagocytosis of these self cells.
Autoantibodies can modulate cell function	Antibodies to certain self cell surface molecules can either interfere with or enhance the functional activity of the cell. For example, Abs to the acetylcholine receptor in myasthenia gravis block their effective interaction with acetylcholine. In Graves' disease, Abs to the TSH receptor overstimulate the thyroid.
Autoantibodies can form damaging immune complexes	Circulating immune complexes, whether composed of autologous or foreign antigens, can result in damage to tissue by complement activation and by triggering release of mediators from Fc receptor-bearing cells (type III hypersensitivity). Immune complexes can deposit in the glomeruli, especially in SLE, leading to kidney damage or, in blood vessels, to vasculitis.
Cell mediated immunity in pathogenesis	Although autoantibodies have been most firmly linked to autoimmune disease, it is clear that cell mediated immunity plays an essential part in pathogenesis in some, if not all autoimmune disorders. Inflammatory T cell infiltrates are a hallmark of organ-specific diseases such as diabetes and multiple sclerosis. Their importance is indicated by studies showing that T cells can transfer particular autoimmune diseases.

Related topics	Phagocytes (B1)	Immune-complex mediated (type
	Functions (F5)	III) hypersensitivity (T4)
	IgM and IgG-mediated type II	Delayed-type (Type IV)
	hypersensitivity (T3)	hypersensitivity (T5)

Tissue damaging reactions in autoimmune diseases

The inflammatory processes underlying the tissue damage that occurs in autoimmune disease are complex and may include all of the components of the immune system. The inflammatory infiltrate usually consists of T cells, macrophages, neutrophils, B cells, mast cells and in some instances plasma cells. However, the nature of the primary insult, whether microbial or other, and site of the target tissue may influence the type of cellular infiltrate. For example, increased numbers of mast cells, eosinophils, lymphocytes and plasma cells may be a feature of gastrointestinal associated autoimmune diseases such as coeliac disease and Crohn's disease, whereas, in the pancreas of the diabetic the cellular infiltrate may be mainly mononuclear cells i.e., lymphocytes and macrophages. Some autoimmune diseases such as Goodpasture's syndrome are caused by autoantibodies to lung and kidney basement membranes which leads to renal failure. Immune complexes become deposited in the kidney also leading to kidney failure in SLE (Topic T4). Paradoxically, immunodeficiency is often associated with an increased incidence of autoimmune disease. Thus, the immune system may be an antagonist as well as a protagonist of autoimmunity. Autoimmune diseases are driven by antigen and when this is removed in experimental animals or man the autoimmune response subsides, e.g. removal of the thyroid gland in Hashimoto's thyroiditis removes the source of autoimmune stimulation and autoantibodies are no longer produced.

Autoantibodies can directly mediate cell destruction

Autoantibodies can bind to self cells and either alone or with complement cause damage. This can be mediated through opsonization via Fc receptors or C3 receptors on phagocytic cells. An example of this is IgG autoantibodies binding to red blood cells in autoimmune hemolytic anemia (AIHA), or to platelets in immune thrombocytopenia purpura (ITP; *Fig. 1*). The Fc mediated mechanism appears to be more important, since successful therapy (e.g. with the immunosuppressive steroid hormones glucocorticoids or corticosteroids) coincides with decreased Fc receptors on monocytes and macrophages, but not with lower autoantibody titers. Furthermore, the injection of high amounts of nonimmune IgG decreased cell destruction, an effect partly due to blocking of the Fc receptors on the body's phagocytes. Autoantibodies can also bind directly to cells in tissues. For example, in Goodpasture's syndrome, IgG antibodies bind to the basement membranes of kidney and lungs attracting phagocytes, which release enzymes that damage these tissues (frustrated phagocytosis).

Autoantibodies can modulate cell function

Antibodies to certain self cell surface molecules can either interfere with or enhance the functional activity of the cell. For example, myasthenia gravis (MG) is characterized by weakened and easily tired muscles. Serum antibodies directed against muscle, and in particular antibodies to the acetylcholine receptor, play a key role. These antibodies not only block the acetylcholine binding sites, but appear to act by cross-linking the receptor so that it becomes non-functional

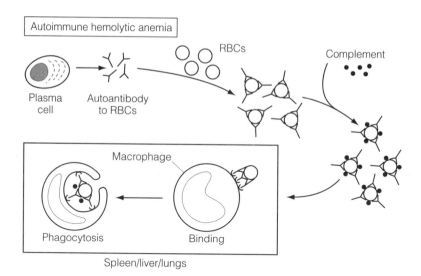

Fig.1. *Autoantibody mediated removal of erythrocytes (AIHA) or platelets (ITP). In autoimmune hemolytic anemia (AIHA), autoantibody to red blood cells (RBCs) binds to the RBC and as these antibody-coated cells pass through the spleen, liver and lungs, they are recognized and bound by Fc receptors for IgG on macrophages in these organs. The RBCs are phagocytosed by these macrophages and destroyed. Similarly, in idiopathic thrombocytopenia (ITP), which is mediated by autoantibody to platelets, the antibody-coated platelets are removed and destroyed. Complement may also play a role in lysing autoantibody coated RBCs or platelets and/or in opsonizing these self cells for phagocytosis by macrophages.*

(Topic T3, *Fig. 2*). This is an example of type II hypersensitivity. The opposite is true in Graves' disease, an autoimmune thyroid disease in which autoantibodies stimulate rather than inhibit receptor function. Both thyroid growth-stimulating immunoglobulin (TGSI: an example of type V hypersensitivity) and thyrotropin binding-inhibitory immunoglobulin (TBII) have been demonstrated. TBII, by binding to receptors for thyroid stimulating hormone (TSH), thyrotropin, stimulates the thyroid gland to make high levels of thyroid hormone resulting in hyperthyroidism. IgG autoantibiodies can cross the placenta and can cause transient hyperthyroidism in the newborns of women who have Graves' disease and MG in the newborns of mothers with MG. It would appear that in MG and Graves' disease, only B-cells specific for a few bodily components are activated. The defect may therefore lie with a very small subset of T or B cells. Since total antibody titer does not correlate well with disease state, antibody class and subclass (e.g. C' binding or nonbinding) may be a crucial consideration.

Autoantibodies can form damaging immune complexes

Circulating immune complexes, whether composed of autologous or foreign antigens, can result in damage to tissue by complement activation and triggering release of mediators from Fc receptor-bearing cells (type III hypersensitivity). Immune complexes may also perturb normal immunoregulation, perhaps through triggering of Fc receptors on lymphocytes. For example, although SLE may involve some target cell-specific autoantibodies (e.g. to erythrocytes), the most life-threatening manifestation of SLE is usually kidney damage, which results from the deposition of soluble immune complexes in the glomeruli. Some immune complexes may deposit in blood vessels leading to vasculitis. Since autoantibodies are produced to many bodily components, there may be a generalized defect in self tolerance similar to the Fas/FasL apoptotic defects seen in certain autoimmune (LPR and GLD) strains of mice. Antibodies to T cells are common as well, and may contribute to progression of the disease.

Cell mediated immunity in pathogenesis

Although autoantibodies have been most firmly linked to autoimmune disease, it is clear that cell mediated immunity plays an essential part in pathogenesis in some, if not all autoimmune disorders. In particular, T cells not only play a helper role in the development of autoimmune disease but also a direct role in tissue inflammation. For example, inflammatory T cell infiltrates are a hallmark of organ-specific diseases such as diabetes and MS, and are also present in skin lesions in SLE. However, a clear understanding of their involvement in autoimmune pathogenesis has been complicated by the MHC restricted nature of T cell recognition and the difficulty in isolating these T cells and in identifying their target antigens. In animal models, using inbred populations, it has been possible to clone autoimmune T cells that are able to transfer the autoimmune disease to other animals. For example, injection of myelin basic protein has been shown to induce experimental allergic encephalomyelitis (EAE) in rats, a disease very like MS in humans. Both encephalogenic and tolerogenic peptides to which T cells bind have been identified and either disease or protection against disease can be transferred to other rats of the same inbred strain with different cloned T cells. In general, clones making Th2 cytokines are protective whereas those making Th1 cytokines elicit disease. Thus, it is clear that T cells play a central role in both pro- and anti-inflammatory aspects of autoimmune disease, and that their MHC restriction, peptide specificity, and Th1/Th2 cytokine profile are important contributors to pathogenesis.

U5 DIAGNOSIS AND TREATMENT OF AUTOIMMUNE DISEASE

Key Notes

Diagnosis

Diagnosis of autoimmune disease is through clinical and laboratory criteria that differ for each disease. Autoantibodies to a variety of autoantigens are detected using tissue sections, immunofluorescence techniques and ELISA. This allows the detection of the IgG Abs to double stranded DNA which are characteristic of SLE, and of rheumatoid factor found in RA patients. Autoantibodies to the acetyl choline receptor or the TSH receptor can be detected by the ELISA.

Replacement therapy

In some cases, critical self antigens are compromised by the autoimmune process and may need to be replaced. In the case of thyroid autoimmunity, the patient is treated with thyroid hormones. In myasthenia gravis, inhibitors of enzymes which break down acetylcholine are given. In diabetes, insulin is given to replace that lost by damage to the islet cells.

Suppression of the autoimmune process

The ideal treatment of an autoimmune diseases is to reinstate specific immune tolerance to self antigen. However, more than one autoantigen is often involved and induction of tolerance is very difficult to achieve during an ongoing immune response. Current treatments are aimed at suppressing the autoimmune response. These include nonspecific aspirin-like drugs (nonsteroidal anti-inflammatory drugs; NSAIDs) or glucocorticoids, used to dampen inflammation, and plasmapheresis to remove autoantibodies. Cytotoxic drugs, cyclosporin and MAbs to T or B cells are also used to modulate or eliminate autoreactive lymphocytes. Drugs targeting cytokines (or their receptors) have also demonstrated considerable promise in RA.

Related topics

Monoclonial antibodies (F6)
Cytokines in the clinic (G3)
Precipitation and
  agglutination (V2)

Immunoassay (V3)
Monoclonal and recombinant
  antibodies (V5)

Diagnosis

Diagnosis of autoimmune diseases is through clinical and laboratory criteria that differ for each disease. In the clinical laboratory, autoantibodies to a variety of autoantigens are detected using tissue sections, immunofluorescence techniques and ELISA (Topic V3). For example, sera containing antinuclear antibodies (ANA), which are characteristic of a number of autoimmune diseases, can be detected on thyroid tissues as can antibodies to thyroid peroxidase which are characteristic of Hashimoto's thyroiditis. Patients with SLE have IgG antibodies to double stranded DNA in their serum, whilst 70% of patients with RA are seropositive for rheumatoid factor – an autoantibody directed to the Fc region of IgG. Autoantibodies to the acetylcholine receptor or the TSH receptor can be detected by ELISA. Antibodies to neutrophil cytoplasmic antigen (ANCA) are detected by immunofluorescence on normal neutrophils, which if present indicates a diagnosis of Wegener's granulomatosis.

Replacement therapy

In some cases the autoantigen that is being removed either directly by the autoimmune response (e.g. pernicious anemia, autoimmune thyroiditis or indirectly by immune damage (e.g. diabetes) may need to be given back to the patient. This includes platelets in autoimmune thrombocytopenias, thyroid hormones in thyroid autoimmunity, B12 in pernicious anemia and insulin in insulin-dependent diabetes.

Suppression of the autoimmune process

The 'Holy Grail' for the treatment of autoimmune diseases is to reinstate specific immune tolerance to the particular autoantigen. However, more than one autoantigen is often involved and induction of tolerance is very difficult to achieve during an ongoing immune response. Therefore, current treatment is essentially aimed at reducing specific inhibition of the ongoing inflammatory response (*Table 1*). Nonspecific aspirin-like drugs (nonsteroidal anti-inflammatory drugs; NSAIDs) or glucocorticoids are often used to dampen inflammation. Removal of autoantibodies and immune complexes from the blood and replacement of patient plasma with plasma from normal donors (plasmapheresis) can be useful but has a short-lived effectiveness. Cytotoxic drugs such as those used to treat tumors are used in severe cases of autoimmune disease to eliminate the autoantigen specific T and B cells which are the origin of the disease. Similarly, lymphoid irradiation has been used to treat drug-resistant RA patients with some success. Drugs that more specifically target immune cells include cyclosporin A, which inhibits cytokine release by T cells, and monoclonal antibodies directed to T cells or B cells, which could eliminate lymphocytes responsible for the disease. However, care has to be taken to avoid elimination of important immune cells leading to secondary immunodeficiency (Topic S3).

Table 1.   *Therapy of autoimmune diseases*

Current	
Replacement of targeted autoantigen	E.g. thyroid hormone for thyroid autoimmune disease; insulin for type II IDDM.
Nonsteroidal anti-inflammatory drugs (NSAIDs) e.g. aspirin, ibuprofen	Inhibit prostaglandins – RA and others
Corticosteroids e.g. prednisone	Anti-inflammatory
Cytotoxic drugs	
Azathioprine	Inhibits cell division, suppresses T cells
Cyclophosphamide	Blocks cell division, inhibits antibody production
Cyclosporin A	Inhibits T cell cytokine IL-2 production
Experimental/in clinical trials	
Monoclonal antibodies to CD4/CD20	In drug-resistant RA
Inhibitors of TNFα	In drug-resistant RA
Antigen given via the oral route to re-establish tolerance	
Myelin basic protein	Treatment of multiple sclerosis
Collagen	Treatment of RA

Drugs targeting cytokines such as inhibitors of IL-1 and monoclonal antibodies to, or soluble receptors for, TNFα have also shown considerable promise in suppressing the inflammatory process in RA and slowing down progression of the disease.

Another approach being developed involves the introduction of antigen via the oral route (mucosal surface) in an attempt to reintroduce specific tolerance (e.g. in RA and MS). There is also experimental evidence that antibodies specific for the autoantibody-producing B cell clones (anti-idiotypic antibodies) may offer effective treatment in the future. Other experimental treatments include targeting the CD40L induced on T cells during cognate interactions with antigen with the idea of removing specific T cell help for autoreactive B cells. This shows promise in re-inducing at least a partial tolerance to the autoantigens.

V1 ANTIBODIES AS RESEARCH AND DIAGNOSTIC TOOLS

Key Note

Antibodies and assays	A variety of assays have been developed which provide specific qualitative and quantitative measurement of Ag or Ab, both of which are often of considerable research and clinical relevance. Ab to an organism in the serum of a patient demonstrates infection by the organism. Ab with defined specificity is used to determine the presence of disease associated antigens in a patient. As tools in molecular and cellular research, Abs permit localization and characterization of Ags.
Related topics	Basic structure (F1) immunodeficiency (S4) Immunization (R2) Diagnosis and treatment of Diagnosis and treatment of autoimmune disease (U5)

Antibodies and assays

Methods for measuring antigen–antibody reactions have been well established and include those that have direct biologic relevance (*Table 1*). The combination of Ab with biologically active Ag (virus, toxin, enzyme and hormone) can be detected by neutralization of the virus infection, toxicity, enzymatic and hormonal activity, respectively. Precipitation and agglutination have also been adapted for development of several useful assays.

A variety of other assays have been developed which provide specific qualitative and quantitative measurement of Ag or Ab for both research and diagnostic purposes. Since the immune system recognizes and remembers virtually all Ags that are introduced into an individual, assays which demonstrate the presence of Ab to an organism in the serum of a patient have become a standard way of determining that the patient has had contact with, was infected by, the organism (e.g. the presence of Ab to HIV in the serum of a patient usually means that the patient has been infected with HIV). Alternatively, Abs with defined specificity (e.g. to Ags associated with cancer cells) can be used to determine the presence of disease associated Ags in a patient. Abs are also extremely important tools in molecular and cellular research as they permit the localization and characterization of Ags.

Table 1.   Effects of combination of antigen and antibody*

Agglutination	Antigenic particle + specific Ab results in aggregation of particles
Precipitation	Soluble Ag + specific Ab results in lattice formation and precipitation
C Activation	Ag in solution or on particle + specific Ab results in activation of C
Cytolysis	Cell + anti-cell Ab + C may result in lysis of the cell
Opsonization	Antigenic particle + Ab + C enhances phagocytosis by Mo, MØ, PMNs
Neutralization	Toxins, viruses, enzymes, etc. + specific Abs may result in their inactivation

* C, Complement; Mo, monocytes; MØ, macrophages; Ab, antibody; PMNs, polymorphonuclear cells

V2 PRECIPITATION AND AGGLUTINATION

Key Notes

Precipitation assays	Combination of Ab with Ag results in lattice formation and precipitation if there is sufficient Ag and Ab (equivalence). These reactions are the basis for qualitative and quantitative assays for Ag or Ab, including radial immunodiffusion and immunoelectrophoresis.
Agglutination assays	The interaction of surface Ags on insoluble particles (e.g. cells) with specific Ab to these Ags results in agglutination of the particles. Agglutination can be used to determine blood types; the presence of Ab to bacteria in serum is an indication of previous or current infection; and in the Coomb's test autoantibodies to erythrocytes can be assayed.
Related topics	Antibody classes (F2) IgM and IgG-mediated type II Transplantation antigens (Q2) hypersensitivity (T3)

Precipitation assays

As previously described (Topic J4), when there is both sufficient Ag and sufficient Ab, the combination of Ag and Ab proceeds until large aggregates are formed which are insoluble in water and precipitate (equivalence). The extent to which a lattice forms depends on the relative amounts of Ag and Ab present.

Lattice formation, and precipitation are the basis for several qualitative and quantitative assays for Ag or Ab. These assays are done in semisolid gels into which holes are cut for Ag and/or for Ab and diffusion occurs until Ag and Ab are at equivalence and precipitate. In **radial immunodiffusion**, Ab (e.g. horse anti-human IgG) is incorporated into the gel and Ag (e.g. human serum) is placed in a hole cut in the gel. Ag diffuses radially out of the well into the gel and interacts with the Ab forming a ring of precipitation, the diameter of which is related to the concentration of the Ag (*Fig. 1*). Similar assays have been developed in which a voltage gradient (electrophoresis) is used to speed up movement of Ag into the Ab containing gel (rocket immunoelectrophoresis).

In **immunoelectrophoresis**, Ags (e.g. serum) are placed in a well cut in a gel (without Ab) and electrophoresed, after which a trough is cut in the gel into which Abs (e.g. horse anti-human) are placed. The Abs diffuse laterally to meet diffusing Ag, and lattice formation and precipitation occur permitting determination of the nature of the Ags (*Fig. 2*).

Agglutination assays

Agglutination involves the interaction of surface Ags on **insoluble particles** (e.g. cells) and specific Ab to these Ags (*Fig. 3*). Ab thus links together (agglutinates) insoluble particles. Much smaller amounts of Ab suffice to produce agglutination than are needed for precipitation. For this reason, agglutination rather than precipitation may be used to determine blood types or if Ab to bacteria is present

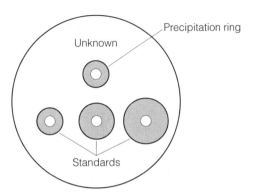

Fig. 1. Measurement of Ag by precipitation in gels. Ab-containing gel is placed on a glass or plastic surface. Holes are cut in the gel and filled with Ag which diffuses radially out of the well and interacts with the Ab in the gel. Soluble complexes are initially formed but as more Ag diffuses equivalence is reached resulting in a lattice and precipitation. The diameter of the precipitation ring is related to the concentration of the Ag and, using known standards, can be quantitated and compared with the levels of Ag in other samples.

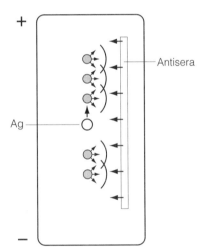

Fig. 2. Identification of antigens using gel electrophoresis. Ag (e.g. serum) is placed in a well cut in a gel and subjected to a voltage gradient which causes the various antigens to migrate different distances through the gel dependent on their charge. After electrophoresis, a trough is cut in the gel into which antibodies (e.g. horse anti-human serum) are placed. The antibodies diffuse laterally from the trough until they meet Ag diffusing from its location after electrophoresis. Again, lattice formation and precipitation occurs and, based on immuno-electrophoresis of defined standards, the identity of the Ag can be determined.

in blood as an indication of infection with these bacteria. Since IgM has 10 binding sites, whereas IgG has two, IgM is much more efficient at agglutinating particles or cells.

Although Abs are frequently used by themselves to assay for the presence of an Ag, a second Ab is sometimes used in what is known as a **Coomb's test**. In some instances, such as when an autoantibody has been produced against a given cell type, the cells will have human Ab bonded to them, and thus can be identified by

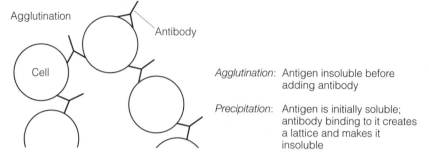

Agglutination: Antigen insoluble before
               adding antibody

Precipitation: Antigen is initially soluble;
               antibody binding to it creates
               a lattice and makes it
               insoluble

Fig 3.   Agglutination.

a second Ab (an Ab to human immunoglobulin) which will cause agglutination of the cells. In an **indirect Coomb's test**, the presence of circulating Ab to a cell surface Ag is demonstrated by adding the patient's serum to test cells (e.g. erythrocytes) followed by addition of Ab to human Ab.

V3 IMMUNOASSAY

Key Notes

ELISA, RIA

The presence and concentration of a specific Ag or of an Ab to a specific Ag in solution can be determined by radioimmunoassays (RIA) or enzyme-linked immunoabsorbent assays (ELISA). Ag attached to a solid surface captures the Ab with which it reacts and is quantitated using a labeled second Ab reactive to the first. These assays permit measurement of a wide variety of Ags as well as the concentration and isotype of Abs specific for a given Ag, such as those reactive with an infectious organism.

Immunofluorescence and flow cytometry

Using a fluorescence microscope and Abs labeled with a fluorescent molecule, tissue sections can be examined for cells expressing particular Ags (e.g. those which are tumor associated). Direct or indirect immunofluorescence techniques permit qualitative and quantitative evaluation of several different cell associated molecules at the same time. Flow cytometers rapidly analyze large numbers of cells in suspension, providing a molecular fingerprint of the cells. Fluorescence activated cell sorters separate cell subpopulations for more detailed study.

Immunoblotting

Immunoblotting is used to assay for the presence of molecules in a mixture. Western blot analysis involves separating molecules by sodium dedecyl sulfate polyacrylamide gel electrophoresis (SDS-PAGE), transferring them to another matrix and detecting the molecule of interest using ELISA or RIA. This assay is often used to confirm the presence of Abs to infectious agents (e.g. HIV) in patient serum. Immunoblotting can also be used to analyze products of single cells (e.g. cytokines) and the nature of the producing cell.

Related topics

Molecules with multiple functions (G1)
The microbial cosmos (O1)
Immunodiagnosis (P4)
Diagnosis and treatment of

immunodeficiency (S4)
IgE-mediated type I hypersensitivity (T2)
Diagnosis and treatment of autoimmune disease (U5)

ELISA, RIA

The presence of Ab to a particular Ag in the serum of a patient can be determined using very sensitive radioimmunoassays (RIA) or enzyme-linked immunoabsorbent assays (ELISA). Such assays (*Fig. 1*) are of particular value in demonstrating Ab to Ags of infectious agents, e.g. virus, bacteria, etc. The presence of an Ab of a particular isotype can also be determined using a modification of these assays. The radioallergosorbent test (RAST) uses as detecting ligand a radiolabeled Ab to human IgE and permits the measurement of specific IgE Ab to an allergen. ELISA and RIA also provide very specific and sensitive measurement of toxins, drugs, hormones, pesticides, etc., not only in

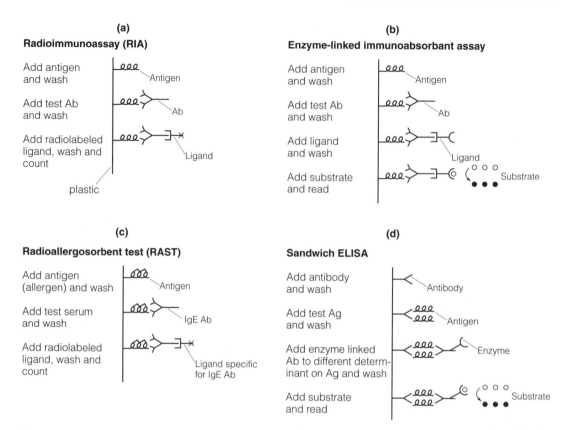

Fig. 1. *(a) Radioimmunoassay (RIA). Antigen is incubated on plastic and small quantities are adsorbed. Free antigen is washed away. Test antibody is added, which may bind to the Ag, and unbound Ab washed away. Ab remaining bound to the Ag is detected by a radiolabeled ligand (e.g. an Ab specific for the isotype of the test Ab, or staphylococcal protein A which binds to the Fc region of IgG). (b) Enzyme linked immunosorbent assay (ELISA). This is similar to RIA except that the ligand (e.g. the Ab that binds the test Ag) is covalently coupled to an enzyme such as peroxidase. This ligand binds the test Ab and after free ligand is washed away the bound ligand is detected by the addition of substrate which is acted on by the enzyme to yield a colored and detectable end product. (c) Radio allergosorbent test (RAST). This measures Ag-specific IgE in an RIA where the ligand is a labeled anti-IgE Ab and is very similar to the standard RIA. (d) Sandwich ELISA and RIA. This is basically the same as described in (a) and (b) except that Ab to the Ag is first used to coat the plastic in order to specifically capture the Ag from a mixture. A second enzyme or radioisotopically labeled Ab, which reacts with an epitope on the Ag which is different from that of the first Ab, is then added for quantitation of the antigen.*

serum, but also in water, foods and other consumer products. Based on these procedures, assays for nearly any Ag or Ab can be readily developed.

Immuno-fluorescence and flow cytometry

Although it is possible to use ELISA and RIA to evaluate the presence of an Ag on a cell, this is usually more conveniently done using Abs to which a fluorescent marker has been covalently attached. Moreover, in most cases a mAb is used and thus is highly specific for a particular molecule and a particular epitope on that molecule. This type of assay can be done using an Ab to the Ag which is directly fluorescent labeled (**direct** immunofluorescence) or by first incubating the unlabeled Ab with the cells (e.g. a mouse mAb to human T cells) and then, after washing away unbound Ab, adding a second fluorescent labeled Ab that reacts with the first Ab (e.g. a goat Ab to mouse immunoglobulin). This **indirect** immunofluorescent assay (*Fig. 2*) has two advantages, it has higher sensitivity and

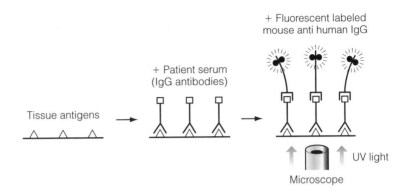

Fig. 2. Indirect immunofluorescence assay. Animal tissues (rat) are frequently used to identify human autoantibodies since the autoantigens recognized are generally conserved across the species. Patient serum is added to the tissue sections and the autoantibodies bind to particular autoantigen(s). After washing, fluorescent antibodies to human IgG are added and viewed under a fluorescence microscope. A green color shows where the human antibodies have bound to the tissue autoantigens.

requires labeling of only one Ab, the second Ab, because, in the example given, it can detect (react with) any mouse Ab.

Fluorescent Abs to cell surface molecules (e.g. those which are tumor associated) are very useful in examining tissue sections for cells expressing the Ag. This assay is done by incubating the tissue section with the labeled Ab (for direct immunofluorescence (IF)) or unlabeled Ab, followed by labeled second Ab and then examining the tissue section using a fluorescent microscope. These microscopes irradiate the tissue with a wavelength of light that excites the fluorescent label on the Ab to emit light at a different wavelength. This emitted light can be directly visualized, photographed and even quantitated. Moreover, it is possible to analyze a tissue sample using several different Abs at the same time, as each Ab could be labeled with a different fluorescent molecule each of which emit light at a wavelength distinct from the others. It is also possible to look for intracellular molecules (e.g. Abs) by first permeabilizing the cells and then doing the staining and fluorescence microscopy. Thus, one can use this approach to develop a molecular fingerprint of the cells associated with a tissue.

Although fluorescence microscopy can be, and is, applied to the analysis of **single cell suspensions**, another rather technologically sophisticated approach, **flow cytometry**, is most often used. This assay uses the same basic staining procedures as described for fluorescence microscopy, followed by automated quantitation of the amount of fluorescence associated with individual cells (*Fig. 3*). In particular, the suspension of stained cells is fed to the flow cytometer which disperses the cells so they then pass single file through a focused laser beam which excites any fluorescent label associated with the cells. Those stained by the fluorescent Ab emit light that is detected and quantitated by optical sensors and the intensity of fluorescence is plotted in histogram form by a computer. This machine can analyze 1000 cells per second and provide quantitative data on the number of molecules of a particular kind on each cell. It can also analyze mixtures of cells and provide data on their size and granularity in addition to their expression of specific molecules. Some versions of this machine (**fluorescence activated cell sorter**) are also able to separate out cells into microdroplets and sort those expressing a selected amount of a particular Ag into a separate tube for further analysis or culture.

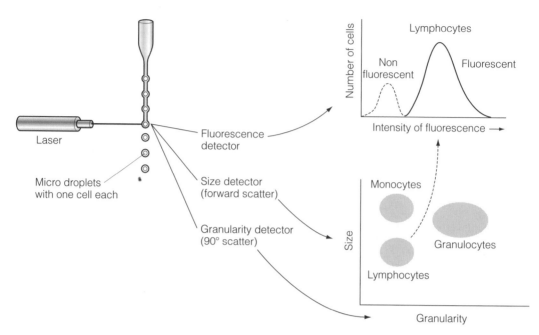

Fig. 3. Flow cytometry. After labeling with fluorescent antibody, cells are passed one at a time through a laser beam. Photodetectors measure the amount of fluorescence which is plotted as a histogram showing the proportion of non-fluorescent (unstained) and fluorescent (stained) cells. Other detectors simultaneously measure scattered laser light, which is used to generate a 'dot blot' in which lymphocytes, monocytes and granulocytes can be discriminated.

Immunoblotting   It is possible to combine various separation and detection procedures for identification and analysis of Ags and for evaluating the expression of molecules by single cells. Western blot analysis involves separating Ags by polyacrylamide gel electrophoresis (PAGE) in the presence of sodium dodecyl sulfate (SDS) which results in separation of molecules on the basis of size. These molecules are then transferred to another matrix (e.g. nitrocellulose) to form a pattern on the matrix identical to that on the gel. Enzyme linked Ab to the molecule of interest is then added, the unbound Ab washed off and substrate added (see ELISA) for visualization. This assay permits specific identification of proteins in a mixture and is also often used to confirm the presence of Abs to certain infectious agents (e.g. HIV) in the serum of patients.

   Immunobloting can also be used to assay for the presence of molecules in a mixture as described for the sandwich ELISA. This has now been extended for analysis of products of single cells. For example, to assay for production of a cytokine, Ab to the cytokine is coated onto the nitrocellulose 'floor' of a special culture well (see sandwich ELISA), the unbound Ab is washed off, and cells are then plated on top of this Ab. After incubation, an enzyme linked Ab to a different determinant on the cytokine is added, followed by washing and substrate addition. Wherever a cell produced the cytokine, it will be captured by the first Ab and will then be detected by the second Ab and its conversion of substrate, forming a colored spot on the nitrocellulose (hence the name ELISPOT assay). The nature of the cell producing the cytokine can also be determined by flow cytometry after staining the cells with a fluorescent labeled cell type specific Ab (e.g. anti-CD4 for T helper cells) and an anti-cytokine Ab labeled with a different fluorochrome.

V4 AFFINITY CHROMATOGRAPHY

Key Note

| Specific purification of Ag and Ab | Ab coupled to an insoluble matrix (e.g. agarose) specifically binds its Ag, which can then be eluted from the Ab yielding relatively pure Ag in one step. Similarly, Ag or protein A coupled to an insoluble matrix permits purification of Ab. |

Related topics   Basic structure (F1)   Pathogen defense strategies (O3)

Specific purification of Ag and Ab

The specificity of Abs is not only important to the development of many research and diagnostic assays, but can, in some instances, be used to purify, or be purified by, interaction with Ag. This is because Abs do not form covalent bonds when they combine with Ag. Ab coupled to an insoluble matrix (e.g. agarose) specifically binds its Ag, removing it from a mixture of other molecules. After washing to remove all unbound molecules, the Ag can be eluted at low pH and/or at high ionic strength, which break the reversible bonds holding it to the Ab. As this can usually be performed without damaging the Ag or Ab, it is possible to obtain relatively pure Ag in one step. Similarly, Ag coupled to an insoluble matrix permits purification of Ab from media or serum. Ab can also be purified based on its binding by proteins (e.g. protein A) isolated from some strains of *Staphylococcus aureus*. Protein A coupled to agarose binds IgG Abs which can be eluted by decreasing the pH and/or by increasing the ionic strength of the eluting buffer, again without damaging the Ab.

Using similar techniques, cell subpopulations with characteristic cell surface molecules (e.g. immunoglobulin on B cells) can also be isolated (positive selection) or removed (negative selection) from a mixture of cells.

V5 MONOCLONAL AND RECOMBINANT ANTIBODIES

Key Notes

Monoclonal antibodies (mAbs)	Standardized procedures involving fusion of an immortal cell (a myeloma tumor cell) with a specific predetermined Ab-producing B cell have been used to create hybridoma cells producing monospecific and monoclonal antibodies (mAbs). These mAbs are standard research reagents with extensive diagnostic and clinical applications.
Humanization and chimerization of mAbs	Most mAbs developed have been mouse, and although useful as research and diagnostic tools, they are not ideal therapeutics because of their immunogenicity in humans. This has been dealt with by humanizing these murine Abs or by making fully human mAbs.
Fv libraries	By randomly fusing heavy (H) and light (L) chain variable (V) region genes from B cells, Fv libraries containing all binding specificities can be generated and used as a source for creation of specific mAbs.
Related topics	Basic structure (F1) IgM and IgG-mediated type II Monoclonal antibodies (F6) hypersensitivity (T3) The cellular basis of the antibody response (J1)

Monoclonal antibodies

In 1975, Kohler and Milstein developed a procedure to create cell lines producing a predetermined, monospecific and monoclonal Ab, for which they received the Nobel Prize. This procedure has been standardized and applied on a massive scale to the preparation of Abs useful to many research and clinical efforts. The basic technology involves creation of a hybrid cell by fusion of an immortal cell (a myeloma tumor cell) with a specific predetermined Ab-producing B cell from immunized animals or people (*Fig. 1*). The resulting hybridoma cell is immortal and synthesizes homogeneous, specific Ab. The utility of this Ab depends on its specificity. Monoclonal Abs (mAbs) can be made in large quantities and against virtually every Ag. Thus, mAbs have become standard research reagents and have extensive diagnostic and clinical applications.

Humanization and chimerization of mAbs

The vast majority of mAbs have been developed in mice, and although useful as research and diagnostic tools, they have not been ideal therapeutic reagents at least partly because of their immunogenicity in humans. That is, a murine Ab introduced into a patient will be recognized as foreign by the patient's immune system and a human anti-mouse Ab (HAMA) response will develop that compromises the utility of therapeutic Ab. This has been dealt with in two basic ways.

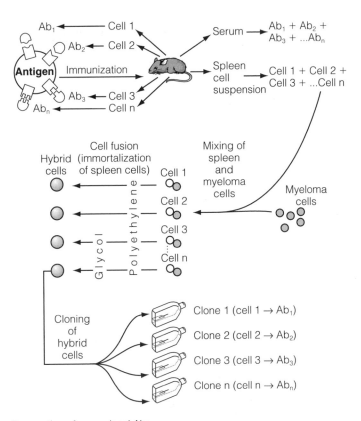

Fig. 1. Preparation of monoclonal Abs.

Humanize murine antibodies

The murine Ab can be genetically modified to be more human (*Fig. 2*). In particular the constant region of the murine IgG heavy (H) and of the murine light (L) chain can be replaced at the DNA level with the constant regions of human IgG1 H and L chains to create a chimeric Ab where only the variable (V) regions are murine. This significantly decreases but does not eliminate the immunogenicity of the Ab. Another approach involves sequencing the V regions of the mouse Ab H and L chains and then inserting the DNA sequences of the hypervariable regions of these chains into human IgG H and L chain genes. The resulting Ab is 95% human with only the binding regions being murine.

Make fully human mAbs

Human Abs have been made by fusing human B cells with myeloma cells, although this has been very difficult and usually requires immortalizing the B cells using Epstein–Barr virus before fusing. This approach is not ideal as a virus is used, the specificity of the mAbs produced is limited and the yield of the Abs produced is poor. More recently, a human antibody mouse has been created by replacing the genes for mouse immunoglobulins with genes for human immunoglobulins. Thus, when the mouse is immunized it makes fully human Abs against the Ag and the B cells making these Abs can be fused with myeloma cells to generate hybridomas making the human mAb.

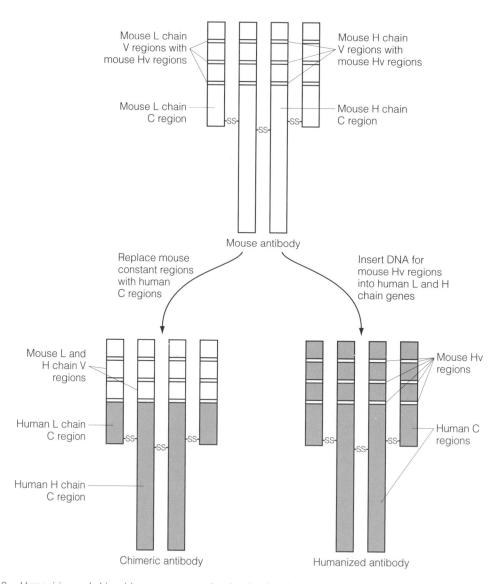

Fig. 2.   Humanizing and chimerizing mouse monoclonal antibodies. Chimeric mAbs are created by replacing the murine genes for the constant region of the light (L) and heavy (H) chain with the corresponding human constant region genes. Humanized mAbs are created by inserting the gene sequences for each of the hypervariable (Hv) regions of the mouse antibody into the corresponding place in the genes for the L and H chains for a human antibody.

Fv libraries   Another way of preparing monoclonal Abs involves Fv libraries (Topic F6). In this approach, the H chain V region genes of a large population of B cells are fused randomly to an equally large number of L chain V region genes to create all combinations and thus a vast number of combining sites (Fv regions). These are cloned into bacteriophage (viruses that infect bacteria) and selected for their specificity. Thus, Fvs can be expressed in a replicating bioform and used as a source from which specific mAbs can be created.

FURTHER READING

A large number of textbooks in immunology are now available which are good reference books for those interested in more detail. In addition, specific detailed information can often be obtained through the WEB and through specialist journal databases, including Medline.

General textbooks

Abbas, A.K., Lichtman, A.H. and Pober, J.S. (1997) *Cellular and Molecular Immunology*, 3rd edn., W.B. Saunders Company, Philadelphia, USA.

Janeway, C.A., Travers, P., Walport, M. and Capra, J.D. (1999) *Immunobiology*, 4th edn., Current Biology Ltd, Garland, London, UK.

Kuby, J. (1997) *Immunology*, 3rd edn., W H Freeman, Oxford.

Peakman, M. and Vergani, D. (1997) *Basic and Clinical Immunology*, Churchill Livingstone, Edinburgh, UK.

Playfair, J. H. L. and Lydyard, P. M. (2000) *Medical Immunology for Students*, 2nd edn. Churchill Livingstone, Edinburgh, UK.

Roitt, I. M. (1997) *Essential Immunology*, 9th edn., Blackwell Scientific, Oxford, UK.

Roitt, I. M., Brostoff, J. and Male, D. (eds.), *Immunology*, 5th edn., Mosby, London, UK.

Sharon, J. (1998) *Basic Immunology*, William and Wilkins, Baltimore, USA.

MULTIPLE CHOICE QUESTIONS

The following pages contain multiple choice questions for self assessment. They are presented in the style of the US Medical Boards part 1 but are used universally in examinations. The questions are based on the material presented in the corresponding Sections into which they are grouped. Answers to these questions can be found on page 311. To make the most effective use of these questions do not try to answer them immediately after reading or reviewing the material on which they are based. Rather, let the knowledge settle overnight and then try the questions. Choose the single best answer.

A–G

1. **Tears contain . . .**

A   IgA
B   IgG.
C   lysozyme.
D   all of the above.

2. **Macrophages . . .**

A   circulate in the blood stream.
B   produce nitric oxide.
C   have receptors for IgM.
D   are the first leukocytes to arrive at the site of a skin infection.
E   are the main immune cells for dealing with viruses.

3. **Phagocytosis . . .**

A   is carried by cells of the adaptive immune system.
B   is restricted to macrophages.
C   is important in bacterial infections.
D   is a process that does not involve energy.
E   results in division of the cell.

4. **Molecules directly involved in NK cell mediated killing include . . .**

A   muramyl dipeptide.
B   granzyme A and B
C   complement.
D   IFNγ.
E   superoxide.

5.   Opsonins include . . .

A   perforin.
B   magainins.
C   C9.
D   IFNγ.
E   C3b

6.   Dendritic cells are characterized by . . .

A   the presence of major basic proteins.
B   expression of CD3.
C   expression of IgM molecules.
D   their ability to release histamine.
E   their interface between the innate and adaptive immune systems.

7.   Both mast cells and basophils . . .

A   are phagocytic
B   circulate in the blood stream.
C   are found primarily in lymph nodes.
D   have receptors for IgM antibodies.
E   release histamine.

8.   Activation of the alternate pathway involves . . .

A   C1.
B   C3.
C   C2.
D   C4.

9.   Control of the activated complement components results from . . .

A   agglutination.
B   immune adherence.
C   instability and inactivation of some of these components.
D   mobility of phagocytes.

10.   All of the following are true about acute phase proteins EXCEPT . . .

A   they include C-reactive protein.
B   they include complement proteins.
C   they are mainly produced in the liver.
D   they function to limit tissue damage.
E   they are not induced by cytokines.

11. **Complement inhibitory proteins include the following EXCEPT . . .**

A   decay accelerating factor.
B   CD59 (protectin).
C   membrane cofactor protein (MCP).
D   ICAM-1.

12. **Helper T cells are distinguished from cytotoxic T cells by the presence of . . .**

A   CD2.
B   CD4.
C   CD3.
D   IL-2 receptor.
E   Class II MHC antigen.

13. **B cells are distinguished from T cells by the presence of . . .**

A   CD3.
B   CD4.
C   CD8.
D   surface Ig.
E   Class I MHC antigen.

14. **T-cells in lymph nodes . . .**

A   occur predominantly in the medullary region.
B   are only of the cytotoxic type.
C   are phagocytic
D   are absent in Di-George syndrome.
E   express surface immunoglobulin.

15. **Lymphocytes of the mucosal immune system . . .**

A   are normally primed in the lamina propria of the intestine.
B   home mainly to mucosal sites and not systemic lymphoid organs.
C   make up less than 10% of the lymphoid tissues in the body.
D   mainly produce IgG antibodies.
E   are only of the T cell type.

16. **Newborns . . .**

A   receive IgM antibodies from the mother through placental transfer.
B   have virtually a full complement of maternal IgG antibodies.
C   have very few lymphocytes in their circulation.
D   respond to antigens as well as adults.
E   receive maternal B cells.

17.   Rearrangement of VH genes begins during . . .

A   the pre-B cell stage.
B   the pro-B cell stage.
C   maturation of B cells into plasma cells.
D   development of dendritic cells.
E   thymus development.

18.   All of the following are true about the development of blood cells EXCEPT . . .

A   cytokines are required
B   IL-7 is involved in T cell development.
C   M-CSF is required for granulocyte development.
D   B cell development takes place mainly in the bone-marrow.

19.   Allotypes are . . .

A   antigenic determinants which segregate within a species.
B   critical to the function of the antibody combining site.
C   involved in specificity.
D   involved in memory.

20.   IgE . . .

A   is bound together by J chain.
B   binds to mast cells through its Fab region.
C   differs from IgG antibody because of its different H chains.
D   is present in high concentration in serum.

21.   Ig heavy chains are . . .

A   encoded by a Constant region exon, Variable exon, Diversity exon, and Joining exon.
B   not glycosylated
C   not important to binding of antigen.
D   expressed by T cells.

22.   The Fab portion of Ig . . .

A   binds to an Fc receptor.
B   contains the J chain.
C   contains the idiotype of the Ig.
D   mediates biological effector functions of Ab molecules (e.g. complement fixation).

23.   Cells destined to become IgA producing plasma cells do not . . .

A   migrate from mucosal areas on stimulation with antigen.
B   home to any mucosal area
C   produce secretory component.
D   produce J chain.

24.   IgA . . .

A   is present in milk and saliva
B   is involved in hay fever.
C   activates complement by the classical pathway.
D   crosses the placenta

25.   Antibody dependent cell mediated cytotoxicity (ADCC) . . .

A   is carried out by B cells.
B   is the main mechanism for killing intracellular microbes.
C   involves Fc receptors on the effector cells.
D   is primarily mediated by IgE antibody.

26.   The Fc region of antibody . . .

A   contains both heavy and light chains.
B   is required for antigen binding.
C   is not a requirement for placental transmission.
D   is not important for triggering of IgE mediated hypersensitivity.
E   generally confers biological activity on the various molecules.

27.   Human IgM . . .

A   crosses the placenta
B   consists of 3 subunits linked together by a J chain.
C   protects mucosal surfaces.
D   is largely restricted to the circulation.
E   is the antibody produced by high affinity plasma cells.

28.   Immunoglobulin light chains . . .

A   are joined to heavy chains by peptide bonds.
B   can be present as both k and l chains as part of a single Ig molecule.
C   are not found in every major immunoglobulin class.
D   all have the same amino acid composition.
E   are present in the Fab fragment of IgG.

29.   The fixation of complement by an antigen-antibody reaction can lead to . . .

A   formation of a factor chemotactic for mononuclear cells.
B   enhanced phagocytosis.
C   activation of T cells.
D   increased synthesis of antibody.

30.   **Both interleukin 1 and 2 . . .**

A   are produced by the same cell.
B   require complement for their biological activity.
C   act on T cells.
D   trigger histamine release.

31.   **Tumor necrosis factor . . .**

A   decreases macrophage effector functions.
B   increases expression of adhesion molecules on endothelial cells.
C   decreases vascular permeability.
D   decreases blood flow.

32.   **IFNγ . . .**

A   is produced by all nucleated cells of the body.
B   induces Th2 responses.
C   can activate macrophages.
D   was discovered because of its effect on tumors.

33.   **Viral replication within cells is inhibited by . . .**

A   IL-13.
B   IL-1.
C   IFNα
D   TNFα
E   IL-4.

34.   **Cytokines that directly elevate body temperature include . . .**

A   IL-10.
B   TGFβ
C   IL-4.
D   IL-5.
E   IL-6.

H–N

35. **A B cell can express on its cell surface . . .**

A   membrane IgM and IgD at the same time.
B   both types of light chain.
C   secretory component.
D   IgG that can bind several different unrelated antigens.

36. **Cytotoxic T cells generally recognize antigen in association with . . .**

A   class II MHC determinants.
B   class I MHC determinants.
C   class III MHC determinants.
D   HLA-DR determinants.

37. **The T cell antigen receptor . . .**

A   recognizes epitopes on linear peptides associated with MHC determinants.
B   has Ig light chains.
C   is made up of a heavy chain and $\beta2$ microglobulin.
D   recognizes conformational epitopes on the native antigen.

38. **TCR gene rearrangement . . .**

A   takes place primarily in the bone marrow.
B   is antigen independent.
C   involves immunoglobulin.
D   requires costimulation by antigen presenting cells.

39. **The class I MHC processing pathway primarily . . .**

A   processes antigens that are present in the cytosol.
B   processes antigens from the extracellular environment.
C   generates peptides, complexes them with class I MHC molecules for presentation to helper T cells.
D   generates peptides, complexes them with class I MHC molecules for presentation to NK cells.

40. **All of the following are true about receptors of the innate immune system, EXCEPT that they .**

A   include those of the Toll family.
B   recognize molecular patterns associated with groups of microbes.
C   include CD14 and scavenger receptors.
D   include MHC molecules.
E   do not include Igα and Igβ.

41.   On the B cell surface, receptors for antigen are associated with . . .

A   CD3γ chains.
B   Igα and Igβ.
C   MHC class II molecules.
D   MHC class I molecules.
E   Toll receptors.

42.   The endogenous pathway of antigen presentation involves . . .

A   mostly peptides derived from extracellular pathogens.
B   presentation of antigen on MHC class II molecules.
C   presentation of antigen to cytolytic T cells.
D   presentation of antigen to Th1 cells.
E   presentation of antigen to B cells.

43.   Potent chemotactic factors (chemotaxins) for neutrophils include . . .

A   C-reactive protein.
B   C3b.
C   arachidonic acid.
D   LTB4.
E   IFNα.

44.   Direct causes of inflammation include . . .

A   TGFβ.
B   histaminase.
C   ICAM-1.
D   VCAM.
E   LPS.

45.   Which of the following is a known inhibitor of inflammation . . .

A   TNFα
B   nerve growth factor.
C   protein C.
D   neuropeptide Y.
E   reactive oxygen species.

46.   Clonal selection . . .

A   necessitates that proteins are multideterminant.
B   requires that each antigen reactive cell have multiple specificities.
C   involves binding of Ab Fc regions to mast cells.
D   explains specificity and memory in immunity.

47. All of the following are true about class switching of antibodies EXCEPT that . . .

A   particular Th subsets are required.
B   it occurs in germinal centers of lymph nodes.
C   cytokines are required.
D   it occurs in patients with Di George syndrome.
E   it does not occur in patients with a genetic defect in CD40L.

48. The following are required for, or are sequelae of clonal selection EXCEPT . . .

A   recognition of antigen by specific antigen receptors on lymphocytes.
B   proliferation of cells triggered by specific antigens.
C   activation of T lymphocytes by superantigens.
D   generation of T cell dependent B cell memory responses.

49. T cells do not . . .

A   make IL-2.
B   respond to IL-4.
C   respond to IL-2.
D   mediate their functions solely by cell to cell contact.

50. Th1 cells do not . . .

A   express CD4.
B   produce IFNγ.
C   activate macrophages.
D   bind soluble antigen.

51. CD8 positive cells . . .

A   can be classified into Th1 and Th2 subgroups based on their biological function.
B   do not produce IFNγ.
C   can recognize and kill virus infected cells.
D   can bind free virus.
E   do not require direct cell to cell contact with their targets for killing.

52. CTL . . .

A   do not mediate cytotoxicity of other T cells infected with virus.
B   mediate killing by insertion of perforin into the membrane of the target cell.
C   do not need to recognize MHC antigens on the target cell to kill.
D   recognise antigens with MHC class II antigens.
E   normally help B cells to make antibodies.

53. **Stimulation of B cells to proliferate and differentiate requires . . .**

A   B cell Immunoglobulin binding of peptide in association with T cell MHC class II.
B   binding of CD40 on B cells by its ligand on T cells.
C   IFNγ.
D   B cell surface antibody binding to C3b.

54. **Superantigens . . .**

A   activate large numbers of T cells by directly binding to the TCRβ chain and class II MHC
B   are high molecular weight antigens that can trigger T cell proliferation in the absence of antigen-presenting cells.
C   can activate all B cells by binding to IgM.
D   can only trigger CD8⁺ T cells.

55. **Type 1 thymus - independent antigens characteristically are . . .**

A   small peptides.
B   bacterial proteins.
C   viral nucleic acids.
D   bacterial polysaccharides.
E   haptens.

56. **Molecules involved in lymphocyte activation include all of the following EXCEPT . . .**

A   CD3.
B   CD79b
C   CD14.
D   lck.
E   CD28.

57. **Stimulation of antigen-specific T cells by appropriately presented antigen alone results in . . .**

A   induction of cytotoxicity.
B   production of IL-2 but not other cytokines.
C   activation resulting in cell division.
D   anergy.

58. **The stage in B-cell development at which tolerance can be most easily induced is . . .**

A   memory B.
B   pre-B.
C   immature B.
D   mature B.
E   plasma cell

59. **Mechanisms whereby peripheral tolerance may be maintained include all of the following EXCEPT ...**

A   the absence of co-stimulation by CD80 or CD86.
B   treatment with glucocorticoids.
C   failure of cytokine signalling.
D   apoptosis of activated T cells induced by Fas ligand on other cells.
E   the absence of co-stimulation by CD154.

60. **Properties of antigen that may influence its role in the induction of tolerance include ...**

A   its nature.
B   its route of administration.
C   the dose of antigen.
D   maturity of the immune system.
E   all of the above.

61. **The process involved in allowing T cells to survive in the thymus is ...**

A   positive selection.
B   negative selection.
C   apoptosis.
D   necrosis.
E   complement inactivation.

62. **For adjuvants to be effective, they need to do all of the following EXCEPT ...**

A   prolong antigen exposure.
B   induce high affinity responses.
C   increase quantitative response.
D   induce release of TGFβ

63. **Central tolerance takes place in ...**

A   lymph nodes.
B   thymus.
C   spleen.
D   liver.
E   pancreas.

64.   Among the steps of maturation of a pre-B cell to a plasma cell, the only one that does not require antigen is . . .

A   affinity maturation.
B   development of memory.
C   clonal selection or tolerance.
D   recombination of the Ig gene loci.
E   tolerance.

65.   One reason why different individuals can mount T cell responses to specific peptides and others cannot is because . . .

A   they lack the expression of class I or class II MHC molecules on specific cell types.
B   the peptides that can be presented by the MHC molecules that a person inherited are limited
C   of an imbalance in the CD4/CD8 T cell ratio.
D   of mutations in the constant region of MHC class I genes.

66.   An anti-idiotypic antibody was infused into a patient with autoimmune hemolytic anemia. This treatment improved the anemia for 2 days, followed by recurrence of the anemia. The improvement was most likely related to binding of anti-idiotypic antibody to . . .

A   the B-cells making the autoantibody.
B   plasma cells making the autoantibody.
C   autoantibody specific T helper cells.
D   circulating serum autoantibody alone.

67.   Cytokines responsible for immunosuppression include . . .

A   IL-1.
B   IL-2.
C   IFNγ.
D   IL-10.
E   TNFα

O–R

68.   Which of the following cell types (or their products) is least effective against extracellular bacterial pathogens?

A   B cells.
B   cytotoxic T cells.
C   helper T cells.
D   neutrophils.
E   macrophages.

69. **Complement components facilitate immunity to extracellular pathogens by all of the following mechanisms EXCEPT . . .**

A   opsonizing the pathogen.
B   mediating the chemotaxis of inflammatory cells to the site of infection.
C   increasing vascular permeability to increase access to the site of infection.
D   binding to T cells inducing their activation.

70. **Extensive cooperation between phagocytes and lymphocytes is essential *in vivo* for . . .**

A   elimination of inert carbon particles (e.g. a splinter).
B   elimination of non-encapsulated bacteria (e.g. *S. epidermidis,* a normal skin bacterium).
C   NK cell killing of tumor cells.
D   elimination of encapsulated bacteria (e.g. pneumococci).

71. **A tetanus booster shot results in the increased production of . . .**

A   tetanus-specific NK cells.
B   T cells that recognize tetanus toxoid but not tetanus toxin.
C   antibodies which neutralize tetanus toxin.
D   T-cells which kill *Clostridium tetani.*

72. **For adjuvants to be effective, they need to do all of the following EXCEPT . . .**

A   prolong antigen exposure.
B   enhance release of TGFβ
C   induce high affinity responses.
D   increase quantitative response.

73. **Tumors induced by chemical carcinogens . . .**

A   express unique TSA
B   express TSA that are the same for all tumors induced by the same carcinogen.
C   do not usually express MHC antigens.
D   can be treated by immunosuppression.

74. **Host antibody against a tumor would most likely be directed against . . .**

A   MHC class II antigens.
B   viral antigens.
C   differentiation antigens.
D   MHC class I antigens.

75. **Tumor immune surveillance may be mediated by ...**

A mast cells.
B neutrophils.
C Langerhans cells
D NK cells.

76. **The HLA typing in a paternity case is as follows:**

mother: A8 B3 C2 DR10
                    A23 B8 C4 DR5
potential father #1:   A2,3; B8,27; C2,11; DR3,9
child: A3,23; B8,27; C2,4; DR5,10

Based on this information potential father #1 should ...

A be convinced that the child is his because a crossover generating a recombinant
    maternal haplotype explains the only discrepancy.
B sue the hospital for mixing up newborns because the child cannot belong to either him or the
    mother.
C review his knowledge of immunogenetics and determine his haplotypes from his previous
    children's HLA types because without this information he cannot be sure if he is the father of this
    latest child.
D determine the HLA type of potential father #2.

77. **Graft survival can be enhanced *without* generalized immunosuppression by ...**

A matching for HLA antigen.
B anti-thymocyte globulin.
C cyclosporin A therapy.
D steroids or cytotoxic drugs.

78. **The mixed lymphocyte reaction ...**

A can be used to determine if two individuals have HLA-D differences.
B if carried out with the cells of identical twins, would show a marked increase in proliferation
    because the cells are antigenically compatible.
C is carried out with the cells from both individuals treated with mitomycin C or X-ray to eliminate
    extraneous proliferation.
D is assayed by measuring cell lysis.

79. **Immunosuppression is not induced by ...**

A antihistamines.
B removal of lymphoid tissue.
C use of anti-lymphocyte antibodies.
D cytotoxic drugs.

80. **Bone marrow engraftment is a unique type of organ transplantation because . . .**

A   MHC differences are not recognized.
B   minor histocompatibility differences are the only antigenic differences that can lead to rejection.
C   graft versus host disease may occur.
D   immunosuppression is never required.

81. **A major transfusion reaction may occur if the recipient . . .**

A   has antibodies to transfused cells.
B   has T cells reactive to blood group antigens.
C   is RhD compatible.
D   is AB positive.

82. **The most acute form of graft rejection (termed hyperacute rejection) results from . . .**

A   occlusion of blood vessels by proliferating endothelial cells.
B   killing of grafted tissue by cytotoxic T cells.
C   occlusion of blood vessels as a result of coagulation.
D   attack by natural killer cells.

83. **In some instances, a graft made between two unrelated donors, who are perfectly matched at HLA-A, B, C, and D, is still rejected. The possible cause of this rejection is . . .**

A   β2-microglobulin differences.
B   mismatching of immunoglobulin allotypes.
C   prior sensitization to major histocompatibility antigens.
D   minor histocompatibility differences.

84. **The immune effector system responsible for acute graft rejection is . . .**

A   cytotoxic T lymphocytes.
B   mast cells.
C   activated macrophages.
D   complement.

85. **An HLA haplotype is . . .**

A   the total set of MHC alleles present on each chromosome.
B   a specific segment of the MHC locus.
C   genes outside the MHC locus that contribute to rejection.
D   one allele of HLA-B

86.   Graft rejection ...

A   occurs between identical twins.
B   rarely involves T lymphocytes.
C   can be accelerated by a previous graft from the same donor.
D   can be prevented by immunostimulation.
E   is mainly prevented by matching at the HLA A, B or C loci.

87.   DNA vaccines can be effective if they ...

A   can be engineered to contain DNA motifs that have an adjuvant effect.
B   encode expression of antigen.
C   encode expression of appropriate cytokines.
D   all of the above.

88.   The antigenic component of a vaccine for melanoma is a 20 amino acid peptide. This
       peptide ...

A   could induce both T cell tolerance and T cell activation.
B   would be expected to work for most people.
C   would be expected to work for a subset of people.
D   items A and C only.

89.   Polysaccharides are rarely effective vaccines by themselves because they ...

A   have repeating B cell epitopes.
B   lack classical T cell epitopes.
C   only induce CTL responses.
D   are usually the same in people and bacteria

90.   Vaccines may fail to induce a protective response because they induce ...

A   humoral immunity when cell mediated immunity is needed
B   IgM but not IgG or IgA
C   production of IL-4 when IFNγ is needed
D   all of the above.
E   items A and B only

91.   An antibody to CD40 would be expected to enhance vaccine effectiveness by ...

A   blocking CD40 signalling on dendritic cells.
B   activating CD40 signalling on dendritic cells.
C   linking dendritic cell CD40 to lymphocyte CD154 (CD40 ligand).
D   inducing dendritic cell apoptosis.
E   none of the above.

S–V

92.   The presence of 70% CD3 positive lymphocytes in the peripheral circulation of a patient indicates that the patient has normal . . .

A   humoral immunity.
B   cellular immunity.
C   numbers of B lymphocytes.
D   numbers of T lymphocytes.

93.   HIV infects all of the following EXCEPT . . .

A   monocytes.
B   T cells.
C   macrophages.
D   B cells.

94.   The receptor through which HIV infects is . . .

A   CD2.
B   CD3.
C   CD4.
D   CD5.

95.   Immunoglobulin deficiency can be detected by . . .

A   flow cytometry.
B   DTH skin test.
C   mixed lymphocyte response (MLR).
D   serum protein electrophoresis.

96.   Cell-mediated immune responses are . . .

A   enhanced by depletion of complement.
B   suppressed by cortisone.
C   enhanced by depletion of T cells.
D   suppressed by antihistamine.
E   enhanced by depletion of macrophages.

97.   Treatments for immunodeficiency would not include . . .

A   antibiotics.
B   bone marrow transplantation.
D   interleukins.
E   anti-CD4 antibody.

98.   Immediate hypersensitivity usually involves . . .

A   mast cells.
B   antibodies to mast cells.
C   platelets.
D   IgG.

99.   Mast cell products mediate some of the symptoms of immediate hypersensitivity by increasing . . .

A   IgE receptors.
B   secretion of IgE
C   capillary leakage.
D   secretion of IgG.

100.   Therapy for immediate hypersensitivity includes injection of antigen (allergen) to . . .

A   induce wheal and flare.
B   increase T cells making IL-4.
C   cause anaphylaxis.
D   increase T cells making IFNγ.

101.   Slow-reacting substance of anaphylaxis (SRS-A) constricts airways and arteries and increases bronchial mucus production. The chemical nature of SRS-A is . . .

A   histamine.
B   leukotrienes.
C   prostaglandin D2.
D   thromboxane.
E   chondroitin sulfates.

102. The predominant antigen presenting cell in contact hypersensitivity (e.g. poison ivy) is the . . .

A   T lymphocyte.
B   B lymphocyte.
C   basophil.
D   Langerhans cell.
E   NK cell.

103.   The cutaneous response of delayed hypersensitivity . . .

A   can be passively transferred by antibody.
B   shows erythema (redness) and induration 1–2 days after injection of the antigen.
C   depends upon the attachment of IgE antibody to mast cells.
D   is mediated by B lymphocytes.

104. **Anti-RhD antibody ...**

A   is not given to RhD negative mothers after birth of an RhD positive infant.
B   does not react with RhD antigens on RBC
C   does not block the development of active immunity to RhD antigen.
D   is obtained from RhD negative women.

105. **Inflammation resulting from IgG-antigen complexes ...**

A   requires IgM to activate complement.
B   involves complement activation.
C   produces the rash of poison ivy.
D   requires T cells.

106. **Immune complex disease ...**

A   requires cytotoxic T cells.
B   requires neutrophils.
C   usually involves IgE
D   usually involves IgA

107. **Serum sickness occurs only ...**

A   when anti-basement-membrane antibodies are present.
B   in cases of extreme excess of antibody.
C   when IgE antibody is produced
D   when soluble immune complexes are formed
E   in the absence of neutrophils.

108. **Both immune complex disease and delayed type hypersensitivity involve ...**

A   phagocytic cells.
B   IgG or IgM antibodies.
C   NK lymphocytes.
D   B cells.

109. **Hemolytic disease of the newborn due to RhD incompatibility depends upon the ...**

A   mother possessing RhD antigens not present on the baby's red cells.
B   inability of the baby to react against the mother's red cells.
C   transplacental passage of IgM anti-RhD antibodies.
D   transplacental passage of IgG anti-RhD antibodies.
E   production of cytotoxic antibodies by the baby.

110. Delayed hypersensitivity as typified by the Mantoux reaction to tuberculin is mediated by . . .

A   lymphocytes.
B   polymorphonuclear cells.
C   anaphylactic antibodies.
D   complement binding antibodies.
E   antigen-antibody complexes.

111. Complement receptors on red blood cells and Fc receptors on platelets probably facilitate . . .

A   immune phagocytosis of immune complexes by red blood cells and platelets.
B   immune pinocytosis of immune complexes by red blood cells and platelets.
C   the synthesis of gamma interferon by the platelet.
D   the elimination of immune complexes by phagocytic cells.

112. The broad spectrum of autoantibody formation in patients with systemic lupus erythematosus is probably indicative of . . .

A   excess production of macrophages.
B   failed regulation of a multi-specific B-cell clone.
C   the presence of many auto-reactive B-cell clones.
D   heterozygosity at the HLA B locus.

113. The clinical disease most likely to involve a reaction to a hapten in its etiology is . . .

A   systemic lupus erythematosus after treatment with glucocorticoids.
B   hemolytic anemia after treatment with penicillin.
C   juvenile diabetes after treatment with insulin.
D   rejection of kidney graft after treatment with cyclosporin.

114. IgG antibodies against "self" proteins . . .

A   are only found in patients with tumors.
B   are only produced in the spleen
C   can cross the placenta
D   are more common in men.

115. Goodpasture's disease involving lesions in the kidney and in lung alveoli is caused by . . .

A   deposition of soluble antigen-antibody complexes.
B   cell mediated hypersensitivity to kidney antigens.
C   IgE antibodies to proximal tubules.
D   antibodies to basement membranes.
E   non-specific reactions due to a high level of serum IgG.

116. **Major histocompatibility antigens are not . . .**

A   linked with a number of autoimmune diseases.
B   important for interactions between T and B cells during an immune response.
C   the only antigens which result in graft rejection.
D   important for graft versus host reactions.

117. **HLA disease association . . .**

A   means that the particular HLA antigen or haplotype involved causes the disease.
B   may in some instances be useful in diagnosis.
C   means that every person with that HLA type will contract the disease.
D   may suggest that genes near the MHC locus code for T cell antigen receptors specific for self antigens.

118. **Reaction between an IgG anti-albumin monoclonal antibody and albumin might result in . . .**

A   precipitation.
B   lattice formation.
C   agglutination.
D   complex formation.

119. **ELISA assay . . .**

A   results in cell lysis.
B   uses a radiolabeled second antibody.
C   involves addition of substrate which is converted to a colored end-product.
D   requires sensitized red blood cells.

120. **Monoclonal antibodies produced by hybridoma technology . . .**

A   are usually of human origin.
B   are each the result of immortalization of a single monocyte.
C   usually have specificity predetermined by prior immunization.
D   are prepared by fusion of T lymphocytes and myeloma cells.

ANSWERS

1.	D	41.	B	81.	A
2.	B	42.	C	82.	C
3.	C	43.	D	83.	D
4.	B	44.	E	84.	A
5.	E	45.	C	85.	A
6.	E	46.	D	86.	C
7.	E	47.	D	87.	D
8.	B	48.	C	88.	D
9.	C	49.	D	89.	B
10.	E	50.	D	90.	E
11.	D	51.	C	91.	B
12.	B	52.	B	92.	D
13.	D	53.	B	93.	D
14.	D	54.	A	94.	C
15.	B	55.	D	95.	D
16.	B	56.	C	96.	B
17.	B	57.	D	97.	D
18.	C	58.	C	98.	A
19.	A	59.	B	99.	C
20.	C	60.	E	100.	D
21.	A	61.	A	101.	B
22.	C	62.	D	102.	D
23.	C	63.	B	103.	B
24.	A	64.	D	104.	D
25.	C	65.	B	105.	B
26.	E	66.	D	106.	B
27.	D	67.	D	107.	D
28.	E	68.	B	108.	A
29.	B	69.	D	109.	D
30.	C	70.	D	110.	A
31.	B	71.	C	111.	D
32.	C	72.	B	112.	C
33.	C	73.	A	113.	B
34.	E	74.	B	114.	C
35.	A	75.	D	115.	D
36.	B	76.	D	116.	C
37.	A	77.	A	117.	B
38.	B	78.	A	118.	D
39.	A	79.	A	119.	C
40.	D	80.	C	120.	C

INDEX